Sick Note

Sick Note

A History of the British Welfare State

GARETH MILLWARD

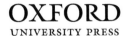

OXFORD
UNIVERSITY PRESS

OXFORD
UNIVERSITY PRESS

Great Clarendon Street, Oxford, OX2 6DP,
United Kingdom

Oxford University Press is a department of the University of Oxford.
It furthers the University's objective of excellence in research, scholarship,
and education by publishing worldwide. Oxford is a registered trade mark of
Oxford University Press in the UK and in certain other countries

First Edition published in 2022

Impression: 2

Published in the United States of America by Oxford University Press
198 Madison Avenue, New York, NY 10016, United States of America

British Library Cataloguing in Publication Data
Data available

Library of Congress Control Number: 2021951712

ISBN 978-0-19-286574-8

DOI: 10.1093/oso/9780192865748.001.0001

Printed and bound by
CPI Group (UK) Ltd, Croydon, CR0 4YY

For Emma

Acknowledgements

The research that went into writing this book was funded by a Wellcome Trust Humanities Fellowship (grant number WT208075/Z/17/Z). I wish to thank Dan O'Connor and Tom Bray at the Wellcome Trust, the interview panel, and anonymous peer reviewers for giving me the opportunity to complete this work. I am especially thankful that the Trust extended my funding during the pandemic, making the completion of this book possible. Thanks, too, to The National Archives, Modern Records Centre, and Albert Sloman Library for access to their manuscript holdings, as well as the British Library's web and oral history archives. I am also indebted to the organizers and participants at various conferences and seminar series at which I was able to present and discuss preliminary findings. This includes the Body Self Family group at the University of Essex, the North American Conference on British Studies conferences in Vancouver, the Modern British Studies conferences in Birmingham, the BodyCapital group at the University of Strasbourg, the History of Philosophy and Science seminar series at the University of Cambridge, the Life Cycles seminar series at the Institute of Historical Research, the Society for the History of Medicine Conference in Liverpool, and the European Association for the History of Medicine and Health Conference in Birmingham. Special thanks go to the editorial team at Oxford University Press and the anonymous readers whose kind-yet-critical comments have improved the quality of this text no end.

This research was completed at the Centre for the History of Medicine at the University of Warwick. Mathew Thomson has been an excellent mentor, offering supportive critical feedback throughout. So too has Roberta Bivins, whose *Cultural History of the NHS* project with Mathew provided the perfect venue for collaborative teaching and research. I thank Jenny Crane, George Gosling, Jane Hand, Nathalie Jones, and Jack Saunders for feedback on my funding application and companionship during the beginning of the project. Hilary Marland and Angela Davies were tremendously supportive as heads of the CHM, as was feedback on chapter drafts from Centre members Rachel Bennett, Andrew Burchell, Fabiola Creed, Rosemary Cresswell, Becky Crites, Ed Devane, Sophie Greenway, Samir Hamdoud, Katey Logan, Louise Morgan, Beccy Rutherford, Claire Shaw, Chris Sirrs, Elise Smith, John Wilmott, and many others who have passed through the Centre and the Department of History over the years. I am especially grateful for the administrative assistance from Sheilagh Holmes, Michelle Nortey, and Claudia Gray, without whom this novice grant holder would have been completely lost. It must also be noted that early career researchers require time and resources beyond their initial contracts to fully complete works like this book. For this reason (and many others) I am grateful to the *Border Crossings* team of Bernard Harris, Martin Gorsky, John Mohan, and Ellen Stewart for hiring me as a research fellow at the University of Birmingham and allowing me the flexibility to complete manuscript revisions alongside my new duties.

This work would also not have been possible without the encouragement and guidance of Alex Mold at the London School of Hygiene and Tropical Medicine. Her mentorship has been invaluable and can never be repaid. The feedback and encouragement on early drafts of this book and on the original funding application from Alex's *Placing the Public in Public Health* project (including Peder Clark, Hannah Elizabeth, Ingrid James, and Daisy Payling) were vital, and my thanks also go to the wider Centre for History in Public Health at LSHTM. Martin Moore and Harriet Palfreyman have been a constant source of advice, some of which was solicited. I am very grateful to PhD students George Severs, Sarah Dorrington, and Adrian Kane-Galbraith for sharing their inspiring research, and I hope I have neither misrepresented them nor underplayed their contributions. Martin Johnes deserves thanks for introducing me to the work of Max Boyce. I must also thank Martin Gorsky and Claudia Stein for continuing to guide my career, as well as Jane Winters for introducing me to, and continuing to fuel my curiosity in, internet archives. Much of the research in Chapter 7 would have been impossible without her.

Emma, mom, dad, and Aidan and the clique have looked after me over the past few years, and I must also thank all those 'key workers' at the University of Warwick and across the country that made it possible for me to work from home and write the manuscript that became this book. I am acutely aware of the privileged position I was in to be able to produce this work during a global pandemic and the devastation COVID-19 has caused to so many excellent research projects. As the Conclusion makes clear, many people will face professional and financial hardship over the coming years as a result of the dislocation caused by the epidemic and the deliberate choices of governments at the local, national, and international levels. I hope this book can provide some perspective on the past and future of the British welfare state—but it cannot escape the conditions in which it was written.

Contents

List of Figures

List of Abbreviations

BAMS	Benefit Agency Medical Service
BMA	British Medical Association
CBI	Confederation of British Industry
CEGB	Central Electricity Generating Board
CPAG	Child Poverty Action Group
DA	Disability Alliance
DHSS	Department of Health and Social Security
DIG	Disablement Income Group
DSS	Department of Social Security
DWP	Department for Work and Pensions
ESA	Employment and Support Allowance
GMSC	General Medical Services Committee
GP	General Practitioner
HNCIP	Housewife's Non-contributory Invalidity Pension
HR	Human Resources
JCC	Joint Co-ordinating Committee
ME	Myalgic Encephalomyelitis
MPNI	Ministry of Pensions and National Insurance
MRC	Modern Records Centre, University of Warwick
NCB	National Coal Board
NCIP	Non-contributory Invalidity Pension
NHI	National Health Insurance
NHS	National Health Service
PAYE	Pay as You Earn
PMT	Pre-menstrual Tension
PTC	Peter Townsend Collection, University of Essex
PTSD	Post-traumatic Stress Disorder
ROF	Royal Ordinance Factory
SBC	Supplementary Benefits Commission
SSP	Statutory Sick Pay
TNA	The National Archives
TUC	Trades Union Congress
UBI	Universal Basic Income
WRAG	Work Related Activity Group

1

Introduction

Darren Anderton played 30 times for the England men's national football team and made 299 Premier League appearances for Tottenham Hotspur. To fans of a certain age, he is known by another name: 'Sicknote'. 'I had a migraine and was throwing up before a Portsmouth game', recounted Anderton in 2016, some eight years after his final Football League match. 'The next day at training, someone laughed, "Oh, Sicknote's here." Nothing came of it until I joined Spurs and had that first groin problem three or four years later. One of the press boys who had covered Pompey picked up on it and that was it.'[1]

The nickname resonated because it meant something to 1990s' British football fans. Just as everyone knew what sort of character Bert Quigley was when he was introduced as 'Sicknote' in ITV's 1980s' serial drama *London's Burning*. He was, according to the fan-edited 'Wiki' entry about the show, 'thin-skinned, pompous… a chronic hypochondriac, and constantly moaned about his ailments, from toothache to backache, which earned him his nickname.'[2] For both Quigley and Anderton, the moniker could be deployed to attack a supposed moral failing in the individual. As a firefighter and a professional footballer respectively, there was a sense that both ought to remain physically robust and be willing to function through pain, injury, and illness. At the same time, there was something endearing about the two characters. Everyone, after all, gets sick.

This book is a history of the welfare state told through the lens of the sick note. These slips of paper, signed by a doctor, were used by employers and government authorities as evidence that an individual was incapacitated for work. In this way, they provide a unique vantage point on postwar British social policy. They sit at the intersection between employment, health, and social security—three of Beveridge's solutions to the 'five giants' that had ravaged interwar Britain.[3] Through exploring the major policy changes around medical certification (as well as the political, social, and cultural shifts that inspired them), *Sick Note* shows the contrasts between the welfare state's complex design and its ability to operate in

---

[1] Andrew Murray, 'A warning for Mourinho? Anderton bemoans having to pay through injury', *Four FourTwo*, 9 November 2016, accessed 31 January 2019, www.fourfourtwo.com/features/be-careful-forcing-players-play-through-injury-mou-darren-anderton-told-us.

[2] The show ran from 1986 to 2002. 'Bert 'Sicknote' Quigley', Fandom—London's Burning Wiki, accessed 31 January 2019, https://londons-burning.fandom.com/wiki/Bert_%27Sicknote%27_Quigley.

[3] Nicholas Timmins, *The Five Giants: A Biography of the Welfare State*, 2nd edn (London: Harper Collins, 2001).

practice. Employers, workers, doctors, civil servants, and politicians all had intimate experience of using, writing, or receiving medical certificates—and all expressed frustration that sick notes did not always suit their needs. Still, all needed some way to prove—or, indeed, *disprove*—that an individual was 'really' sick. These arguments exposed how the various parts of the welfare state interconnected, how they were designed to work, how they operated in practice, and what different constituencies hoped they might one day become. Because, despite their flaws, sick notes remained. They worked well enough in just enough areas to be a more attractive proposition than any realistic alternative. In this sense, they were a perfect metaphor for the welfare state itself.

What Is a Sick Note?

There is a long history of people providing evidence of sickness to avoid obligations. Katherine Foxhall's work on migraine since the Middle Ages shows correspondence between individuals apologizing for missing important social events due to severe headaches.[4] James Riley demonstrates that mutual funds for sick workers in the early-modern era would require paperwork detailing symptoms. By the mid-nineteenth century, the verification of such symptoms and diagnoses increasingly fell on the shoulders of licensed physicians.[5] Medical certificates of this kind, for reasons that will be explored below and in Chapter 2, flourished across the nineteenth and twentieth centuries. Doctors were asked to pronounce: the time and cause of death; the mental fitness of an accused person to stand trial; suitability for recruitment to the armed forces; the extent of industrial injuries; whether a person should receive more rations or access to restricted goods in wartime; and much more besides.[6]

Sick Note is interested in a specific form of medical testimony, one that came to be known colloquially in Britain as 'the sick note': the National Insurance medical certificate. Across the postwar period, this was the type of certificate that general practitioners (GPs) were asked to write most frequently. They acted as the formal

---

[4] Katherine Foxhall, *Migraine: A History* (Baltimore: Johns Hopkins University Press, 2019), esp. pp. 61–2.

[5] James C. Riley, 'Sickness in an early modern workplace', *Continuity and Change* 2, no. 3 (1987): pp. 363–85; James C. Riley, *Sick, Not Dead: The Health of British Working Men During the Mortality Decline* (Baltimore: Johns Hopkins University Press, 1997); Charles Hardwick, *The History, Present Position, and Social Importance of Friendly Societies* (London: Routledge, Warne and Routledge, 1859).

[6] On some of these types of certification and their historical uses, see: Ian A. Burney, *Bodies of Evidence: Medicine and the Politics of the English Inquest, 1830-1826* (Baltimore: Johns Hopkins University Press, 1999); Janet Weston, 'Managing mental incapacity in the 20th century: A history of the Court of Protection of England & Wales', *International Journal of Law and Psychiatry* 68 (2020); Emma Newlands, *Civilians into Soldiers: War, the Body and British Army Recruits, 1939–45* (Manchester: Manchester University Press, 2014); Kirsti Bohata, Alexandra Jones, Mike Mantin, and Steve Thompson, *Disability in Industrial Britain* (Manchester: Manchester University Press, 2020).

gateway to state sickness benefits and were co-opted as a mechanism for employers to police absenteeism. As such it was a document created out of negotiations between the Ministry of Health, Ministry of National Insurance, business groups, the medical profession, trades unions, and the other government departments. It entered circulation on the Appointed Day of 5 July 1948; and, despite several reforms to its name and format, it remained until the creation of the 'fit note' by the New Labour government in 2010. Still, 'the sick note' lived on in common parlance and in the fit note's de facto operation.

As British welfare systems expanded in the late-nineteenth and early-twentieth centuries, so did gatekeeping systems and the need for sick notes. This became most acute after the introduction of National Insurance in 1911, which brought millions of workers under the purview of a system that provided access to primary care and sickness benefits.[7] Claims under the Workmen's Compensation Act 1897 for industrial injuries also used medical evidence, as was the case with its predecessor, the Employer's Liability Act 1880.[8] It must be stressed, however, that these developments were not driven simply by 'the government'. Even before 1911, mutualist friendly societies and sickness clubs had relied upon evidence of incapacity. While many funds continued to use other forms of validation, such as sick visitors to assess a claim in person, this was not always practical in the larger friendly societies, even less so in private for-profit insurance firms or, after 1911, National Insurance.[9] The note became a useful proxy, endorsed by a medical professional—even if, as discussed in Chapter 2, it had its drawbacks.

Employers were also concerned with medical surveillance. 'Industrial medicine' became an increasingly important medical specialism during the interwar years, drawing both on epidemiological approaches to accidents and providing surveillance and medical care through 'the works' doctor'.[10] Coalmine owners used such physicians to certify fitness for work, reduce absenteeism, and to cajole employees back to the pit.[11] The introduction of the National Health

---

[7] Michael Heller, 'The National Insurance Acts 1911–1947, the Approved Societies and the Prudential Assurance Company', *Twentieth Century British History* 19, no. 1 (2008): pp. 1–28; Jackie Gulland, 'Extraordinary housework: Women and claims for Sickness Benefit in the early twentieth century', *Women's History Magazine* 71 (2013): pp. 23–30. See also Chapter 2.

[8] Robert Asher, 'Experience counts: British workers, accident prevention and compensation, and the origins of the welfare state', *Journal of Policy History* 15 (2003): pp. 359–88; Audrey C. Giles, 'Railway accidents and nineteenth-century legislation: "Misconduct, want of caution or causes beyond their control?"', *Labour History Review* 76, no. 2 (2011): pp. 121–42. On the use of medical evidence in liability and compensation cases more generally, see Deborah A. Stone, *The Disabled State* (Philadelphia: Temple University Press, 1984).

[9] Riley, 'Ill health'; Martin Gorsky, 'The growth and distribution of English friendly societies in the early nineteenth century', *Economic History Review* 51 (1998): pp. 489–511.

[10] Vicky Long, *The Rise and Fall of the Healthy Factory: The Politics of Industrial Health in Britain, 1914–60* (Basingstoke: Palgrave Macmillan, 2010); 'Industrial medicine: A report by the Social and Preventive Medicine Committee of the Royal College of Physicians of London', *British Journal of Industrial Medicine* 2, no. 1 (1945): pp. 51–5.

[11] The loss of works' doctors (and legal recourse) after 1948 was lamented in the National Coal Board files. See Chapter 3 and The National Archives (hereafter TNA): COAL 26/170, Cabinet,

Service lessened the need for the direct provision of medical care, leading the specialism to focus more on what would become known as 'health and safety'.[12] But the need for medical expertise to gatekeep the boundary between sickness absence and other forms of leave remained. This was true of *both* public and private institutions, before and after the Second World War.

This book argues that sick notes came to represent medical gatekeeping in the welfare state. The perceived need to delineate capacity from incapacity never went away, even if the specific form of the sick note evolved over time. Complaints and jokes about sick notes reflected inadequacies in gatekeeping systems—whether they let 'undeserving' people through or denied 'deserving' cases access to support. Successive governments tweaked medical certification rules, but they were unable to grapple with the underlying social, economic, cultural, and bureaucratic structures that had created and upheld Britain's sickness system. These structures continued to change over the postwar period. Yet the sick note was able to adapt to these changing circumstances. It provided forms of gatekeeping that were acceptable enough to all the various interconnected parts of the welfare state, surviving by being a more cost-effective, practical, and understood technology than any realistic alternative.

To tell this political and cultural history, this book uses 'the sick note' in three ways. First, it traces the form itself, showing how it circulated around public and private benefit systems. It considers how the layout of the note changed, how the regulations around its use were modified, and how the diagnoses written on these notes differed across time and place. Second, 'the sick note' is seen as a representation of the bureaucratic structures that upheld its use. Political discourse around sick notes therefore offers a reflection of wider anxieties about the welfare state, the workforce, the economy, labour conditions, and much more besides. Third, and finally, 'the sick note' is also shown to be a *driver* of policy change. By tracing its day-to-day operation through the welfare state and how others discussed its meaning, we see that policy evolved beyond policy makers' original design and intentions because of how the sick note was actually used. It is therefore through medical certificates and the popular discourse around them that we can understand the history of the British welfare state and the constituencies it attempted to serve.

Committee on Involuntary Absenteeism in the Coalmining Industry, Memorandum by Ministry of Fuel and Power, 7 September 1949.

[12] Ronnie Johnston and Arthur McIvor, 'Marginalising the body at work? Employers' occupational health strategies and occupational medicine in Scotland c. 1930–1974', *Social History of Medicine* 21, no. 1 (2008): pp. 127–44; A. Meiklejohn, 'Doctor and workman', *British Journal of Industrial Medicine*, 7, no. 3 (1950): pp. 105–16; Christopher Sirrs, 'Accidents and apathy: The construction of the "Robens Philosophy" of occupational safety and health regulation in Britain, 1961–1974', *Social History of Medicine* 29, no. 1 (2016): pp. 66–88; Long, *The Rise and Fall of the Healthy Factory*.

What Is Sickness?

How the specific post-1948 National Insurance sick note emerged, evolved, and differed from the plethora of other medical certificates will be explored in Chapter 2 and throughout this volume. But there is a more fundamental question that arises from this: what is 'sickness'?

First, it must be noted that there is a difference between 'sickness' in a cultural sense and 'sickness' as a bureaucratic category. On the cultural side, Talcott Parsons' 'sick role' is the classic sociological theory. Parsons argues that illness is a form of social deviance. Society expects people to be healthy, but individuals cannot always live up to this ideal. Sickness provides a culturally acceptable form of deviance from 'normal' behaviour, giving someone the time and resources to return to fitness. In return, individuals must do their utmost to recover and seek instruction from medical authorities.[13] Simon Williams has shown how sociologists of illness have thoroughly critiqued this 'sick role' since the 1950s. Parsons placed too much emphasis on a consensual relationship between the individual and medical authorities, did not fully explore the differences between acute and chronic illness, did not account for those who were incapable of recovery, and did not engage with 'class, gender, age and ethnicity'.[14] Meanwhile, historians have stressed that sickness is relative and socially constructed, problematizing the idea that the 'sick role' existed at all times and in all contexts. That is not to say that viruses, bacterial infections, injuries, organ dysfunction, and pain are irrelevant—rather, the meanings attached to symptoms, diagnoses, treatments, and patient behaviour are deeply rooted in cultural assumptions about sickness and health.[15] By extension, the roles performed by the 'sick' and the 'well' are not static.

While Parsons' work is therefore limited in understanding how concepts of sickness circulate within society, it is still useful in understanding *bureaucratic* definitions of sickness. This is because Parsons' approach recognizes that there is a difference between an 'illness' and a socially recognized state of 'sickness'. When defining a person as sick for bureaucratic purposes, a person might be ill—i.e., he or she might have a legitimate medical condition—but this alone is not enough to qualify for a financial benefit or legal rights. For National Insurance benefits alone, employment status, citizenship, contributions records, gender, and age could all affect whether 'being ill', even with a doctor's note, would translate into actual benefit payments. Applying 'the sick role' to bureaucratic procedures therefore allows us to interrogate how institutions set medical criteria, what they

---

[13] Talcott Parsons, *The Social System* (Glencoe: Free Press, 1951), esp. ch. 10.

[14] Simon J. Williams, 'Parsons revisited: From the sick role to…?', *Health* 9 (2005): pp. 123–44.

[15] Michel Foucault, *The Birth of the Clinic: An Archaeology of Medical Perception* (London: Tavistock, 1973).

provided to people who did qualify, and what instructions they expected claimants to follow.

Deborah Stone's *The Disabled State* remains the most illuminating example of
how this analysis can be done. Using Poor Law and disability schemes from the
early modern period to the 1980s in Britain, North America, and West Germany,
Stone shows how states created complex legal frameworks to provide benefits to
citizens deemed sick, but that this status often required the forfeiture of certain
rights.[16] Stone and disability studies scholars have argued that this became
necessary because industrialization increased people's reliance upon waged
labour. Poverty relief for those unable to work, particularly after the Victorian
Poor Law, was built on the premise of 'less eligibility'. Welfare was provided at
deliberately low and degrading levels so that waged labour would always appear
more attractive. This was designed to instil work ethic in the working classes
under the Malthusian belief that the poor would remain idle if given the
opportunity to be so.[17] Christian values of charity and disability led authorities
and citizens to recognize some as 'deserving poor', such as those unable to work
due to age, infirmity, or disease.[18] At the same time, resources were finite and the
work ethic of healthy individuals had to be maintained. Thus, there was a need to
set a level of 'incapacity' above which it was morally and legally acceptable to
receive support; and to create a gatekeeping procedure that could accurately
measure who fell on which side of this dividing line.[19] Not all illnesses—and not
all citizens—would meet this threshold. The perceived need to measure incapacity
has continued into the twenty-first century, as has the 'sick role' obligation to
recover by following the doctor's (or the state's) orders.[20]

These ever-shifting cultural and bureaucratic definitions of sickness make it
difficult to compare quantifiably across time. This matters because various
commentators concerned themselves with aggregate and relative rates, despite
the fundamental incompatibility of the subjective state of sickness and objective
measures of 'true' incapacity.[21] Businesses, of course, have long managed medical
absenteeism for disciplinary purposes and to extract the most possible from

[16]   Stone, *The Disabled State*.
[17]   David Feldman, 'Migrants, immigrants and welfare from the Old Poor Law to the welfare state',
Transactions of the Royal Historical Society 13 (2003): pp. 79–104; Rodney Lowe, *The Welfare State in
Britain since 1945* (Basingstoke: Palgrave Macmillan, 2005).
[18]   George Sher, 'Health care and the "deserving poor"', *The Hastings Center Report* 13 (1983):
pp. 9–12; Robert F. Drake, 'Charities, authority and disabled people: A qualitative study', *Disability &
Society* 11 (1996): pp. 5–23.
[19]   Deborah A. Stone, 'Physicians as gatekeepers', *Public Policy* 27 (1979): pp. 227–54; Stone, *The
Disabled State*; Michael Oliver and Colin Barnes, *The New Politics of Disablement* (Basingstoke:
Palgrave Macmillan, 2012); Jane Campbell and Michael Oliver, *Disability Politics: Understanding Our
Past, Changing Our Future* (London: Routledge, 1996).
[20]   Jackie Gulland, *Gender, Work and Social Control: A Century of Disability Benefits* (London:
Palgrave Macmillan, 2019).
[21]   Ibid.

their labour.[22] Trades unions have used various measures of sickness to monitor workplace safety and general working conditions. Both these groups, alongside the National Insurance authorities, friendly societies, and other insurance companies, have been providers of sick pay and other benefits at different points over the twentieth century. They have therefore had an interest in monitoring sickness levels to ensure schemes remain viable.[23] Finally, researchers have used measures of sickness to determine present-day trends to inform workplace and public health policies, as well as seeking out historical data to tell us more about experiences of sickness in the past.[24]

But all these groups had different ways of defining and measuring sickness, which were in turn different to the definition required for a sick note to excuse a patient from work. Because of that, there was little reliable data for sickness on the population level, creating plenty of room for contestation—especially when the very act of measuring sickness in the first place was tied to wider political concerns. Chapter 3, for example, discusses the myriad interpretations of involuntary absenteeism statistics in the 1950s and how they reflected contemporary anxieties about the economy and British society. Chapter 6 demonstrates how increasing rates of Incapacity Benefit were used as justification for stricter policies on disability claims. Both these 'problems' were caused by (as authorities saw it) 'too many' people receiving sick notes which gave them medically approved time away from paid work.

However, this world view relies on a notion that there is somehow a 'real' level of sickness in society that is significantly lower than the number of benefit claims being filed. Whether true or not, commentators had little substantive, long-term, commensurate evidence to go on. The postwar Survey of Sickness provided some identification of the 'real' level of sickness for the population, but it was only run once between 1943 and 1952 and therefore was not useful for tracking trends.[25] Health Survey for England has more comparable data over time, but it only began 1991.[26] There is a longer run of data for notifiable diseases, but this covers a very narrow range of conditions and does not include some of the usual suspects for absenteeism—most notably, common colds. Individual surveys of absenteeism would be published from time to time, as seen by the growth in this 'industry' in Chapter 7; but for the most part benefit claims were the easiest, most directly comparable, and most visible metric. This is partly why 'sick note' became a proxy

---

[22] Phil Taylor, Ian Cunningham, Kirsty Newsome, and Dora Scholarios, '"Too scared to go sick" – Reformulating the research agenda on sickness absence', *Industrial Relations Journal* 41, no. 4 (2010): pp. 270–88.

[23] See Chapters 2 and 3.   [24] See Chapter 2 and Riley, *Sick, Not Dead*.

[25] Stephen Taylor, 'The Survey of Sickness, 1943–52: Was our survey really necessary?', *The Lancet* 271, no. 7019 (1958): pp. 521–3.

[26] NHS Digital, 'Health survey for England – Health social care and lifestyles', *NHS Digital*, 2 March 2021, accessed 17 August 2021, https://digital.nhs.uk/data-and-information/areas-of-interest/public-health/health-survey-for-england—health-social-care-and-lifestyles.

for discussing absenteeism, disability, and other health-related issues in postwar Britain. Yet, as should now be clear, the slipperiness of the term 'sick' also allowed actors to express a wealth of other concerns about British society about and through discourse around the sick note.

With these caveats in mind, however, it is possible to do some work with the historical data to get a picture of British society in the past. Changes in sickness claim behaviours reflect not just shifts in disease patterns but also shifts in Britons' attitudes towards work and ill health. After all, absence from work remains one of the few proxies available in significant numbers for different regions and historical periods. One of the best examples is James Riley's work on the records of the Ancient Order of Foresters in the late-nineteenth and early-twentieth centuries, which demonstrated that both life expectancy and sickness increased over time.[27] S. Ryan Johansson attributed Riley's morbidity findings to a 'cultural inflation' of sickness, implying that societies became more tolerant (and more capable) of allowing people time off work for minor diseases that in generations past would not have led to absenteeism. How else can one explain a nation getting healthier (i.e., dying later) and yet taking more time off work with sickness?[28]

Martin Gorsky, Aravinda Guntupali, Bernard Harris, and Andrew Hinde, however, argue that the growing number of people over the age of 50 in the membership of the Ancient Order accounts for most of this increase. As more people lived to a point where their working capacity would be diminished by chronic injuries, disease, and general ageing, so they would have to claim more sickness benefits to support their families through periods of worklessness. If there was any cultural inflation amongst younger cohorts, it was offset by better health among the population.[29] Regardless of what 'really' happened, it is evident throughout *Sick Note* that postwar commentators also questioned the extent to which 'cultural inflation' was an inherent by-product of the 'generosity' of Britain's welfare state; while others paid closer attention to the significant demographic shifts in the country, including (but not limited to) greater female participation in the workforce, part-time work, migration, declining infectious disease relative to chronic conditions, and an ageing population.

Given contemporaries' interest in sickness data, then, it is worth briefly explaining what can be said about sickness in the postwar period. Changes in National Insurance benefits, the effective privatization of sickness benefit in the early 1980s, and the way data were reported make it difficult to give precise,

[27] Riley, *Sick, Not Dead.*

[28] S. Ryan Johansson, 'The health transition: The cultural inflation of morbidity during the decline of mortality', *Health Transition Review* 1, no. 1 (1991): pp. 39–68. See also discussion of 'moral hazard' in Chapter 2.

[29] Martin Gorsky et al., 'The "cultural inflation of morbidity" during the English mortality decline: A new look', *Social Science & Medicine* 73, no. 12 (2011): pp. 1775–83; Bernard Harris et al., 'Long-term changes in sickness and health: Further evidence from the Hampshire Friendly Society', *The Economic History Review* 65, no. 2 (2012): pp. 719–45.

comparable figures, but there is enough to show broad trends. Two series are most helpful. The first is the average number of claims to UK sickness benefit across the year, supplied by the Department of Health and Social Security and its predecessors. This is reasonably reliable up to the introduction of Statutory Sick Pay in the early 1980s as sickness benefit was used as the gateway to occupational sick pay and leave for those with an adequate National Insurance contributions record.[30] The introduction of Invalidity Benefit complicates the totals somewhat, but since this was effectively a replacement for long-term claims to sickness benefit, especially for unemployed claimants, it remains useful as a general indicator.[31] The second series is the Labour Force Survey which began tracking absenteeism from 1993 to the present day. Here, we find indicators of the amount of labour hours lost to sickness as well as the number of days missed per spell of incapacity.

Figures 1.1 and 1.2 show these series across time. They demonstrate that there was no great surge in sickness benefit claims in the earlier period, although there is a noticeable increase across the 1960s and 1970s, especially in long-term benefit claims once the two become disaggregated. Yet the general population was also growing and included more older people (Figure 1.3). For the later period, absenteeism remains relatively stable until the late 2000s, at which point the amount of time lost and the average spell of incapacity both begin to drop steadily. On these metrics at least, there does not seem to have been a great increase in sickness or in the willingness to claim sickness benefits at the national level. Indeed, in many instances it is clear that cultural reactions to sick notes had a tenuous relationship with any quantifiable data on medically verifiable morbidity or claims to sickness-based benefits. For instance, the discourse around 'sick note Britain' outlined in Chapter 7 occurred at precisely the moment that the data in Figure 1.2 suggest that absenteeism was on the decline. Responses to sick notes were therefore bound up in other economic, political, and cultural concerns.

Sick notes were, however, not only written for short-term absence from work. Doctors were also involved in certifying disability and long-term incapacity. Here, there were significant changes in claim patterns. As is discussed in more detail in Chapters 6 and 7, localized economic shocks in the 1980s and 1990s as well as national policies towards unemployment meant that there was a significant increase in claims to Incapacity Benefit over the 1980s (see Chapter 6 and Figure 6.1). 'Sickness'—in bureaucratic terms—was therefore experienced in different ways, by claimants, doctors, administrators, businesses, and politicians.[32] Again, *Sick Note* does not attempt to analyse the extent to which these changes

[30] The relationship between National Insurance and occupational sickness benefits is discussed in Chapters 3 and 5 especially.
[31] These developments are discussed in more detail in Chapters 5 and 6.
[32] Gulland, *Gender, Work and Social Control.*

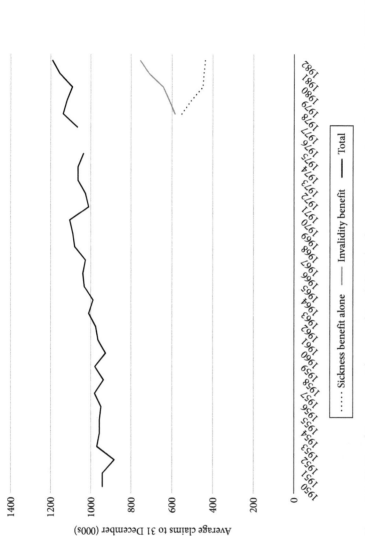

Figure 1.1 National Insurance sickness and invalidity benefits average annual number of claimants, 1950–1982. No data for 1976 due to industrial action.

Sources: 1950–53: Central Statistical Office, Annual Abstract of Statistics, No. 92 (London: HMSO, 1955), Table 42, p. 48; 1954–59: Central Statistical Office, Annual Abstract of Statistics, No. 102 (London: HMSO, 1965), Table 52.ii, p. 54; 1960–62: Central Statistical Office, Annual Abstract of Statistics, No. 105 (London: HMSO, 1968), Table 43, p. 49; 1963–65: Central Statistical Office, Annual Abstract of Statistics 1971, No. 108 (London: HMSO, 1971), Table 43, p. 50; 1966–69: Central Statistical Office, Annual Abstract of Statistics 1974 (London: HMSO, 1974), Table 3.16, p. 56; 1969–71: Central Statistical Office, Annual Abstract of Statistics 1977 (London: HMSO, 1977), Table 3.16, p. 67; 1972–74: Lawrence Ethel (ed.), Annual Abstract of Statistics 1980 (London: HMSO, 1980), Table 3.16, p. 68; 1975 and 1977: Lawrence Ethel (ed.), Annual Abstract of Statistics 1983, No. 119 (London: HMSO, 1983), Table 3.15, p. 54; 1978–82: Department for Work and Pensions, 'Spring budget 2020: Expenditure and caseload forecasts', gov.uk, 20 March 2020, accessed 13 July 2021, https://www.gov.uk/government/publications/benefit-expenditure-and-caseload-tables-2020.

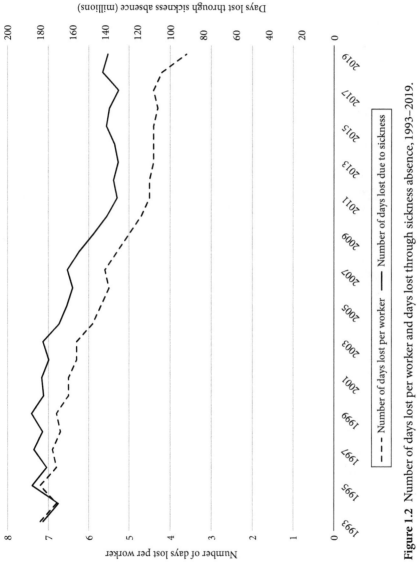

Figure 1.2 Number of days lost per worker and days lost through sickness absence, 1993–2019. 2020 not included because the COVID-19 'furlough' scheme renders data incomparable.

Source: Office for National Statistics, 'Sickness absence in the UK labour market', gov.uk, 3 March 2021, accessed 13 July 2021, https://www.ons.gov.uk/employmentandlabourmarket/peopleinwork/employmentandemployeetypes/datasets/sicknessabsenceinthelabourmarket.

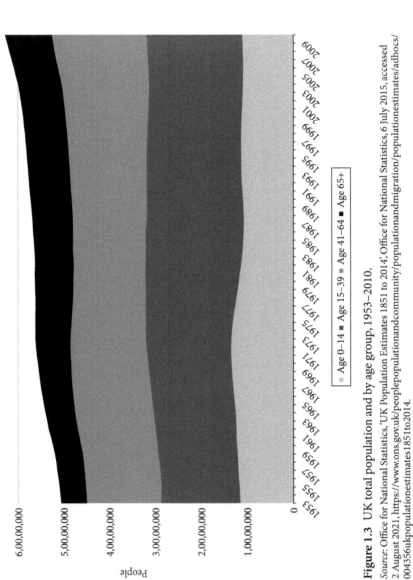

Figure 1.3 UK total population and by age group, 1953–2010.

Source: Office for National Statistics, 'UK Population Estimates 1851 to 2014'; Office for National Statistics, 6 July 2015, accessed 2 August 2021, https://www.ons.gov.uk/peoplepopulationandcommunity/populationandmigration/populationestimates/adhocs/004356ukpopulationestimates1851to2014.

were 'really' happening. But it is concerned with how these changes—experienced through subjective interactions, selectively reported aggregate data, or rigorous academic analysis—reflected and helped shape Britain's relationship to the sick note. In doing so, we see the broader relationships to the British welfare state and the changing composition of the British population.

'Sick Note Britain'?

The research presented in this book was prompted in part by a series of newspaper headlines from the 1990s onwards, beginning with the *Daily Mail*'s 1998 story 'Sign up here for Sick-note Britain'.[33] More recently, occupational health practitioner Adrian Massey has written a book called *Sick-Note Britain* criticizing the concept of medical certification.[34] This volume is therefore not concerned simply with the sick notes themselves but with the endurance of an idea. 'Sick note' came to mean much more than simply medical certification. It was conflated with absenteeism, worker behaviour, NHS doctors, welfare payments, business practices, and economic performance. These types of investigations can provide fertile ground for social historians. Lauren Pikó's work, for example, demonstrates that Milton Keynes' cultural legacy is just as much about how the North Buckinghamshire town lived in the public imagination as the 'real' bricks and mortar.[35] The continued use of the term 'sick note' in common parlance in the 2020s (a decade after the New Labour government replaced it with the 'fit note') says much about how the concept has endured in the national consciousness.[36]

Besides, any project that focused solely on the physical note would be short-lived. Doctor–patient confidentiality and research ethics necessarily limit the number of completed certificates available to historians. When they do appear, they do so in the specific context of administrative irregularities and tribunals.[37]

---

[33] David Jones, 'Sign up here for Sick-note Britain', *Daily Mail*, 14 April 1998, pp. 22–3. See also Chapter 7 and examples such as: TUC, 'Countering an urban legend: Sicknote Britain?', TUC, 7 January 2005, accessed 2 September 2020, archived 8 November 2005, http://web.archive.org/web/20051108200505/http://www.tuc.org.uk/welfare/tuc-9208-f0.cfm; WalesOnline, '"Rip up sick-note Britain"', Wales Online, 13 November 2007, accessed 23 November 2020, https://www.walesonline.co.uk/news/wales-news/rip-up-sick-note-britain-2217280; Laura Donnell, 'The "terrible legacy" of sick-note Britain', *Daily Telegraph*, 9 March 2008; Maria Tadeo, 'Sick note Britain: Employees face four week health check under new scheme', *Independent*, 13 February 2014, accessed 23 November 2020, https://www.independent.co.uk/news/business/news/sick-note-britain-employees-face-four-week-health-check-under-new-scheme-9126201.html.

[34] Adrian Massey, *Sick-Note Britain: How Social Problems Became Medical Issues* (London: Hurst Publishers, 2019).

[35] Lauren Pikó, *Milton Keynes in British Culture: Imagining England* (Abingdon: Routledge, 2019).

[36] See Chapters 7 and 8 and: Carol Mary Black and David Frost, *Health at Work: An Independent Review of Sickness Absence* (London: TSO, 2011).

[37] For this reason, this book anonymizes individuals where actual medical records are used. Full references are given to archival files for scholars interested in the details, provenance, and context. This emulates the approach taken by Roberta Bivins in her work on sensitive health issues around

Instead, it is more productive to follow the archival trail that emerges from them and debates surrounding them. As discussed, sick notes sit at the confluence of employment, social security, and health policy. The evidence from newspapers, government documents, trades union archives, business confederation archives, archived oral histories, comedy shows, web archives, and contemporary research reveal these three worlds, the connections between them, and their significance within (and to) wider British society. Building on Alex Mold's recent project on 'the public in public health', this history traces how publics 'spoke back' to policy makers through their active and passive engagement with sickness welfare systems.[38] This approach offers a break from 'statist' or 'top-down' histories of Whitehall-dictated law by focusing on implementation and reception.[39] Recent works such as Guy Ortolano's study of Milton Keynes, Peter Mandler's volume on state education or Jennifer Crane's investigation of child protection show how rich histories of a period and a nation can be drawn from what might, at face value, seem like narrow microhistories.[40] This book uses 'the sick note' in this way. A single object reproduced in multiple places across different areas of the welfare state, it offers a long-term view of the postwar welfare state in terms of its design, evolution, day-to-day operation, and cultural meaning to the various constituencies that funded, used, and benefited from it.

In doing so, we gain insight into how various constituencies understood the welfare state. Inevitably, the stories uncovered in sick note regulations and public discourse foreground the disputes rather than the many thousands of interactions with the state that have passed without hassle or comment. Following the work of Daisy Payling, these complaints offer a window onto the state's failings—but they also give various actors the opportunity to articulate visions of what the state ought to be.[41] Historians of emotion have brought these stories to the fore

migrant health. Roberta E. Bivins, *Contagious Communities: Medicine, Migration, and the NHS in Post-War Britain* (Oxford: Oxford University Press, 2015), p. 115, esp. note 2.

[38] Alex Mold, Peder Clark, Gareth Millward, and Daisy Payling, *Placing the Public in Public Health in Postwar Britain* (London: Palgrave Macmillan, 2019).

[39] On the criticism of 'statist' approaches, see: B. J. Gleeson, 'Disability studies: A historical materialist view', *Disability & Society* 12 (2010): pp. 179–202. For newer policy histories focusing on wider policy-making processes and health, see for example: Virginia Berridge, *Marketing Health* (Oxford: Oxford University Press, 2007); Sally Sheard, *The Passionate Economist: How Brian-Abel Smith Shaped Global Health and Social Welfare* (Bristol: Policy Press, 2013); Alex Mold, *Making the Patient-Consumer: Patient Organisations and Health Consumerism in Britain* (Manchester: Manchester University Press, 2015); Bivins, *Contagious Communities*; Jameel Hampton, *Disability and the Welfare State in Britain: Changes in Perception and Policy 1948–1979* (Bristol: Policy Press, 2016); Martin D. Moore, *Managing Diabetes, Managing Medicine: Chronic Disease and Clinical Bureaucracy in Post-War Britain* (Manchester: Manchester University Press, 2019).

[40] Jennifer Crane, *Child Protection in England, 1960–2000: Expertise, Experience, and Emotion* (London: Palgrave Macmillan, 2018); Guy Ortolano, *Thatcher's Progress: From Social Democracy to Market Liberalism through an English New Town* (Cambridge: Cambridge University Press, 2019); Peter Mandler, *The Crisis of the Meritocracy: Britain's Transition to Mass Education since the Second World War* (Oxford: Oxford University Press, 2020).

[41] Daisy Payling, '"The people who write to us are the people who don't like us:" Public responses to the government Social Survey's Survey of Sickness, 1943–1952', *Journal of British Studies* 59 (2020):

(such as Stephen Brooke's study of voluntary organizations in 1980s London); as have investigations into marginalized functionaries within state institutions (such as Julian Simpson's oral history of South Asian doctors).[42] Disputes are therefore useful not necessarily because they are statistically representative of the typical interaction between the 'normal' citizen and the state (although they might be)— their significance lies in the underlying common-sense discourses that are articulated in the archives in response to perceived injustices.[43]

While this is a story of conflict, it should not be read as a story of decline. These narratives do exist in the material, such as employer and media dismay at a supposed declining British work ethic, and in this sense they add to those found in other postwar social histories: a perceived loss of traditional gender roles;[44] of relative imperial power;[45] of working-class certainties in a post-Fordist economy;[46] of public accountability at the expense of private profit;[47] of welfare state protections against the rise of 'Thatcherite' or 'neoliberal politics'.[48] No doubt these helped actors 'interpret' the statistics presented earlier around absenteeism and disability as well as colouring historians' views of the period.[49] Nevertheless, while the perception of decline informed responses to change, historians do not have to reify it. As Florence Sutcliffe-Braithwaite shows in her insightful analysis of the way English people talked about and understood traditional class divides,

pp. 315–42. Payling builds on the work of Julian Baggini, *Complaint: From Minor Moans to Principled Protests* (London: Profile, 2010); John Clarke, 'Going public: The act of complaining', in *Complaints, Controversies and Grievances in Medicine: Historical and Social Science Perspectives*, edited by Jonathan Reinartz and Rebecca Wynter (London: Routledge, 2014), pp. 259–69.

[42] Stephen Brooke, 'Space, emotions and the everyday: The affective ecology of 1980s London', *Twentieth Century British History* 28, no. 1 (2017): pp. 110–42; Julian M. Simpson, *Migrant Architects of the NHS: South Asian Doctors and the Reinvention of British General Practice (1940s–1980s)* (Manchester: Manchester University Press, 2018). See also: Hannah J. Elizabeth, 'Love carefully and without "over-bearing fears": The persuasive power of authenticity in late 1980s British AIDS education material for adolescents', *Social History of Medicine* (2020); Michael Lipsky, *Street-Level Bureaucracy: Dilemmas of the Individual in Public Services* (New York: Russell Sage Foundation, 1980).

[43] Pat Thane, 'Family life and "normality" in postwar British culture', in *Life after Death: Approaches to a Cultural and Social History of Europe During the 1940s and 1950s*, edited by Richard Bessel and Dirk Schumann (Cambridge: Cambridge University Press, 2003), pp. 193–210; G. Millward, '"A matter of commonsense": The Coventry poliomyelitis epidemic 1957 and the British public', *Contemporary British History* 31 (2017): pp. 384–406.

[44] Helen McCarthy, 'Women, marriage and paid work in post-war Britain', *Women's History Review* 26, no. 1 (2017): pp. 46–61.

[45] David Edgerton, *The Rise and Fall of the British Nation: A Twentieth-Century History* (London: Allen Lane, 2018).

[46] Jim Tomlinson, 'De-industrialization not decline: A new meta-narrative for post-war British history', *Twentieth Century British History* 27, no. 1 (2016): pp. 76–99.

[47] Janet Newman and John Clarke, *Publics, Politics and Power: Remaking the Public in Public Services* (London: Sage, 2009).

[48] Stuart Hall, 'The great moving right show', in *The Politics of Thatcherism*, edited by Stuart Hall and Martin Jacques (London: Lawrence & Wishart, 1983), pp. 19–39; Taylor et al., '"Too scared to go sick"'.

[49] On trends in welfare state historiography mirroring contemporary politics, see: Bernard Harris, *The Origins of the British Welfare State: Society, State and Social Welfare in England and Wales, 1800–1945* (Basingstoke: Palgrave Macmillan, 2004).

class did not go away in the 1990s. Rather, it was remoulded alongside other cultural shifts across several decades.[50] Jim Tomlinson has similarly demonstrated using the concept of 'de-industrialization' that Britain's economy, politics, and society underwent profound changes, the details and significance of which are lost if seen solely through the lens of 'decline'.[51] This book is informed by such analyses, using the persistence of different forms of 'the sick note' across the postwar period to show *change* in the welfare state—not necessarily *decline*.

This gives insight into attitudes towards welfare in Britain. Yet the following chapters also make it clear that there was no singular 'the welfare state' or 'the government' across the entirety of the period. Indeed, none of the constituencies discussed here—including doctors, workers, and employers—were homogenous. Differing political positions and life experiences coloured the testimony left by these actors in the historical record. For 'the government', departments responsible for employment, health, social security, economic output, and the Treasury all had a stake in the operation of medical certification. But each had different incentives for reform and different organizations lobbying them. There were therefore many competing power dynamics between various institutions, and these changed significantly over time. The concept of welfare regimes has been used by historians and political scientists to explain these processes over an entire welfare state. However, even if, as Gøsta Esping-Andersen does, one categorizes the United Kingdom as a 'liberal' welfare state with (relatively) low taxation and means-tested benefits, this obscures the dynamism of other welfare logics flowing through Britain across the postwar period.[52] As James Vernon demonstrates through his analysis of the business and employment practices of Heathrow Airport, it is through the operation of policy that we can see a concept such as 'neoliberalism' emerging well before its supposed 'introduction' under Margaret Thatcher in the 1980s.[53] *Sick Note* does not make any claims about if or when Britain was a 'social democratic' or a 'neoliberal' welfare state. Rather, it shows that at different points and in certain circumstances there was a greater or lesser importance of certain *logics* of welfare that guided the principal actors and policy outcomes.[54] That is not to deny, for example, that neoliberalism was in general more dominant in policy design and operation after the International Monetary

---

[50] Florence Sutcliffe-Braithwaite, *Class, Politics, and the Decline of Deference in England, 1968-2000* (Oxford: Oxford University Press, 2018).
[51] Tomlinson, 'De-industrialization'.
[52] Gøsta Esping-Andersen, *The Three Worlds of Welfare Capitalism* (Cambridge: Polity, 1990). On the potential flattening effects of broad regime labels, see: Peter Baldwin, *The Politics of Social Solidarity: Class Bases of the European Welfare State 1875-1975* (Cambridge: Cambridge University Press, 1990); Kees van Kersbergen and Barbara Vis, *Comparative Welfare State Politics: Development, Opportunities, and Reform* (Cambridge: Cambridge University Press, 2014), esp. pp. 53–77.
[53] James Vernon, 'Heathrow and the making of neoliberal Britain', *Past & Present* (2021).
[54] On 'logics' as analytical frames and heuristic devices for analysing welfare state activity, see van Kersbergen and Vis, *Comparative Welfare State Politics*, esp. pp. 31–52. On contested periodization in the UK and in other welfare states, see: Frank Nullmeier and Franz-Xaver Kaufmann, 'Post-war welfare state development', in *The Oxford Handbook of the Welfare State*, edited by Francis G. Castles,

Fund loan in 1976.[55] Rather, it is to say that neoliberalism was not the only welfare logic in operation in this era and that its seeds were detectable far earlier. It further allows us to move beyond these economic frames and consider welfare logics understood through other critiques of power. It opens discussions about, as Jane Lewis has described it, the 'breadwinner welfare regime' centred on the male head of a nuclear family; 'chauvinism', and the denial of support to those considered as 'immigrants'; or the 'ableism' inherent to 'biopsychosocial' models of disability and welfare provision.[56] Each existed in different forms across the entire period. It is by focusing on the implementation of policy and its cultural reception that *Sick Note* shows these processes in action.

We see, too, that the immediate postwar welfare state was not just, as Marxist historians might view it, a corporatist bargain by the forces of capital to secure the cooperation of labour in rebuilding the postwar economy.[57] The insurance nature of Beveridgean social security reveals how the welfare state was also built around the rise of 'risk' as a lens through which social policy and governance were constructed.[58] Employers, employees, and government bodies benefited from the collectivized nature of sickness benefit and National Insurance, as shown in the debates over sick note policy.[59] The risks of sickness were spread across industrial sectors, helping those businesses engaged in more dangerous work or employing demographics more prone to ill health. Small and large organizations alike benefited from the absentee monitoring procedures and tribunals built into the certification and National Insurance system. The relative role of public, private, collective, and individual responsibility for sickness would change across the postwar period but debates about these central welfare state principles recur throughout this book.

Stephan Leibfried, Jane Lewis, Herbert Obinger, and Christopher Pierson (Oxford: Oxford University Press, 2010), pp. 81–102.

[55] A traditional dividing line between the 'Thatcherite' and 'classic welfare state'. See: Matthew Hilton, Chris Moores, and Florence Sutcliffe-Braithwaite, 'New Times revisited: Britain in the 1980s', *Contemporary British History* 31, no. 2 (2017): pp. 145–65; Hampton, *Disability and the Welfare State in Britain*; Lowe, *The Welfare State in Britain since 1945*; Anne Digby, *British Welfare Policy: Workhouse to Workfare* (London: Faber, 1989).

[56] Jane Lewis, 'Gender and the development of welfare regimes', *Journal of European Social Policy* 2, no. 2 (1992): pp. 159–73; Jeroen van Der Waal, Willem de Koster, and Wim van Oorschot, 'Three worlds of welfare chauvinism? How welfare regimes affect support for distributing welfare to immigrants in Europe', *Journal of Comparative Policy Analysis: Research and Practice* 15, no. 2 (2013): pp. 164–81; Tom Shakespeare, Nicholas Watson, and Ola Abu Alghaib, 'Blaming the victim, all over again: Waddell and Aylward's biopsychosocial (BPS) model of disability', *Critical Social Policy* 37, no. 1 (2017): pp. 22–41.

[57] Ian Gough, *The Political Economy of the Welfare State* (London: Macmillan, 1979); Lowe, *The Welfare State in Britain since 1945*, pp. 37–40.

[58] Mary Douglas and Aaron Wildavsky, *Risk and Culture* (Berkeley: University of California Press, 1983); Jakob Arnoldi, *Risk: An Introduction* (Cambridge: Polity, 2009); Ulrich Beck, *World at Risk* (Cambridge: Polity, 2009).

[59] On the role of industry and business leaders in driving welfare state formation and policy, see: Jeppe Nevers and Thomas Paster, 'Business and the Nordic welfare states, 1890–1970', *Scandinavian Journal of History* 44, no. 5 (2019): pp. 535–51; Vernon, 'Heathrow'.

Despite these narratives of change, *Sick Note* is also a story of remarkable continuity. The sick note endured. As demonstrated throughout, authorities regularly found that sick notes did not solve the administrative complexities of determining incapacity, controlling claimant behaviour, and ensuring optimal use of resources. Massey is merely the latest to 'discover' this in a long line of medical, employment, citizen, and government commentators.[60] That they remained, despite the profound economic, political, and social changes across postwar Britain, says something about the endurance of the welfare state, as well as its ability to adapt and entrench itself through its everyday operation. Proponents of 'liberalism', 'social democracy', 'neoliberalism', and 'the Third Way' all needed a gatekeeping device. The sick note was dynamic enough to meet the needs of all— at least well enough to survive to the next crisis. This endurance had cultural ramifications, further embedding its position. Just as Mike Savage's work on social science has shown how the British public came to understand itself in sociological terms through becoming subjected to repeated measurement and social surveys, so too did British workers and institutions become bound to the sick note as the primary mode of understanding paid work, ill health, and sickness-related benefits.[61]

Chapter Plan

To tell this history, the rest of *Sick Note* is broken into six main chapters following a broadly chronological structure. Chapter 2 shows how the 1948 National Insurance sick note—the 'Med 1'—was born. It explains the form of the certificate, what it was used for and how it fit into the wider plans for the postwar welfare state. It is this 'sick note' (and its descendants) that remains central to the rest of the book. But while the 'Med 1' was created specifically for the new National Insurance system, much like the 'birth' of the welfare state, this chapter shows that it is also important to acknowledge the deeper roots of medical certification before 1945. This does not just apply to the bureaucratic act of a GP writing a note; it also pertains to the relationships that had long existed between sickness benefit providers, the medical profession, employers, and employees. Furthermore, these experiences directly informed how the relationship between National Insurance and the National Health Service was designed to operate. The Beveridge Report's blueprint for the welfare state imagined that universal health services and social security would provide the basis for rebuilding the economy, but only if gatekeeping procedures were robust enough to deal with demand.

---

[60] Massey, *Sick-Note Britain.*
[61] Michael Savage, *Identities and Social Change in Britain since 1940: The Politics of Method* (Oxford: Oxford University Press, 2010).

Because of this longer history of medical certification, the Med 1 was controversial. By following doctors' complaints about workloads and expectations, a more nuanced picture of the negotiations between the British Medical Association (BMA) and the Ministry of Health around the National Health Service acts emerges than existing narratives that focus primarily on pay and conditions.[62] Anxieties about the potential loss of professional autonomy within a state-controlled service were sincere. Crucially, these events exposed how reliant the postwar welfare state would be upon medical expertise, even if it could not necessarily be easily co-opted in a way that was immediately useful or efficient for bureaucrats, citizens, and practitioners alike. Doctors would continue to insist that they did not possess the right type of expertise to judge incapacity for work, nor had they any desire to be the gatekeepers of private and public welfare. Though these arguments would change in intensity, they informed the BMA's actions for decades to come.

Chapter 3 analyses the problem most associated with sick notes: absenteeism. From the very beginning of National Insurance, right-wing critics and business leaders argued that increased availability of sickness benefits encouraged employees to take too much time off work. This analysis recurs throughout the book. However, the specific circumstances of the 1940s and 1950s intensified the criticism and its political significance. Labour and Conservative governments set targets for rebuilding the economy after the war to reset the balance of payments and pay off the large war debts owed to the United States. At the same time, nationalization had created and expanded UK-wide organizations that produced large amounts of data on worker absence across time. These statistics showed that absenteeism had indeed increased since 1948. The government invested in research into the problem and how it might be solved, but the answers from medical sociologists, trades unions, and management were unsatisfying. The sick note could not eliminate absenteeism, though it worked well enough for the government's purposes that it remained in use. Ultimately, the absenteeism problem faded not so much because the 'real' amount of sick leave dropped, but because its political salience had declined in the face of other economic and social priorities. Absenteeism would remain a background concern throughout the postwar period, flaring up when wider anxieties about Britain's relative place in the global economy emerged.

Chapter 4 considers groups who were not central to this discourse. Using files from the National Assistance Board and debates about married women's benefits from the 1940s to the 1970s, it shows that there were other gatekeeping procedures to deny sickness-related benefits to certain types of claimant. Those who did not

---

[62] Such as: Rudolf Klein, *The New Politics of the NHS*, 7th edn (London: CRC Press, 2013); Charles Webster, *National Health Service: A Political History*, 2nd revised edn (Oxford: Oxford University Press, 2002).

fit the model of the British-born male 'breadwinner' were often categorized in ways that minimized or eliminated the relevance of medical certification, even in cases where the National Insurance sick note would otherwise have been the central question of eligibility for support. The sick note—or, rather, the ignoring of its importance in these specific cases—uncovers the racist, ableist, and sexist assumptions built into welfare state's administration from the 1940s, the echoes of which continued into the twenty-first century. It shows how and why the medical status of women and Commonwealth migrants intersected with deeper concerns about Britain's national identity, employment policy, domestic labour, and traditional gender roles. But rather than being a new problem in the 1960s, when civil rights and equalities politics became more visible in the media and national political discourse, Britain's changing demographics had caused administrative confusion from the very beginning. This would only increase as the country's workforce became ever more non-white and non-male.

However, Chapter 5 shows that the welfare state *could* adapt its day-to-day operations in certain circumstances. In the 1980s, the Thatcher government introduced Statutory Sick Pay. This began the process of effectively privatizing sickness benefit, passing the responsibility for administration to employers. These reforms gave the BMA an opportunity to press for self-certification for workers whose illnesses lasted less than one week. This chapter shows how privatization rhetoric accelerated in the late 1970s, but that employers had always played a key role both as beneficiaries and providers of sickness-related welfare. Similarly, it demonstrates that the Thatcherite reforms were only made possible by the changing structure of the welfare state explored in the previous chapters. Gradual reform of medical certification—such as the replacing of the 'Med 1' with the 'Med 3' in 1966—could only happen when those with grievances about sick notes were able to take advantage of simultaneous weaknesses in employment, health, and social security policy. The sick note remained for longer-term sickness and would continue to be a central part of British employment. Indeed, the changes here informed the different directions that short-term absenteeism management and chronic disability benefit policy would develop from the late 1990s and into the new millennium.

Chapter 6 continues this theme by focusing on the rise of 'sick note' as a short-hand for several sickness-related anxieties in the British media from the 1980s onwards. As businesses became increasingly responsible for managing short-term sickness, they complained at the loss of collectivized protection against absence. Simultaneously, they intensified their absenteeism disciplinary machinery. Meanwhile, the government sought reform of its gatekeeping procedures for long-term sickness benefits. As a result of expanded welfare for disabled people in the 1970s and increased unemployment in the 1980s, expenditure on Incapacity Benefit had risen dramatically. New capacity tests were designed to redefine the boundaries between sickness and unemployment and reduce demand, built on new theories of disability and employment. Contemporaneously, the media reflected a new, humorous discourse around sick notes that reflected cultural shifts over the postwar period and scepticism about gatekeeping procedures. The phrase could be used as a nickname (for men like Darren Anderton and Bert Quigley) as well as indicating deeper misgivings with social policy and the welfare state. Overall, it seemed that the British people expected the sick note to remain as a defence against overzealous employers or government agencies that would deny rights to pay and leave; yet they were keenly aware of the faults in the system.

Finally, Chapter 7 takes these arguments into the New Labour era and shows how Conservative sickness and disability policies were reformed under 'Third Way' logic around welfare and employment. Sick-note discourse in the media expanded from discussion about absenteeism and humorous jibes at sport stars to visceral attacks on the largesse of welfare. As Labour committed to tackling the perceived problems of 'scroungers' and worklessness, business groups continued to produce statistics and drive a narrative that absenteeism was hampering Britain's ability to compete in a globalized economy. Absenteeism policing increased in the workplace and the government put tougher conditions on disability benefits; though both tempered this with the offer of rehabilitative options for those willing and able to access them. This 'active labour market' logic manifested in the 'fit note' in 2010, which finally replaced the 'Med 3' with a statement on what a claimant *could* do in the workplace rather than what they could not. While de-industrialization, declining union power, and 'flexible' employment practices had reduced organized resistance to these trends, the World Wide Web provided new opportunities for communities of individuals with similar experiences to share information and provide support. New discourses emerged around the sick note that reflected these changes. Thus, even though the fit note had replaced it, the idea of the sick note lived on. Just as 1948 had not truly represented the sick note's 'birth', 2010 was not really its 'death' either.

The book concludes with the shorter Chapter 8, bringing these arguments together and reflecting on what 'sick note Britain' looks like in the 2020s. Precarious employment, the gig economy, automation, presenteeism, and zero-hours contracts concerned political commentators and economists in the 2010s. And then came COVID-19. The pandemic exposed the limitations of a system reliant upon stable employment provided by solvent private businesses with sickness spread sparsely through the population. Direct illness from the virus coupled with self-isolation protocols and 'lockdowns' wrought havoc on privatized welfare systems and overwhelmed the remaining public ones. In this discussion, the book resists simple narratives of decline and nostalgia. After all, the 1940s' sickness system failed many who did not fit the model of the British-born male breadwinner. Still, it examines how an unprecedented crisis might affect the way sickness gatekeeping operates in the short and long term.

2

The 'Birth' of the Sick Note

The 'sick note' was born on 5 July 1948. Or at least the National Insurance sick note was born on this Appointed Day. The repeal of the Victorian Poor Law and its replacement with the National Health Service, National Insurance, and National Assistance was revolutionary in many ways. And yet, it was also clearly an evolution from systems that had developed out of the late-nineteenth century and through the interwar period. The 'Med 1' (which forms the basis of discussion across the rest of this book) was a new certificate born here. Yet it was built on a logic of medical certification that had been practised for decades, retaining many of the idiosyncrasies that had frustrated workers, doctors, and administrators alike. Much like the 'death' of the sick note in 2010, it is clear that the idea of sick notes lived well before and well after the 'Med 1' and its successor the 'Med 3' were in official circulation.

One cannot understand the postwar evolution of the sick note and the way various institutions and individuals understood medical certification without first understanding earlier developments. As Chris Renwick describes it, borrowing from Beveridge's description of a 'British Revolution', the welfare state was '150 years in the marking'.[1] The sick note also had a long lineage, and many of the doubts expressed about their utility in 1948 had been circulating in previous decades. The 'Med 1' relied upon the expertise and labour of doctors but was in no way a scientific assessment of an individual's capabilities relative to their usual work duties. Authorities knew that gatekeeping procedures would have to consider more than just the evidence of the sick note, and yet insisted on such certificates in almost every instance. This mattered because the new welfare state envisioned by Lord Beveridge and the incoming Labour government after the Second World War was built around an overarching system coordinating employment, health, and social security, held together by medical certification.

This chapter introduces the key 'flaws' in the sick note system through the lens of the debates between doctors and the government over the foundation of the NHS. This is instructive, because even though there were clear weaknesses in the medical certification system, these were not considered so insurmountable that sick notes were abandoned. Doctors' views had been heavily informed by experiences of the 1911 National Health Insurance system. Although the primary

---

[1] Chris Renwick, *Bread for All: The Origins of the Welfare State* (London: Penguin, 2018), p. 4.

arguments with the Ministry of Health in the 1940s had been over remuneration and financial independence, a key battleground centred on professional autonomy. If doctors were to be required by law to write sick notes, and if they were to be, in effect, state employees, how could the medical profession ensure its neutrality? Given that family physicians, upon whom the greatest burden would be placed, were not experts in occupational health, were they the best people to write sick notes? If these certificates were simply 'ipse dixit'—Latin for 'he/she said it', no more than an acknowledgement that 'the patient says they cannot work'—were they not a waste of time? It is within these battles over the scope and function of medical certification, that wider concerns about the system were expressed. Many of these were longstanding, with the specific historical circumstances of the mid-1940s amplifying their importance.

In spite of these well-known flaws, the sick note was repurposed and remained the keystone of sickness benefit gatekeeping for the next 60 years. Doctors did not all have the same opinion on sick notes, and through their disputes it becomes clear that there were perceived benefits to the system. Although it did place a burden on GPs, the workload was not considered unbearable. Besides, encouraging workers to go to the GP when sick would allow them to be assessed and given treatment if necessary; and prescribing rest could well be part of the therapy in itself. For authorities, the sick note worked in the majority of cases and was administratively simple. In those instances where there were doubts, other gatekeeping mechanisms could be deployed on top of the medical certificate. Perhaps as importantly as any of these reasons, the historical precedent of sick notes for National Health Insurance and the Approved Societies meant that doctors, patients, and benefit providers could all work within a familiar system. The way prewar medical certification practices could be adapted to the needs of the postwar welfare state ensured their survival. Sick notes were not perfect; but they did appear to be the workable, least terrible option available.

The main body of this chapter begins by explaining the relationship between the NHS, National Insurance, and National Assistance. While the Labour government did not follow William Beveridge's blueprint for a postwar welfare state[2] to the letter, the fundamental principles of a health service and social security system working together to reduce sickness, idleness, and want remained critical. Certification was integral to this new structure, explaining why the sick note was so important in the decades that followed. The second section then examines doctors' complaints expressed in the medical journals prior to the creation of the NHS. Here we see that GPs' anxieties were tied to wider apprehensions about the place of the medical profession in a new, centralized health service. The peculiar position of GPs (as independent contractors almost

---

[2] William H. Beveridge, *Social Insurance and Allied Services (Cmd. 6404)* (London: HMSO, 1942).

entirely dependent upon the state for their income) meant that sick notes were emblematic of the ties, new and old, between the state and physicians. As the primary providers of sick notes, GPs had a particular interest in how this new system would work and how it would affect their ability to practice. In the final section, we see the compromises reached between the Ministry of Health and the British Medical Association (BMA). The Safford Report of 1949 exposed the extent of and problems with medical certification that went well beyond National Insurance sick notes; but while government departments in Whitehall and Edinburgh made commitments to reduce their reliance upon such certificates, the sick note itself remained. As an extant technology that performed enough tasks with competence, it remained a better and cheaper option than any alternative. With light adaptation, sick notes could continue to serve the state's purposes and those of the other constituencies that had come to rely upon them.

In combination, these sections introduce the long-running issues that recur throughout the rest of this volume. One cannot understand or analyse these without appreciating the historical context in which the 1948 sick note was born. Although the sick note would change over the decades—and although evolving social, cultural, economic, and political circumstances would lead some flaws to be more pertinent as times than others—it is here that a coherent idea of 'the sick note' began.

First, Intermediate, Final

Before discussing the Beveridge plan, however, it is worth explaining what 'the sick note' studied across this volume was. Most of the discussion around medical certificates in the postwar period focused on the 'Med 1' National Insurance certificate, also known as a 'First' certificate (Figure 2.1). It was used by a patient to provide evidence of incapacity for a sickness benefit claim. Available from the third day of sickness, it would be sent to the local National Insurance office to collect benefit; although in practice many workers would also send a copy to their employer or friendly society to demonstrate their entitlement to sick leave or benefits under those organizations' policies.[3] It marked the beginning of the sickness process, the main 'gate' into the system. Although it could be challenged, in the majority of cases this was the point at which a person's status within the welfare state changed to 'sick'. Therefore, as we will see throughout this book, it was the most meaningful for patients, employers, and government officials.

---

[3] The National Archives (hereafter TNA): PIN 7/368, Ministry of Health and Department of Health for Scotland, 'Report of the Inter-Departmental Committee on Medical Certificates', 1949.

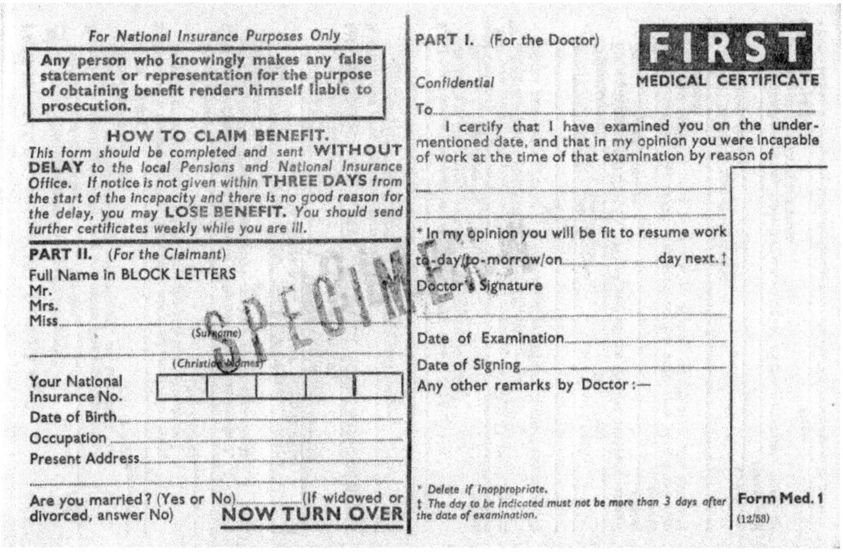

For National Insurance Purposes Only

Any person who knowingly makes any false statement or representation for the purpose of obtaining benefit renders himself liable to prosecution.

HOW TO CLAIM BENEFIT.

This form should be completed and sent **WITHOUT DELAY** *to the local Pensions and National Insurance Office. If notice is not given within* **THREE DAYS** *from the start of the incapacity and there is no good reason for the delay, you may* **LOSE BENEFIT.** *You should send further certificates weekly while you are ill.*

PART II. *(For the Claimant)*

Full Name in BLOCK LETTERS

Mr.

Mrs.

Miss........................

(Surname)

....

(Christian Names)

Your National Insurance No. | | | | | |

Date of Birth........................

Occupation........................

Present Address........................

....

Are you married? (Yes or No)..............(If widowed or divorced, answer No)

NOW TURN OVER

PART I. (For the Doctor)

FIRST

MEDICAL CERTIFICATE

Confidential

To........................

I certify that I have examined you on the under-mentioned date, and that in my opinion you were incapable of work at the time of that examination by reason of

....

....

* In my opinion you will be fit to resume work to-day/to-morrow/on..............day next.†

Doctor's Signature

....

Date of Examination........................

Date of Signing........................

Any other remarks by Doctor:—

** Delete if inappropriate.*

† The day to be indicated must not be more than 3 days after the date of examination.

Form Med. 1

(12/58)

SPECIMEN

Figure 2.1 Ministry of National Insurance, Med. 1, front (1953).
TNA: PIN 35/100. In circulation 1948 to 1966.

The process of ‘signing off’ a person from work can be traced to this note, even after changes to the forms in the 1960s.[4]

These notes followed a similar pattern throughout the postwar period. The doctor would fill out his or her details in ‘Part 1’, often including a rubber stamp with the address of the surgery. In ‘Part 2’, the claimant was asked to provide the key National Insurance information such as name, sex, marital status, address, and National Insurance number. There was also a signature to declare that the information being provided was, to the best of the claimant’s knowledge, truthful. On the back (Figure 2.2) came the more specific details about past claims, whether the claim was for sickness or industrial injury, the time of the claim (down to the hour to take into account shift work, especially if it spanned midnight), the dependents in the household, and other particulars that could affect the rate of payment.

The ‘Med 1’ held the most meaning because of its position at the start of what could be a long bureaucratic process. However, there were two other certificates that were generally lumped into the common understanding of ‘the sick note’. One determined whether a patient was *still* sick; the other that it was safe for a claimant to return to work. The ‘Med 2A’—or ‘Intermediate’—and ‘Med 2B’—or ‘Final’—served these purposes. Broadly in the same format as the Med 1, they were vital parts of the gatekeeping machinery. Intermediate certificates were

[4] See Chapter 5.

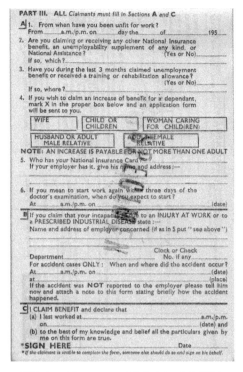

Figure 2.2 Ministry of National Insurance, Med. 1, back (1953).
TNA: PIN 35/100. In circulation 1948 to 1966.

required weekly in the early stages of illness, before becoming less frequent for longer spells.[5] The 'Final' certificate was designed to protect the worker's safety and economic productivity. To return to work early could risk relapse or, particularly in the case of heavy industrial labour, could be dangerous. Employers also had an incentive to allow sick workers time to recuperate fully so that they would be more productive when they returned. Additionally, the use of a 'Final' certificate could allow workers to seek a return to employment when they were ready, rather than 'waiting out' the full length of previous certificates. The odd day here and there soon added up for an economy in desperate need of the labour hours.[6] Both notes were collected in the same way as the 'Med 1' and, for the patient and doctors alike, represented the same type of duty on both to gather or provide medical evidence in support of a claim.

But while the 'Med 2' forms did encourage patients to keep in contact with a doctor throughout their sickness and ensure proper treatment was provided, in

---

[5] The duration of these certificates and changes made to regulations over time are covered in more detail in Chapter 5.
[6] See Chapter 3.

many cases such surveillance was unnecessary. Technically, a doctor needed to provide two consultations for a patient who requested a note for a minor ailment on the third day of their absence from work; one for a 'First' certificate and another for a 'Final'. In practice, doctors and patients were able to fudge this, but it was a bureaucratic load for all concerned.[7] Similarly, 'Intermediate' certificates were needed in the early stages of sickness regardless of a diagnosis. For conditions with a relatively standard prognosis—such as a broken arm—or with slim chance of recovery, this was medically unnecessary.[8]

There were 'Convalescent', 'Monthly', and 'Voluntary' certificates in 1948, but these do not appear regularly in the record.[9] Any additional details that might be required could be provided on the 'Supplemental' certificate, or 'Med 5'. This might include providing a case history if the patient needed evidence that they were sick before being able to procure a 'Med 1' (or fit enough to return before obtaining a 'Med 2B').[10] A 'Med 6' allowed doctors to provide additional details on a patient in confidence to the National Insurance office, such as when a diagnosis might cause difficulties for a patient with an employer due to stigma or prejudice.[11] It should also be noted that certificates for confinement and maternity were covered under the same regulations as National Insurance sick notes, as will be explored in more detail in Chapter 4.[12] Although maternity was not 'sickness' per se, complications arising from pregnancy fell into a hinterland; and it was considered 'common sense' that women would be unable to work (or should not be expected to work) in the final weeks of pregnancy.[13]

Nevertheless, when talking about 'the sick note' that emerges over the following decades the focus was on 'Med 1' and 'Med 2'. To emphasize the similarity in their bureaucratic function as well as their status in the eyes of claimants, these forms

---

[7] Doctors would find ways to effectively mark a single consultation as two consultations held back-to-back. The Ministry knew about this practice but was content to let it continue providing it was not abused. See evidence throughout the early postwar period, but esp.: TNA: MH 135/743, British Medical Association, Statement of the Association's Evidence to the Departmental Committee on Medical Certification (attached to letter 17 June 1948); PIN 35/150, Medical Certificates for National Insurance Purposes, memorandum attached to letter dated 23 March 1965.

[8] See later in this chapter, Chapter 5 and TNA: MH 135/741, Press cutting, W. R. Lord (King's Norton), letter to *Birmingham Mail*, 9 March 1949.

[9] Anon, 'The Act in Action', *The Lancet* 252, no. 6534 (November 1948): pp. 823–5. These were so rare that by 1952 the Ministry of National Insurance did not even mention them in its list of certificates. TNA: PIN 52/3, Medical certificates etc., for National Insurance Purposes, February 1952.

[10] TNA: PIN 52/3, Medical certificates etc., for National Insurance Purposes, February 1952.

[11] Ibid. On stigma, see especially Chapter 6.

[12] Ministry of National Insurance, *National Insurance (Medical Certification) Regulations, 1948 (HC 149 (1947–48))* (London: HMSO, 1948); National Insurance Advisory Committee, *National Insurance (Maternity Benefit) Regulations 1948: Report (HC 147 (1947–48))* (London: HMSO, 1948).

[13] Anon, 'The panel conference', *The Lancet* 246, no. 6378 (November 1945): pp. 684–6; Anon, 'Towards Social Security', *The Lancet* 247 (1946): p. 356. On 'common sense' as evidence in policy making, see: Gareth Millward, '"A matter of commonsense": The Coventry poliomyelitis epidemic 1957 and the British public', *Contemporary British History* 31, no. 3 (2017): pp. 384–406.

would eventually become merged into a single 'Med 3' in 1966.[14] Various other changes to the regulations would come as a result of negotiations between business groups, unions, voluntary organizations, the BMA, and government departments to reduce the need for certificates in certain circumstances. In 1948, however, this was the state of play, designed to fit the needs of the new Beveridgean welfare state's social security and health services.

The 'Health Service'

While the Appointed Day for the new National Health Service has survived in the popular memory—most notably in 2018's *#NHS70* 'celebrations'[15]—two other central parts of the Beveridgean welfare state launched on 5 July 1948: National Insurance and National Assistance. Neither endured in the same way as the NHS. National Assistance would become Supplementary Benefit in 1968 and then abolished entirely in 1988, while the importance of National Insurance as a qualifying criterion for pensions, unemployment, and sickness benefits would decrease as the 'insurance principle' was undermined by successive reforms to the social security system.[16] The GPs and the hospitals, however, remained and took on the status as 'the closest thing the English have to a religion.'[17] The history of the 'sick note' helps to explain how and why these institutions should be considered as a package. It also shows that while a new sick note was born in 1948 to help manage them, it was a document built upon foundations that went much deeper into the past of how British citizens accessed health care from their GP.

The Beveridge Report was clear that the three institutions were inseparable.[18] As a unit, universal health care and social security would eventually reduce the burden on the state of the 'five giants'.[19] This 'productionist' approach to medicine was tied to economic output.[20] Access to medical care would keep workers fitter for longer across their life cycles, as well as interacting with rehabilitative services to return citizens to capacity after injury or illness. Universal access, without the

---

[14] See Chapter 5.

[15] A project at the University of Manchester collecting and analysing oral histories of people who have worked or been treated in the NHS since 1948 has approach the 70th anniversary from a more critical gaze. See Stephanie Snow and Angela Whitecross, 'Connecting voices in a time of crisis: NHS at 70 and Covid-19', *Oral History Review*, 5 May 2020, accessed 17 September 2020, http://oralhistoryreview.org/current-events/nhs-70-covid-19/; and the project website: 'NHS at 70', accessed 17 September 2020, www.nhs70.org.uk.

[16] Rodney Lowe, *The Welfare State in Britain since 1945* (Basingstoke: Palgrave Macmillan, 2005).

[17] Nigel Lawson, *The View from No. 11: Memoirs of a Tory Radical* (London: Bantam, 1992), p. 613.

[18] *Cmd. 6404.*

[19] Want, disease, ignorance, squalor, and idleness. Nicholas Timmins, *The Five Giants: A Biography of the Welfare State*, 2nd edn (London: Harper Collins, 2001).

[20] John Pickstone, 'Production, community and consumption: The political economy of twentieth-century medicine', in *Medicine in the Twentieth Century*, edited by R. Cooter and J. Pickstone (Abingdon: Routledge, 2003), pp. 1–20.

patient having to worry about cost or availability, would mean health problems would be seen quicker and long-term incapacity would be reduced across the population.

Such services would only be accessible, however, if citizens could afford to take enough time off work and rest to stop minor conditions becoming serious, seek treatment, and convalesce fully to prevent relapse. The provision of adequate sickness benefit would allow and encourage recuperation. Industrial injuries benefits would perform a similar role, with the hope that this would also encourage businesses to improve safety as they would have to insure themselves against liability.[21] National Insurance and National Health would therefore keep the costs of each other manageable. Workers who were in a safe environment, well-rested, and taking responsible prophylactic action would not get to the point of needing invasive, expensive treatments for injuries and diseases; while properly treated patients would return to work quicker, reducing their demands on social security. So inseparable were these services that, in the early years, some referred to National Insurance benefits and the NHS interchangeably as 'the health service'.[22]

Meanwhile, National Assistance would deal with the remaining citizens who, for whatever reason, could not build an adequate National Insurance record, such as the very young, the old, or the chronically sick and disabled. Providing a subsistence income, National Assistance was designed to alleviate absolute poverty but to still provide an incentive to work and protect oneself against the risks of sickness through state, mutual, and private forms of insurance. As we will see, especially in Chapter 4, Beveridge and the postwar Labour government underestimated how many people would fall under this category, including misjudging the number of single parents, the extent of disability, and the arrival of non-British-born migrants.[23]

In many ways, these plans reflected the prewar status quo. The National Health Insurance system (hereafter NHI to distinguish it from postwar National Insurance) had been established by the Liberal government as part of a series of reforms to provide industrial injury protection, old age pensions, access to health

---

[21] Ministry of Reconstruction, *Social Insurance Part II: Workmen's Compensation. Proposals for an Industrial Injury Insurance Scheme (Cmd. 6551)* (London: HMSO, 1944). On occupational health and safety, see: Christopher Sirrs, 'Accidents and apathy: The construction of the "Robens Philosophy" of occupational safety and health regulation in Britain, 1961–1974', *Social History of Medicine* 29, no. 1 (2016): pp. 66–88.

[22] TNA: CAB 129/35/12, Ministry of Fuel and Power, 'Effect of new sickness and injury benefits upon absenteeism in coal mines' (31 May 1949), para 6. See Chapter 3.

[23] This realization became politically influential during the 'rediscovery of poverty' in the 1960s. See: Brian Abel-Smith and Peter Townsend, *The Poor and the Poorest: A New Analysis of the Ministry of Labour's Family Expenditure Surveys of 1953–54 and 1960* (London: Bell, 1965); Rodney Lowe, 'The rediscovery of poverty and the creation of the Child Poverty Action Group', *Contemporary Record* 9 (1995): pp. 602–11; John Viet-Wilson, 'The National Assistance Board and the "rediscovery" of poverty', in *Welfare Policy in Britain: The Road from 1945*, edited by Helen Fawcett and Rodney Lowe (Basingstoke: Macmillan, 1999), pp. 116–57.

care, and unemployment and sickness insurance. It formalized, financially protected, and increased access to a network of sickness and medical benefit providers across the United Kingdom who took on the status of 'Approved Societies'. Many of these organizations were mutualist friendly societies which provided sick pay and access to a General Practitioner for their members, though trades unions and for-profit insurance companies also performed these functions for certain professions and individuals.[24] It had been customary for friendly societies to pay doctors a 'capitation fee' for their services—regular payments based on the number of society members on the doctor's list. In return, doctors would provide consultations, treatments, prescriptions, and, when required, medical certificates so that the patient could claim sick pay from the society.[25] National Insurance adopted this capitation method for paying GPs. As will be discussed later, this arrangement continued after 1948 (albeit not without a fight).[26] The capitation system produced long-standing grievances between approved societies, doctors, and claimants. Historians have discussed the adequacy of such payments and the restrictions they could impose upon doctors at length.[27] For the story of the sick note, however, the centrality of certification to the relationship between Approved Societies' administrators and members created tensions that continued into the postwar era.

A key issue was what economists refer to as 'moral hazard'. Friendly societies were not always financially stable and had to restrict access to health-related benefits to keep their funds solvent. Even larger, more stable funds and for-profit insurance companies had to be mindful of their margins to ensure continued survival and/or surpluses. Trades unions, especially those representing professions with high sickness or injury rates, often found themselves unable to compete in this marketplace because their sick pay expenditure left little for providing medical benefits.[28] The moral hazard was that if sickness benefits were too 'generous' and too easy to acquire, fund members would choose to extend their convalescence beyond what they might otherwise have done rather than return to work and resume paying their membership fees.[29] The pressure was on

[24] William H. Beveridge, *Voluntary Action: A Report on Methods of Social Advance* (London: George Allen & Unwin, 1948); Martin Gorsky, 'The growth and distribution of English friendly societies in the early nineteenth century', *Economic History Review* 51 (1998): pp. 489–511; Lowe, *The Welfare State in Britain since 1945*.

[25] Frank Honigsbaum, *The Division in British Medicine: A History of the Separation of General Practice from Hospital Care 1911–1968* (London: Kogan Page, 1979).

[26] Charles Webster, *National Health Service: A Political History*, 2nd revised edn (Oxford: Oxford University Press, 2002).

[27] Honigsbaum, *The Division in British Medicine*; Andrew Morrice, '"Strong combination": The Edwardian BMA and contract practice', in *Financing Medicine: The British Experience since 1750*, edited by Martin Gorsky and Sally Sheard (London: Routledge, 2006), pp. 165–81.

[28] Honigsbaum, *The Division in British Medicine*, esp. pp. 219–23.

[29] Martin Gorsky et al., 'The "cultural inflation of morbidity" during the English mortality decline: A new look', *Social Science & Medicine* 73 (2011), 1775–83; Deborah Stone, 'Behind the jargon: Moral hazard', *Journal of Health Politics, Policy & Law* 36 (2011): pp. 886–96.

doctors, therefore, to keep certification to a minimum. After the introduction of NHI, many more workers, including those in lower-paid manual professions, gained access to GPs and therefore to certificates. The NHS expanded these liabilities still further.

Thus, to ensure the new system remained affordable and protected from abuse, Beveridge asserted that access to sickness-related benefits would have to be restricted.

> The measures for control of claims to disability benefit – both by certification and by sick visiting – will need to be strengthened, in view of the large increases proposed in the scale of compulsory insurance benefit and the possibility of to this substantially through by voluntary insurance through Friendly Societies.[30]

Strong gatekeeping systems would protect the National Insurance fund and, by extension, the NHS and the entire welfare state project. That gatekeeping would come in large part from the certificates written by a medical profession ever more tightly bound to the state through the NHS. The connection between sickness benefits, sick notes, and the medical profession was to become even stronger, mutually reinforcing the importance of all three. This had significant repercussions for government departments, doctors, patients, and employers.

The bitter experience of certification under NHI informed Beveridge's thinking. The system described above meant that patients and doctors were very familiar with the ritual of seeking and providing sick notes.[31] So too were administrators. After repeated complaints from Approved Societies and the government that the number of claims to sickness benefit had increased substantially since NHI had begun, a Departmental Committee investigated in 1914. The final report detailed several contributing factors to the growth in claims, many of which also applied in the 1940s.[32]

Witnesses to the Committee hinted at what Johannson, as discussed in the previous chapter, calls a 'cultural inflation of morbidity'.[33] Outlining the 'moral hazard' economic incentives for both GPs and patients, witnesses compared the NHI system unfavourably with what it had replaced. For GPs, especially in working-class districts, a significant proportion of their reliable income was dependent upon the capitation payments coming from the number of NHI

---

[30] *Cmd. 6404*, p. 58.

[31] This familiarity was played on in information films about the new system in 1948. See: Ministry of National Insurance, 'Industrial Accidents – Trailer', British Pathé, 1948, accessed 20 February 2021, https://www.britishpathe.com/video/industrial-accidents-trailer.

[32] Claud Schuster, *Report of the Departmental Committee on Sickness Benefit Claims Under the National Insurance Act (Cd. 7687)* (London: HMSO, 1914), p. 4.

[33] S. Ryan Johansson, 'The health transition: the cultural inflation of morbidity during the decline of mortality', *Health Transition Review* 1 (1991): pp. 39–68.

patients on their lists.[34] While many workers continued their coverage and arrangements—friendly society membership totalled around 6.6 million in 1910—for a significant proportion of others the 1911 Act provided affordable access to a GP and sick pay for the first time.[35] In turn, the new patients created demand for new doctors. NHI made opening a GP's surgery in deprived areas more financially viable as the panel system provided a steady stream of income. The number of NHI GPs increased from around 15,000 to 19,000 between 1913 and 1938.[36] Their de facto patron was now the state rather than any individual friendly society.[37]

According to GPs and administrators, an important direct relationship with friendly societies had therefore been lost. In the old system, a society would know the details of the worker's job, past claim history, and the reputation of the GP. Witnesses argued that all knew their responsibilities to the fund: workers would not claim unless they really needed it, and doctors would not sign off unless they were convinced the sickness merited treatment and rest. Under the new, faceless, NHI system, such relationships were more impersonal—and in many cases had not existed before NHI made it possible for the doctor to find work and the patients to access a doctor. The report cautioned against blind nostalgia, noting that societies often contested the GP's statement or the patient's case history, and had other actuarial tools for assessing the legitimacy of a claim.[38] Such narratives of a decline of a 'voluntary' or communal spirit and the dangers of state intervention were not uncommon throughout the period and reflected political anxieties as much as an actual change in collective behaviour.[39] At the same time, the volume of claims from newly insured persons (backed by sick notes from a new tranche of doctors who had limited experience of doing work for Approved Societies), for benefits that were higher in value than in generations past, created economic pressures that the sick note was not equipped to defend against. Something must have led to this, reasoned the government, even if the decline of voluntarism were discounted.

The Commission's answers to this question will become very familiar to readers by the end of this book. Doctors were, apparently, too willing to write sick notes. For the cynic in Whitehall, they had a habit of prioritizing the care of their patient

---

[34] Noel Whiteside, 'L'assurance sociale en Grande Bretagne: La genèse de l'état providence', trans. N. Whiteside, in *Les assurances sociales en Europe*, edited by Michel Dreyfus (Rennes: Presses Universitaires de Rennes, 2009), pp. 127–58.

[35] *Cd. 7687*, pp. 6–17. Estimates of membership from Beveridge, *Voluntary Action*, p. 328. By contrast, 13.7 million were insured under NHI in 1914. Anne Digby and Nick Bosanquet, 'Doctors and patients in an era of national health insurance and private practice, 1913–1938', *Economic History Review*, 41, no. 1 (1988): pp. 74–94.

[36] Digby and Bosanquet, 'Doctors and patients'.

[37] Honigsbaum, *The Division in British Medicine*, esp. pp. 15–16.   [38] *Cd. 7687*, p. 9.

[39] Geoffrey Finlayson, 'A moving frontier: Voluntarism and the state in British social welfare 1911–1949', *Twentieth Century British History* 1, no. 2 (1990): pp. 183–206.

rather than the Treasury. GPs' notes were not considered the most scientific or binding form of evidence, yet they were deemed almost essential to every single claim to benefit, increasing the workload of everyone involved in a claim. Patients, now able to afford to take time off (and access medical care), took advantage of increased benefit rates, which lead them to seek more sick notes. For some, NHI, Approved Societies', occupational, and trades unions' sick pay schemes meant that, in certain circumstances, patients would accrue more take-home pay by staying at home sick rather than working. For this and other reasons, workers were chastised for not making enough effort to *return* to work, even if there was no disputing the legitimacy of the original malady. Authorities hoped citizens would be more responsible and warned of the 'Danger of Development of Valetudinarian Sprit'.[40] Simultaneously, they did not want to return to a time when 'presenteeism'[41] saw sick people working through injury and illness, becoming more unproductive and taking more time off in the long run. The government did not want to attribute these problems to a 'real' rise in 'malingering' but could not find evidence of a 'real' rise in morbidity, suggesting a 'cultural inflation of morbidity'.[42] The system appeared designed for the majority of anticipated cases, from regularly employed male manual workers who would only have occasional needs to draw on funds—and yet there was no standardized definition of 'incapacity' to give consistent decisions from one worker, one diagnosis, or one industrial sector to the next.[43] To emphasize this miscalculation, the architects had been surprised by the particular needs of, and the extent of demand from, women.[44]

GPs and Sick Notes

While none of these problems were new to 1948, 5 July did change their importance and scale. Everybody could now access an NHI 'panel' GP, not just insured workers. The insured population in 1936 was estimated to be 19.2 million (or 54 per cent of the adult population), of which 17.6 million were registered with a GP.[45] In 1948, there were an estimated 38.1 million adults living in Great

---

[40] Section subheading in *Cd. 7687*, p. 16.
[41] Not a contemporary phrase, but a concept that has gained attention since the 1990s. See Chapters 7 and 8 and Gunnar Aronsson, Klas Gustafsson, and Margareta Dallner, 'Sick but yet at work. An empirical study of sickness presenteeism', *Journal of Epidemiology & Community Health* 54, no. 7 (2000): pp. 502–9.
[42] See Chapter 1 and: Johansson, 'The health transition'.
[43] On this specific question across the twentieth century, see: Julie Gulland, *Gender, Work and Social Control: A Century of Disability Benefits* (London: Palgrave Macmillan, 2019).
[44] All outlined in the first part of *Cd. 7687*, pp. 1–17.
[45] Digby and Bosanquet, 'Doctors and patients'.

Britain and Northern Ireland.[46] The connection to the wider benefits system also meant that sick notes would be available to more than just insured workers. For example, unemployed sick National Assistance claimants required evidence that they were unwell so that they would not be forced to seek work.[47] In the late 1940s, rationing was still in place, creating a different form of certification workload provided for free by the NHS.

To explore this further, and to emphasize the significance of the Appointed Day, these issues are best explored through doctors' complaints about sick notes, highlighted in the debates between the Ministry of Health and the BMA over the creation of the NHS. Such complaints are a window onto how doctors believed systems ought to work and where the Ministry's proposals did not meet this ideal. They also expose areas upon which doctors themselves did not agree.[48] Here, we see that arguments about medical certification cannot be separated from wider anxieties about the place of the medical profession in the new Beveridgean welfare state. Sick notes emblemized the role of the GP as a 'gatekeeper' to state benefit, in turn exemplifying the relationship between the medical profession and the Ministry.[49] The functionary nature of the task represented deprofessionalization.[50] Yet, despite the many limitations of sick notes that were freely acknowledged by doctors and government departments—and had been for many decades—the sick note remained central to the welfare system.

The battle between the BMA and Ministry of Health over the NHS is an infamous part of the Service's history. By far the biggest sticking point was money, an aspect that has seeped into the popular memory through the often quoted words of Minister of Health, Aneurin Bevan, that his solution to the impasse with the doctors was to 'stuff their mouths with gold'.[51] Charles Webster and Rudolf

---

[46] Office of National Statistics, 'Mid-1838 to mid-2015 population estimates for United Kingdom and its constituent countries: Total persons, Quinary age groups and Single year of age; estimated resident population', 2016, accessed 9 September 2020, https://www.ons.gov.uk/file?uri=/peoplepopulationandcommunity/populationandmigration/populationestimates/datasets/populationestimatesforukenglandandwalesscotlandandnorthernireland/mid2015/ukandregionalpopulationestimates18382015.zip. See also Figure 1.3.

[47] National Assistance Board, *Report of the National Assistance Board for the Year Ended 31st December 1948 (Cmd. 7767)* (London: HMSO, 1949). See also Chapter 4.

[48] For the use of complaints as historical evidence and their utility for social and cultural histories, see: James G. Hanley, 'The public's reaction to public health: Petitions submitted to Parliament, 1847–1848', *Social History of Medicine* 15, no. 3 (2002): pp. 393–411; Daisy Payling, '"The people who write to us are the people who don't like us:" Public responses to the Government Social Survey's Survey of Sickness, 1943–1952', *Journal of British Studies* 59, no. 2 (2020): pp. 315–42.

[49] Deborah A. Stone, 'Physicians as gatekeepers', *Public Policy* 27 (1979): pp. 227–54; Bjørgulf Claussen, 'Physicians as gatekeepers: will they contribute to restrict disability benefits?', *Scandinavian Journal of Primary Health Care* 16, no. 4 (1999): pp. 199–203.

[50] Marie R. Haug, 'The deprofessionalization of everyone?', *Sociological Focus* 8, no. 3 (1975): pp. 197–213; R. R. Reed and D. Evans, 'The deprofessionalization of medicine. Causes, effects, and responses', *Journal of the American Medical Association* 258, no. 22 (1987): pp. 3279–82.

[51] Brian Abel-Smith recounts that Bevan said this to him in a private conversation, and the aphorism spread over time. Sally Sheard, *The Passionate Economist: How Brian-Abel Smith Shaped Global Health and Social Welfare* (Bristol: Policy Press, 2013), p. 521. For examples of its invocation, see:

Klein have detailed the compromises made to GPs and consultants, allowing them to take private practice work on top of NHS duties.[52] However, disagreements were not solely about remuneration. Frank Honigsbaum's study of the evolution of General Practice from the late eighteenth century, Andrew Morrice's work on the Edwardian BMA's conflicts with the Ministry of Health, and Jane Lewis's analysis of the GP contract negotiations of the 1960s and 1990s show that professional autonomy was consistently defended when state organizations threatened to restrict doctors' ability to practice as they saw fit.[53] Sick notes offer a window onto similar concerns in the 1940s. Doctors feared the workload certification would generate and the threat to their ability to exercise independent judgement if they were reliant upon the state for their income. The ultimately successful battle to retain the independent contractor status of GPs rested, in part, on the demand that doctors should be free to represent their patients and take on a case load of their own choosing rather than having their salary and practice dictated by the Ministry of Health as a direct employer. After the Appointed Day, then, the process of procuring a sick note from the GP was much the same as it had been before 1948—but this only served to continue and exacerbate existing flaws.

The endurance of rationing in the late 1940s meant that GPs understood how government regulations could increase workloads. Patients could use a medical certificate to get special diets or gain access to restricted goods made from scarce materials, such as vacuum flasks and corsets.[54] Doctors expressed that they had been willing to perform this task in wartime as part of their duty to the nation.[55] But with peace achieved, they were not inclined to continue to subject themselves or their patients to 'totalitarian' regimes of certification and surveillance that, 'allegedly, we went to war to abolish.'[56] The Lancet's 'In England Now' sketch column in 1946 lamented that 'doctors never asked to be the controllers of the nation's milk-supply and we would be heartily glad to be rid of the whole

'Bevan +25', The Economist, 7 July 1973, p. 21; Geoffrey Rivett, From Cradle to Grave: Fifty Years of the NHS (London: King's Fund, 1998); Arthur H. Gale, '"I stuffed their mouths with gold"', Missouri Medicine 114, no. 1 (2017): pp. 13–15.
    [52] Charles Webster, 'Doctors, public service and profit: General practitioners and the National Health Service', Transactions of the Royal Historical Society 40 (1990): pp. 197–216; Rudolf Klein, 'The state and the profession: the politics of the double bed', British Medical Journal 301 no. 6754 (1990): pp. 700–2; Webster, National Health Service; Rudolf Klein, The New Politics of the NHS, 7th edn (London: CRC Press, 2013).
    [53] Honigsbaum, The Division in British Medicine; Morrice, '"Strong combination"'; Jane Lewis, 'The medical profession and the state: GPs and the GP Contract in the 1960s and the 1990s', Social Policy & Administration 32, no. 2 (1998): pp. 132–50.
    [54] Anon, 'Medicine and the law', The Lancet 245, no. 6343 (1945): pp. 381–2; Basil S. Kent, 'Medical certification', British Medical Journal 1, no. 4493 (1947): p. 268; R. L. Gibson, 'Medical certification', British Medical Journal 1, no. 4499 (1947): pp. 424–5.
    [55] Anon, 'Medicine and the law';Lennox Johnston and D. A. Scott, 'Indulgent certification', The Lancet 245, no. 6356 (1945): pp. 801–2; L. P. Gray, 'Direction of Labour', British Medical Journal 2, no. 4537 (1947): p. 1007.
    [56] Edward Glover, 'Limits of certification', British Medical Journal 2, no. 4519 (1947): p. 269.

time-consuming and thankless job'.[57] The problem with certificates was that they required patients to present themselves on the basis of the benefit they wanted to claim rather than any acute medical necessity—and it was difficult to dissuade them from doing so. 'When I suggest to a patient that a certain medicine is expensive, or that a certificate of incapacity for work is not a ticket-of-leave-with-pocket-money, the reaction varies from indifference to righteous indignation', wrote one Scottish GP.[58] More benefits to claim would lead to more requests for certificates; and if the NHS were to make everything (appear) free at the point of delivery, this problem would only get worse. A another GP noted, 'each new [wartime] restriction or Government order brought its crop of certificate-addicts to the surgery' hoping to avoid some new imposition on their lives on medical grounds.[59] Employers and businesses added to this workload by demanding proof of illness from workers who were absent or through other amendments to obligations.[60] Doctors proposed charging patients or the agencies requesting sick notes as a way to reduce demand, occasionally adding the threat of strike action as a way to protest the elements of the National Insurance Act that most troubled them.[61] In the end, neither would come to fruition, but it would not be the last time such proposals or actions were taken.[62]

If doctors were to endure an increased workload as the gatekeepers of sickness benefits, for whom were they writing sick notes: the patient or the Treasury? This question had been asked before. Under the NHI's system of 'panel' doctors and 'capitation' fees, authorities believed that doctors were, in general, too lenient on their patients and did not give enough consideration to insurance funds. Because many GPs, especially in urban areas, were reliant upon their NHI patients for a stable income, getting a reputation for being parsimonious with medical certificates could result in losing customers to rival doctors. The accusation was that GPs had an economic incentive to give the benefit of the doubt to their patient, resulting in sick notes that reflected the worker's desire to get sickness benefit rather than the medical reality.[63] This debate intensified in the 1940s, stoked in part by a speech in Parliament by the Lord Chancellor in November 1946 during the third reading of the National Health Service Bill. Lord (William) Jowitt, who had been Minister of National Insurance during the war, caused

---

[57] Anon, 'In England now', *The Lancet* 248, no. 6428 (1946): pp. 691–2.

[58] M. Ludlam, 'Points from letters: Two masters', *British Medical Journal* 1, no. 4554 (1948): p. 758.

[59] Practitioner, 'The doctor's wife', *The Lancet* 251, no. 6508 (1948): pp. 811–12.

[60] Basil S. Grant, 'National Health Service', *British Medical Journal* 1, no. 4544 (1948): p. 273; E. Roland Williams, 'Points from letters: A "medical certificate"', *British Medical Journal* 1, no. 4508 (1947): p. 785.

[61] V. B. Goldman, 'National Health Service', *British Medical Journal* 1, no. 4541 (1948): p. 120; G. S. M. Wilson, 'National Health Service', *British Medical Journal* 1, no. 4547 (1948): p. 414.

[62] See Chapters 5 and 7.

[63] An Insurance Committee Secretary, 'The white paper reviewed', *The Lancet* 243, no. 6289 (1944): p. 350.

offence to GPs when he remarked (in favour of removing the panel system and imposing a salaried service):

> The success or failure of all our schemes depends in a very large measure on our getting satisfactory certification. If we are going to have lax – still more, dishonest – certification, then all our schemes are going to break down on that rock. I have a most profound regard for the medical profession, and for their standard of honour, but I am bound to tell your Lordships that I did come across cases – not many – where there were two competing doctors, where one was strict with his certification and the other was lax. The people who were on the panel of the strict doctor were inclined to leave that panel and to go on the panel of the lax doctor, not because the lax doctor was a better doctor, but because from the lax doctor they could more easily get certificates.[64]

Although the government was still considering a salaried service in late 1946, GPs would eventually succeed in maintaining the status quo of capitation. Depending on one's point of view, either of these outcomes could have helped or damaged the profession. On the one hand, if doctors were salaried it would make it easier for them to be assertive with difficult patients. A doctor's income would not be affected by patients transferring themselves to another GP.[65] On the other hand, if the authority managing the insurance fund was also paying the doctor's wages, would GPs be induced to protect the public purse over the best interests or medical needs of the patient?[66] 'The State or works doctor's job is to keep the man at or get him back to the machine', wrote a GP to *The Lancet* in July 1945, whereas 'the private doctor's job is to get the patient well: these sound much the same but they are not.'[67] This was not a trivial debate. At the BMA's 1945 Annual Representative Meeting the representative from Belfast argued that 'the success or failure of the National Health Service turns on the question of certification. By this terrible burden...the doctor is divorced and held apart from his true work.'[68] Or, as a 1947 letter in the *British Medical Journal* put it:

> Certification is the crux of the problem [with the NHS Acts]. The government is going to control the doctor, because if the doctor were not controlled he might be "lax or dishonest," or, worse still, he might treat his patients with kindness and humanity....And who defines "satisfactory certification"? The Minister of

---

[64] Lord (William) Jowitt, 'National Health Service Bill', *House of Lords Official Report (Hansard)*, 31 October 1946, vol. 143, cc. 924–52 at col. 928.

[65] Johnston and Scott, 'Indulgent certification'.

[66] G. I. Watson, 'The basic salary', *British Medical Journal* 2, no. 4482 (1946): p. 836.

[67] R. E. Clarke, 'Indulgent certification', *The Lancet* 246, no. 6359 (1945): p. 60.

[68] Anon, 'British Medical Association Annual Representative Meeting', *The Lancet* 246, no. 6362 (1945): pp. 148–150, at 148.

Health and his officials. Perhaps when a "production drive" is in progress the Minister of Labour may arrange a further tightening up of certifications.[69]

Another doctor argued that the entire point of the NHS was 'based on the Treasury's urgent desire to control the doctors' and reduce sickness benefit claims.[70] By focusing on the sick note element of this debate on capitation and a salaried service, we see that GPs were not simply clamouring to have their mouths stuffed with gold. There was a fundamental question about whether the doctor was a client of the patient or of the state; an independent expert or a civil servant. In practice, one cannot separate these logics of professionalism entirely—but it would be churlish to dismiss the material impact this issue could have on the doctor's day-to-day to practice.[71] The sick note was a useful example for doctors to demonstrate the legitimacy of their opposition.

Even if the terms of employment could be resolved, there was still a fundamental problem with using GPs as the primary distributor of sick notes. GPs were not occupational health specialists, nor did they have access to sophisticated diagnostic equipment to judge the true extent of a patient's symptoms or their effects on his or her job. Investigations into prewar Workmen's Compensation had shown it would take a specialist with the correct tools around 30 minutes to detect possible malingering, whereas GPs were expected to do the same job with far more limited resources in a 'short 3 to 6 minute' consultation.[72] Meanwhile, it was regularly reported that GPs had misdiagnosed serious industrial injuries and poisonings as minor ailments which turned out to be fatal.[73] Some had hoped that industrial medicine, which had been gaining in prominence during the interwar years, might offer an alternative outlet.[74] But this did not come to pass.[75] Especially in the case of short-term illnesses, aches, and pains, many sick notes had to be written 'ipse dixit'.[76] There was no way for a GP

---

[69] Reginald T. Payne, 'The National Health Service Act', *British Medical Journal* 1, no. 4489 (1947): pp. 102–6.

[70] D. Saklatvala, 'National Health Service', *British Medical Journal* 1, no. 4496 (1947): pp. 308–9.

[71] On logics of professionalism in public/private systems see Mirko Noordegraaf, 'From "pure" to "hybrid" professionalism: Present-day professionalism in ambiguous public domains', *Administration & Society* 39, no. 6 (2007): pp. 761–85; Eliot Freidson, *Professionalism: The Third Logic* (Cambridge: Polity, 2001).

[72] Honigsbaum, *The Division in British Medicine*, pp. 19–20.

[73] Ibid., pp. 219–23.

[74] Anon, 'Industrial medical services', *The Lancet* 248, no. 6418 (1946): pp. 321–2; Vicky Long, *The Rise and Fall of the Healthy Factory: The Politics of Industrial Health in Britain, 1914–60* (Basingstoke: Palgrave Macmillan, 2010). For more on the role of occupational health, see esp. Chapter 7. See also the journal *British Journal of Industrial Medicine* and contemporary professional bodies: Anon, 'Proceedings of the Association of Industrial Medical Officers', *British Journal of Industrial Medicine* 3, no. 1 (1946): pp. 48–54.

[75] For the effects of this, see esp. Chapters 3 and 7.

[76] The phrase is used commonly in the 1960s and 1970s by the BMA and government departments in debates about the worth of medical certification. See Chapter 5 and TNA: PIN 35/150, Hellon to Swift, 23 March 1965.

to tell whether the patient requesting the sick note was genuine, regardless of suspicions one way or the other. As one example given in 1949 put it, a doctor could not, without an unreasonable level of surveillance over a long time—including before the patient suspected illness—take anything other than a woman's word that her symptoms included an irregular period. By the time the 'facts' of the case were established, the patient might have recovered (rendering the need for the sick note moot) or a much bigger problem might have developed than the need to miss a week's work.[77] Sick notes were not scientific 'proof' that a patient was 'really' ill. At best they were, in the words of one correspondent to the *British Medical Journal*, 'testimony': evidence for the authorities to reach their own judgement and nothing more.[78] Besides, the note itself would not be read in the National Insurance offices by a medical professional or occupational health specialist, leaving the evidence shorn of context and incapable of being challenged on scientific grounds without reference to specialists.[79] The existence of sick visiting, specialist medical officers and other checks in the prewar and postwar systems suggested that authorities were well aware that the sick note was not proof, or, on its own, an effective check against abuse. But these other systems were much more expensive to run.[80]

Nevertheless, perfect diagnosis would not reconcile the difference between how doctors understood 'illness' and how insurance authorities defined 'sickness'. The logic of sick notes required a binary status. If a claimant met all other qualifying criteria, either a claimant was sick (and therefore entitled to benefit) or they were not. There was no hinterland to accommodate partial incapacity, reduced duties to prevent a condition getting worse, or convalescence. Again, this was a long-running problem. A doctor had told the 1914 Committee that a sick note 'assumes that illness starts on one day and finishes on another' whereas in reality 'it is the exact opposite; it comes on gradually and declines gradually'.[81] 'We had hoped that the day had passed when administrators viewed statistics on their office desks as if the difference between capacity and incapacity was always the difference between black and white—rather than different shades of grey', lamented a *Lancet* editorial in 1944. While in the past 'the drawing of arbitrary lines was unavoidable' under the heterodox world of NHI and Approved Societies, the author hoped (in vain) that 'the unification of administration' would offer an 'opportunity for a new outlook'.[82] This emphasized the difference between illness (that medical professionals treat) and sickness (as a bureaucratic category

---

[77] TNA: PIN 7/368, Ministry of Health and Department of Health for Scotland, 'Report of the Inter-Departmental Committee on Medical Certificates', 1949, p. 5.

[78] R. S. Brock, 'Disqualification under the Bill', *British Medical Journal* 1, no. 4449 (1946): p. 585.

[79] D. W. Hudson, 'Certificates for soldiers', *The Lancet* 246, no. 6383 (1945): p. 863; Desmond Curran, 'Limits of Certification', *British Medical Journal* 2, no. 4517 (1947): p. 187.

[80] Gulland, *Gender, Work and Social Control*, esp. p. 55.   [81] Cd. 7687, p. 15.

[82] Anon, 'Incapacity for work', *The Lancet* 244, no. 6319 (1944): p. 475.

designed to manage welfare benefits)—but did nothing to help doctors or patients.[83]

If sick notes were unscientific sources of tension between the state, patients, and doctors that increased workloads, then they were, as many GPs complained in the 1940s, a 'waste of time'. This was expressed not just in absolute terms—the total number of hours dedicated to the task—but in relation to other professional duties. Every minute spent writing 'ipse dixit' First and Final certificates for a worker who claimed to have a bad cold the week before was a minute not spent on 'real' work. A group of GPs from Hampshire argued that 'the [NHS] is unworkable because of the greatly increased demand on the practitioner by the minor sick and certification, leaving him insufficient time for adequate treatment of the really ill'.[84] 'Even the least work-shy among us will be breaking under the strain', agreed a Kent physician, and 'what is more, those of our patients who are suffering from serious disorders will suffer from our being unable to give sufficient time to their care'.[85] Such demands on time extended beyond simply filling out forms:

A mother wanting extra coal opens the interview by requesting examination of her baby's chest; only when the child has been stripped and examined is her true purpose disclosed. Others ask quickly enough for the form, and then say: 'While I am here, doctor...' going on to explain some minor disorder which in itself would not warrant their coming to the surgery. There is thus good reason for reducing as far as possible the number of attendances for forms and certificates.[86]

It is here, regardless of salary, capitation, or private practice, that the effect of sick notes on professional capacity was made clear. Doctors objected to the work because it was functionary, mundane, did little to actively cure the patient and required very few of the specialist skills for which they were trained. It also invited other interactions with patients that did not (medically) require urgent attention. They had 'been treated as...technical labour' by the government despite— perhaps even because of—their near 'monopoly in knowledge and understanding of medicine'.[87] We can, in part, bring this back to the debates over money. If GPs were forced to work full time signing sick notes for the government then they could not engage in the activities that had brought them financial reward in the interwar years, such as acting as medical referees, consultants to private

---

[83] For more on the state's management of partial incapacity see Chapter 7 and Gulland, *Gender, Work and Social Control.*

[84] A. W. Harrington et al., 'National Health Service', *British Medical Journal* 1 no. 4541 (1948): p. 120.

[85] M. Curwen, 'National Health Service', *British Medical Journal* 1, no. 4541 (1948): p. 120.

[86] Anon, 'The Act in action'.

[87] Lindsey W. Batten, 'National Health Service', *British Medical Journal* 1, no. 4550 (1948): p. 561.

companies, and part-time medical officer work.[88] But such choices were also about power and professional independence: choosing how and when that money could be made.

Nevertheless, despite this torrent of objections the sick note remained the central plank of the social security system. The prewar system could, with a little adaptation, meet the needs of the postwar era. The National Health Service Acts were passed, and the BMA eventually agreed to the terms of the new Service. One of the compromises involved was that the Ministry of Health would conduct an inquiry into the extent of medical certification and seek to reduce its load to a minimum.[89] Eventually published as the *Report of the Inter-Departmental Committee on Medical Certificates* in 1949, it forced government departments to confront the scale of their demands on the profession.[90] Still, it did not result in any fundamental changes to the system for the 'Med 1' sick note.

The Safford Report

The Inter-Departmental Committee was chaired by Archibald Safford, who had been an adjudicator for appeals in the NHI system.[91] Its report confirmed that doctors had grounds for their complaints about the number of medical certificates they could be compelled to write by Acts of Parliament. 390 types of certificate emerged, covering 27 government departments in England and Scotland. (Although, as shown in Chapter 4, the 27 did not include the National Assistance Board; an oversight with significant consequences for the administration of benefits of some of the country's most marginalized claimants.) Of those nearly 400 certificates, 171 fell under the terms of the National Health Service Act 1946 and therefore had to be provided by doctors on demand for free.[92] The 'form-mongers'[93] concurred that this was excessive and agreed to reduce their number. Any future medical certificates would have to be negotiated with the BMA. Such talks would continue for the rest of the century and are covered in more detail in Chapter 5.

Despite the mountain of forms and reports, certification for National Insurance purposes was by far the most onerous on a quotidian basis.[94] Although Safford's

---

[88] Digby and Bosanquet, 'Doctors and patients'.   [89] See discussions in TNA: PIN 21/86.

[90] TNA: PIN 7/368, Ministry of Health and Department of Health for Scotland, 'Report of the Inter-Departmental Committee on Medical Certificates', 1949.

[91] Archibald Safford, 'The creation of case law under the National Insurance and National Insurance (Industrial Injuries) Acts', *Modern Law Review* 17, no. 3 (1954): pp. 197–210. Discussed in Gulland, *Gender, Work and Social Control*, p. 4.

[92] TNA: PIN 7/368, Ministry of Health and Department of Health for Scotland, 'Report of the Inter-Departmental Committee on Medical Certificates', 1949.

[93] A. R. Eates, 'Certification for extra milk', *British Medical Journal* 1, no. 4383 (1945): pp. 26–7.

[94] It was rivalled only by rationing, which all acknowledged would eventually become unnecessary. TNA: MH 135/743, British Medical Association, Statement of the Association's Evidence to the Departmental Committee on Medical Certification (attached to letter 17 June 1948).

recommendations were not followed through entirely, evidence from the BMA, Trades Union Congress (TUC), employers' federations, and government departments allowed the committee to draw up guidelines for how the technology of the note itself could be improved to reduce the burden upon GPs. Safford recommended forms should have a common layout with clear and uncluttered typefaces so that they were easy to read and understand for doctors and civil servants alike.[95] The committee agreed with the BMA that it would probably be helpful if there was a single form for National Insurance purposes, but it would take nearly 20 years before the 'Med 3' would arrive.[96]

In the deliberations, however, it became clear that sick notes did indeed serve a useful purpose. Despite the protestations from government officials in the 1910s and doctors in the 1940s, medical certification was a practical tool for managing complex bureaucracies. It was impractical to visit every single person who claimed sickness benefit. Not only would it be unaffordable, there would not be enough licensed specialist doctors to perform the task. The Regional Medical Officers in the National Insurance system were better used on specific long-term cases or where a claimant's pattern of behaviour (such as taking repeated short-term bouts of sickness, especially around local holidays, or strike action) necessitated greater surveillance.[97] The government might not have liked it, but even 'lax' certification was better than the alternative. Similarly, workers and businesses knew that sick notes could create problems for them. A letter to the *Birmingham Mail* made plain the absurdity of needing a sick note to sign someone off work (the 'Med 1') and another to allow them to return (the 'Med 2B'):

armed with the two vital documents, which have officially proclaimed [the worker's] fall and rise...he is deemed to have fulfilled his contract to his employer....If he doesn't get them, he loses pay and/or gets marked as AWOL by his employer, which harms his promotion/employment prospects.... Production suffers, wages are sacrificed - but who cares? Industrial bureaucracy has been achieved.[98]

Yet the alternative was also bad for productivity. The TUC and British Employers' Confederation both argued that sick notes could be used to track morbidity and industrial injury better than any other form of evidence. As social scientists began to study ever more closely occupational safety, epidemiology, and absenteeism,

---

[95] TNA: PIN 7/368, Ministry of Health and Department of Health for Scotland, 'Report of the Inter-Departmental Committee on Medical Certificates', 1949, pp. 3–5.

[96] Anon, 'The Act in action'. On how the 'Med 3' was introduced in 1966, see Chapter 5.

[97] Gulland, *Gender, Work and Social Control*, p. 67; TNA: PIN 35/125. See also management of 'repeat short period claimants' in TNA: PIN 35/229 and discussion in Chapter 5.

[98] TNA: MH 135/741, Press cutting, W. R. Lord (King's Norton), letter to *Birmingham Mail*, 9 March 1949.

there was a case for making sick notes even more detailed than they already were.[99] These organizations suggested reviving a wartime form that provided more diagnostic information, but this was rejected in favour of simplicity for doctors and National Insurance staff.[100] Likewise, as seen in Chapter 3, employers did not want to encourage workers to return to work too early and create problems around 'presenteeism'; nor did they want to be too officious and destroy company morale by hectoring otherwise decent employees. The new welfare state was explicitly designed to prevent that. The sick note might not be the most reliable proof of the worker's capacity, but it was better to be safe than sorry.

The sick note was also, in many cases, inseparable from treatment. To provide relief from work and access to sickness benefit could reduce anxiety and allow the patient to focus on recovery. 'The doctor cannot reasonably complain' about filling in a form, argued one GP, 'because he has the power to allay [fears] by a stroke the pen'.[101] Doctors could rebel by charging for certificates or going on strike; but there was a danger that privatizing the sick note would make patients see them as 'a right', regardless of how ill they 'really' were.[102] As dangerous as the workload from sick notes was, would turning access to sickness benefit into a consumer product, create longer queues and set worrying precedents?[103] Indeed, once the new system was up and running, a *Lancet* editorial conceded that 'no serious objection has been voiced against the certificates issuable under the National Insurance Act'—however, GPs remained concerned at the number they were writing for 'clubs and employers', despite the fact they could charge a fee if the authority would not accept a 'Med 1'.[104] The very fact they could charge proved their willingness on some level to perform this function. Employers would take the opportunity to make use of the 'product'.[105]

Above all, the BMA had to be pragmatic. The public supported the NHS and a nationalized system of health care. As Nick Hayes cautions, the idea that there was irresistible demand for a radical new health system has been overestimated in the intervening decades. But it was clear that the British electorate would support governments who would place greater emphasis on state planning and control to

[99] See Chapter 3, especially in relation to absenteeism. On the rise of social science in the postwar period by public and private institutions, see: Michael Savage, *Identities and Social Change in Britain since 1940: The Politics of Method* (Oxford: Oxford University Press, 2010); Payling, '"The people who write to us".

[100] TNA: MH 135/741, British Employers' Confederation, 'Committee on Medical Certificates. Statement of evidence submitted to the Government Committee', 5 March 1949; TNA: MH 135/742, Trades Union Congress, Evidence to Committee on Medical Certificates, 9 December 1948.

[101] Practitioner, 'The doctor's wife'.   [102] Curwen, 'National Health Service'.

[103] Dorothy Porter, *Health Citizenship: Essays in Social Medicine and Biomedical Politics* (Berkeley: University of California Press, 2011); Alex Mold, *Making the Patient-Consumer: Patient Organisations and Health Consumerism in Britain* (Manchester: Manchester University Press, 2015).

[104] Clubs referred to various organizations that provided occupational sick pay, such as trades unions, friendly societies, private insurance companies and the like. Anon, 'The Act in Action'.

[105] This problem recurs throughout this volume but see esp. Chapters 5 and 7.

provide better social security and standards of living.[106] In the brave new world of 'social rights',[107] doctors would have to accept that citizens would expect services from them and they would be obliged to provide. This would include sick notes. This new welfare state 'was produced by a Liberal, taken up by the Conservatives, and actuated by the Socialists', wrote one High Wycombe doctor. 'No party could allow this luscious plum' of the NHS and social security 'to fall outside its vote-catching ambit'.[108] 'Whatever its merits and demerits', noted 'Justinian' in *The Lancet*, 'the old independence of the State from any relationship with individuals (unless he commits a crime) is passing away....In future every patient—and for that matter every doctor—will have a personal interest in cash benefits, and it will no longer be fashionable to affect superiority by disdaining to claim them.'[109] Perhaps it would not be so bad. To imply that it was impossible to give an honest assessment on sickness in a state system was 'a slur on our professional integrity that is unwarranted', chided a Cheshire GP who had seen the advantages in wartime of practising in a system where his patients did not have to worry about how they would pay him.[110] And besides, GPs did not want the task of being the gatekeepers: 'but nobody else is capable of taking it on, so we must make the best of it'.[111]

This reflected the relationship between the state and the medical profession that had built since at least the passing of the 1858 Medical Act.[112] State and medical power had grown hand-in-hand as medicine offered solutions to problems of governance and economic productivity.[113] If *The Lancet* could lament a lost world of 'the old independence', one has to ask when that world ever existed. Doctors had already been providing causes of death on death certificates; acting as expert witnesses in trials; performing compulsory vaccinations; treating troops on the battlefield; and offering solutions to intractable problems of infectious disease in the metropole and in the colonies. Indeed, the very reason the profession had become so indispensable as the gatekeeper to social security was because of the unique expertise that it sold to insurance companies, mutual societies, and

---

[106] Nick Hayes, 'Did we really want a National Health Service? Hospitals, patients and public opinions before 1948', *The English Historical Review* 127, no. 526 (2012): pp. 625–61. For more on re-evaluating support for Labour and the NHS in 1945, see: Steven Fielding, 'What did "the people" want?: The meaning of the 1945 General Election', *The Historical Journal* 35 no. 3 (1992): pp. 623–39; Andrew Seaton, 'Against the "sacred cow": NHS opposition and the Fellowship for Freedom in Medicine, 1948–72', *Twentieth Century British History* 26, no. 3 (2015): pp. 424–49.

[107] T. H. Marshall, *Citizenship and Social Class, and Other Essays* (Cambridge: Cambridge University Press, 1950).

[108] W. J. O'Connor, 'National Health Service', *British Medical Journal* 1, no. 4496 (1947): pp. 307–8.

[109] Anon, 'Towards social security', *The Lancet* 247, no. 6392 (1946): pp. 320–1.

[110] K. Cobban, 'The health service Bill', *British Medical Journal* 1, no. 4451 (1946): p. 659.

[111] Anon, 'In England Now'.   [112] Honigsbaum, *The Division in British Medicine.*

[113] David Armstrong, *Political Anatomy of the Body: Medical Knowledge in Britain in the Twentieth Century* (Cambridge: Cambridge University Press, 1983); Michel Foucault, *Discipline and Punish: The Birth of the Prison* (New York: Pantheon Books, 1977).

the state in being able to diagnose incapacity and offer therapeutics that would return workers and citizens to productivity. The sick note was a problem that the profession had caused for itself.

Conclusion

While the 'Med 1' was 'born' on 5 July 1948, then, the concept of 'the sick note' had a much longer history. And despite the many problems with them, they remained. Administratively simple and cheap, especially compared to the alternatives, they were not such an egregious imposition that doctors could not overcome their reservations. Small changes to forms and procedures could allow the concept of medical certification to survive the Second World War and, as we will see, myriad other developments in Britain's welfare state and economy over the rest of the century. They were enough of a curb on absenteeism and provided enough epidemiological data to outweigh the cynicism of businesses and government officials about their objective scientific truth claims. They were also *there*. There was no need to create elaborate new systems of gatekeeping and surveillance when the existing one did an adequate job. Just as the new NHS had built itself around the existing hospital and GP architecture rather than building new hospitals and health centres *en masse*, doctors, patients, employers, and governments could live with the old sick note system with a few tweaks to take into account the new health and social security services.[114]

This is not to say the adoption of the sick note in the form of the 1948 'Med 1' was inevitable; nor was it the bureaucratic equivalent to the QWERTY keyboard, a relic of the nineteenth century that survived despite its inefficiencies because nobody could agree on a single alternative.[115] Rather, an element of 'path dependence' can be seen which increased the opportunity cost of choosing a different direction.[116] The sick note performed its many required tasks with enough competence enough of the time for enough people to remain in place. As seen in the following chapters, however, there were points where this positive side of the ledger would be temporarily forgotten. Employers would complain about how sick notes were not an effective curb on absenteeism; officials and claimants would discover that sick notes did not always work well for those who did not fit the British masculine ideal of the non-disabled worker; doctors would continue

---

[114] See: Ed Devane, 'Pilgrim's Progress: The Landscape of the NHS Hospital, 1945–70', *Twentieth Century British History* (2021).

[115] This is a very crude summation of the debate on path dependency and market failure in science and technology studies. See S. J. Liebowitz and Stephen E. Margolis, 'The fable of the keys', *The Journal of Law & Economics* 33, no. 1 (1990): pp. 1–25.

[116] Paul Pierson, 'Increasing returns, path dependence, and the study of politics', *The American Political Science Review* 94 (2000): pp. 251–67.

to show the wasted resources medical certification caused in an already-stretched health system. Governments would eventually come to find new ways of determining access to disability and sickness benefits based on degrees of incapacity and functioning tests rather than the scrawl of the doctor's pen—but by that point the idea of 'the sick note' had become so ingrained that the media had dubbed the nation 'Sick-note Britain'.[117] It is to these issues that the book now turns. Through detailing these changes, we see how the specific form of arguments against medical certification evolved according to contemporary economic context and public attitudes towards work, medicine, and their relationship to authorities.

---

[117] David Jones, 'Sign up here for Sick-note Britain', *Daily Mail*, 14 April 1998, pp. 22–3.

3

Absenteeism and Postwar Rebuilding

'Every miner who steals a day's holiday hurts not only his own pit and his own mates but every fellow-citizen', cautioned a *Manchester Guardian* editorial in 1953.[1] Dr Leslie Hunter, the Bishop of Sheffield warned that absenteeism 'could mean the end of the welfare state.... Absenteeism in a nationalized industry and slack working in general are one example of an irresponsible attitude to the State which is widely shared by all classes. Tax evasion, cheating the railway, trying to get more than one needs and more than a fair share out of the welfare services, are some forms of this irresponsibility.'[2] Had the new 'health services', as some had come to call the package of universal health care and social security instituted on 5 July 1948, caused all this shirking?[3]

If they had, the timing was unfortunate. Britain needed all the labour it could muster in order to rebuild the country's infrastructure and economy. Every hour lost in British mines, factories, and offices made it all the more difficult to produce the exports vital to managing the nation's balance of payments and service the large debts accrued during the war. While sick notes and absenteeism were rhetorically intertwined throughout the entire period covered in this book, the years immediately following the introduction of the 'Med 1' provide useful insight into how such concerns could be explicitly linked to contemporary economic anxieties.

Sick notes were important to this story because the majority of absenteeism was due to medical leave and, to qualify, workers had to convince their employers that they were actually sick. For many occupational sick pay schemes one had to provide a certificate after the third day of illness—and since the new National Insurance system also required and provided such notes, a significant proportion of absenteeism was accompanied by Med 1s and Med 2s.[4] But while 'genuine' sickness was accepted as a legitimate reason for not working, the government and bosses were sceptical about the 'genuineness' of all cases. After 1948, absenteeism rose significantly in some nationalized industries, yet other statistical returns suggested that there had been no accompanying rise in 'real' morbidity or injury. As authorities placed the blame on individual behaviour, the sick note was

---

[1] 'Stolen holidays', *Manchester Guardian*, 9 July 1953, p. 4.
[2] '"Ruin if we slack like miners"', *Daily Mail*, 29 July 1953, p. 3.
[3] The National Archives (hereafter TNA): CAB 129/35/12, Ministry of Fuel and Power, 'Effect of new sickness and injury benefits upon absenteeism in coal mines' (31 May 1949), para 6.
[4] On these forms see Chapter 2.

representative of poor discipline, malingering, and 'abuse' of the new welfare systems that were designed to increase health and productivity.

Still, while the rhetoric could conflate sick notes and absenteeism, they were
not the same thing. As authorities began to investigate the causes of and solutions
to their absence problems it became increasingly clear that tightening certification
regulations would cause more problems than it would solve. Just as the doctors
and the ministries had elected to keep the sick note in 1948 for want of a better
alternative to managing the new National Insurance bureaucracy, so too did
employers begrudgingly accept that other more pressing structural issues would
have to be overcome before it was worth considering an alternative to sick notes.
For while sickness certification was the first suspect whenever absenteeism rate
increased, attention quickly—and sometimes embarrassingly—turned to pay,
conditions and the relationship between management and staff.

This chapter explores absenteeism through four 'public-sector' industries in
the first ten years of National Insurance: Royal Ordinance Factories (ROFs); the
coalmines of the National Coal Board (NCB); the Metropolitan Police; and
the Post Office. These organizations employed thousands of people in a range of
occupations across the entire United Kingdom, making repeated references to
how the changing class, age, and gender demographics of their workforce had
affected their management practices and ability to function. Given how certain
industries were brought into public ownership and the growth in public-sector
employment after 1945, it also serves to highlight the similarities and differences
in how workers were seen and disciplined in contrast to the 'private sector'.[5]

Further, this time period is instructive because it shows just how quickly the
'health services' and other welfare-state policies such as full employment were
criticized for their effects on absenteeism. The specific ways in which prewar
statistics were analysed and compared to postwar output were not simply
products of the rise of technocratic approaches to knowing and managing the
state.[6] Political imperatives were just as important. Labour and Conservative
governments had to manage the need to repay huge wartime debts and rebuild
the economy on the one hand with the necessity to maintain good labour relations
and electoral viability on the other. Sick notes and absenteeism were therefore
representative of fundamental tensions in the logic of the new welfare state regime—
one designed to help capital advance the nation's economic power while also

---

[5] The number of people employed in the 'public sector' increased from 1.8 million in 1939 to 6
million by 1951. See Figure 7.2 and Blessing Chiripanhura and Nikolas Wolf, 'Long-term trends in UK
employment: 1861 to 2018', Office of National Statistics, 29 April 2019, accessed 24 November 2020,
https://www.ons.gov.uk/economy/nationalaccounts/uksectoraccounts/compendium/economicreview/
april2019/longtermtrendsinukemployment1861to2018.
[6] On technocracy and economic planning after 1945 see: David Edgerton, 'C. P. Snow as anti-
historian of British science: Revisiting the technocratic moment, 1959–1964', History of Science 43, no.
2 (2005): pp. 187–208; Michael Savage, Identities and Social Change in Britain since 1940: The Politics
of Method (Oxford: Oxford University Press, 2010).

providing social rights and protections to the workers the state desperately needed to be productive.

Absenteeism

'Is it not a fact that we know a little too much about absenteeism?', sniped Horace Holmes on the Committee of Public Accounts in 1950.[7] Holmes, a Labour MP in a mining constituency, was no doubt exasperated at the stream of press coverage and political hand wringing over manpower efficiency in the recently-nationalized coalmines.[8] It was certainly true that the NCB spent a great deal of time and money talking about and investigating absenteeism. But even in the third decade of the twenty-first century, and despite multiple reports from business and human relations think tanks of the detrimental economic effects of absence, there is little definitive understanding the phenomenon.[9] As Chapter 1 made clear, measures consistently change, as do the political meanings ascribed to the data.

Absenteeism is a measure of the time an employee does not work compared to his or her contracted hours.[10] It is used by businesses and economists to determine the efficiency of labour usage. Statistics at the level of a single employee, a workplace, sector-wide, region-wide, nationwide, or internationally have been a core part of managerial practice and public economic, labour, and public health policy. On their own, these numbers mean very little. They take on a subjective and moral significance when the data are used to develop and justify attempts to reduce absenteeism from a level deemed 'too high'.[11] For businesses, absenteeism represents waste and inefficiency. The utopian level is therefore zero per cent. In reality, most accept that this will never be possible; and, indeed, attempts to ensure

[7] Committee of Public Accounts, *First, Third and Fourth Reports from the Committee of Public Accounts Together with the Proceedings of the Committee, Minutes of Evidence, Appendices and Index (HC 71-I, 78-I, 138-I (1950))* (London: HMSO, 1950), p. 254.

[8] Holmes represented Hemsworth in West Yorkshire.

[9] See Chapter 7 and S. Bevan and S. Hayday, *Costing Sickness Absence in the UK* (Brighton: Institute for Employment Studies, 2001), p. 70; Centre for Economics and Business Research, *The Benefits of Early Intervention and Rehabilitation* (London: Centre for Economics and Business Research, September 2015); Chartered Institute of Personnel Development, *Health and Well-Being at Work* (London: Chartered Institute of Personnel Development, April 2019); PwC, 'Rising sick bill is costing UK business £29bn a year – PwC research', PwC, 15 July 2013, accessed 19 July 2019, https://pwc.blogs.com/press_room/2013/07/rising-sick-bill-is-costing-uk-business-29bn-a-year-pwc-research.html.

[10] Though this is not a simple measure. For example, from the 1930s, coalmines measured absenteeism as 'shifts lost [through non-attendance] as a percentage of "possible" shifts' (F. D. K. Liddell, 'Attendance in the coal-mining industry', *The British Journal of Sociology* 5, no. 1 (1954): pp. 78–86 at p. 78). However, from 1954 this was changed to another measure around typical working weeks and contracted hours (L. J. Handy, 'Absenteeism and attendance in the British coal-mining industry: An examination of post-war trends', *British Journal of Industrial Relations* 6, no. 1 (1968): pp. 27–50).

[11] Phil Taylor et al., '"Too scared to go sick"—reformulating the research agenda on sickness absence', *Industrial Relations Journal* 41, no. 4 (2010): pp. 270–88.

perfect attendance are likely to destroy morale, reduce productivity, increase long-term sickness, lead to the resignation of key staff, be a public-relations nightmare, and, ultimately, prove self-defeating.[12] A balance 'must be struck. As the head of North East Division of the NCB noted in 1958, 'nothing is to be gained and much is to be lost by phrases like "get tough" and slanted sneers at a fine body of men'.[13]

Absenteeism is therefore usually subdivided for management purposes between 'voluntary' and 'involuntary', with verified sickness absence categorized as the latter. But 'involuntary' did not mean 'unavoidable'; and while direct disciplinary measures were easier to impose upon the worker who had simply breached the terms of his or her employment by not turning up, the worker with a sick note was not necessarily immune to management pressure. Sickness was the biggest burden in terms of time lost and in pay, even when taking into account industrial action, especially after the growth in occupational sick schemes after the war.[14] As seen in the previous chapter, bosses often doubted the legitimacy of sick notes, concerned that doctors were too willing to write them and patients too eager to seek them. If workers could be encouraged to take sick leave less often, by carrot or by stick, absenteeism would be reduced.

Government departments were similarly concerned with absenteeism. They were employers in their own right, but also had a stake in overall economic output. Departments therefore produced myriad reports with varying degrees of emphasis depending on contemporary managerial or economic anxieties. Trades unions also kept a close eye on absenteeism statistics so they could hold employers to account. High absenteeism could demonstrate the strain certain industries or companies put on their members' health, while lower figures could represent good employer-employee relations and exemplary health and safety practice.[15] Most importantly for understanding the general rhetoric around sick notes and absenteeism, these reports, statistics, and anxieties did not remain siloed in policy meetings away from public discourse. They often made their way into the press, presented in ways that emphasized what Britain could achieve if only unnecessary absenteeism could be eliminated.[16] Thus, absenteeism could be measured in cash or coal, despite the 'lost' hours never having 'really' existed.[17]

---

[12] John Treble and Tim Barmby, *Worker Absenteeism and Sick Pay* (Cambridge: Cambridge University Press, 2011), p. 3.

[13] 'Yorkshire miner "not lazy"', *Manchester Guardian*, 16 January 1958, p. 2.

[14] On the relative burden of sickness absence versus other forms of absence—including strikes – see: J. P. W. Hughes, 'Sickness Absence Recording in Industry', *British Journal of Industrial Medicine* 9, no. 4 (1952): pp. 264–74; Magnus Henrekson and Mats Persson, 'The effects on sick leave of changes in the sickness insurance system', *Journal of Labor Economics* 22, no. 1 (2004): pp. 87–113.

[15] TNA: MH 135/742, Trades Union Congress, Evidence to Committee on Medical Certificates, December 1948.

[16] William David Ross, *Royal Commission on the Press 1947–1949. Report (Cmd. 7700)* (London: HMSO, 1949), pp. 112–13.

[17] Examples include: '300,000 tons of coal lost', *The Times*, 31 August 1949, p. 4; 'Days off – in tons', *Daily Mail*, 24 April 1950, p. 5; 'Coal production (absenteeism)', *House of Commons Official Report (Hansard)* (hereafter *Hansard [Commons]*), 12 March 1956, vol. 550, col. w64.

Perhaps the most critical aspect for understanding absenteeism in this chapter and the rest of this volume is its relativity. Absenteeism could be 'higher' or 'lower' than some other place at some other time. It could even be 'too high'. But this was not against some absolute value. As discussed below with regard to the coalmines and ROFs, the problem for the Cabinet sub-committee was not how high the line on a chart went but whether it was travelling upwards or was higher than the line produced by another sector. The production of such statistics that were comparable across time and industry (at face value, if not scientifically) allowed the problem to be 'seen', yet they also constructed the problem by driving demand for new investigations and the production of more statistics.

This chapter discusses in detail who went looking for absenteeism and why, but it is important to stress that the political and historical significance of any given measure of overall absenteeism or sickness absence will be inevitably linked to wider economic concerns. This is not to say, as sociologist Phil Taylor and colleagues have done, that the ways in which experts measure absenteeism has changed according to the demands of economic planners and business managers (although of course they have).[18] It is to say that the relative priority political actors assigned to absenteeism was tied as much to historical conditions as any 'real' level of absence, relative or absolute. Despite the consistent background level worries about economic output and productivity it was during specific crises around the viability of the welfare state project that absenteeism was a greater political priority. The analysis of absenteeism in this chapter, therefore, is not interested in whether British public sector workers were 'really' getting sicker or if there was a 'cultural inflation of morbidity'.[19] Rather, it is through examining how contemporaries discussed absenteeism as a concept that we understand something about how sickness and sick notes were understood and how this reflected the British welfare state's particular anxieties in the 1940s and 1950s.

Royal Ordnance Factories

The problem of managing sickness absence was put bluntly by the civil servants investigating absenteeism in the ROFs. 'There is a widespread impression among local representatives that the [sick pay] scheme is being abused', they reported, drawing on the subjective experience of managers in the organizations, 'but little

---

[18] Taylor et al., 'Too scared to go sick'.
[19] See Chapter 1 and Martin Gorsky et al., 'The "cultural inflation of morbidity" during the English mortality decline: A new look', *Social Science & Medicine* 73 (2011): pp. 1775–83; S. Ryan Johansson, 'The health transition: The cultural inflation of morbidity during the decline of mortality', *Health Transition Review* 1 (1991): pp. 39–68.

concrete evidence of this has been produced.'[20] Like many employers in the postwar period, ROFs began to offer their 'industrial' employees the same sick pay rights as 'white-collar' civil servants.[21] The new scheme effectively replaced the worker's earnings when sick for the first 13 weeks of absence by paying the worker's normal rate wage, minus what they could claim from National Insurance. For a further 13 weeks they would pay at half rate. This meant that a worker had to apply for both benefit from the state and sick pay from the employer, though he or she could use the same National Insurance sickness certificate for both purposes.[22]

The rate of absenteeism immediately increased by 130 per cent.[23] The Ministry of Supply and the Treasury—responsible for paying the wages of the 60,000 or so workers covered by the scheme—estimated that this cost them £300,000 a year 'for no return in work.'[24] The ROFs were already under threat, with the House of Commons Select Committee finding that over two-thirds of their capacity were not being used. The Ministry of Supply wanted to accept more civil contracts to make better use of the factories, but they were hampered by a lack of skills, experience, or equipment to radically change the work that could be done.[25] Absenteeism was a problem for the future of many of the ROFs because of inefficiency, the need to produce goods and materiel in postwar reconstruction, and for the poor publicity that would come from inefficient use of public funds. The Ministry called for an investigation.[26] In doing so, they pre-empted Cabinet, who also asked for an inquiry but were content with waiting for the Ministry's findings.[27]

The Cabinet had expected an increase in sickness absence. Similar trends had been seen in the 1910s with the introduction of National Health Insurance.[28] After all, the entire point of the new scheme was to give people enough time to

[20]   TNA: T 217/52, Secret—Joint Co-ordinating Committee for Government Industrial Establishments, Report of the Sub-committee on Absence from Work Attributed to Sickness, 2 January 1950.
[21]   For the increase in the number of work-place sick pay schemes being introduced for industrial workers in the years immediately following the war, see the collection of sick pay regulation booklets and research by the Transport and General Workers Union: Modern Records Centre (hereafter MRC): MSS 126/TG/RES/M/18, files A, 1, 2 and 3. On the growing interest of businesses as providers of welfare in a historical context, see: Jeppe Nevers and Thomas Paster, 'Business and the Nordic welfare states, 1890–1970', *Scandinavian Journal of History* 44, no. 5 (2019): pp. 535–51.
[22]   TNA: T 217/47, Joint Co-ordinating Committee for Government Industrial Establishments, Scheme for Paid Sick Leave for Government Industrial Employees, 28 July 1948.
[23]   This was on average. The Royal Air Force, for example, reported an increase of over 180 per cent. TNA: T 217/47, Air Force to Lees, 30 March 1949.
[24]   TNA: COAL 26/170, Cabinet, Committee on Involuntary Absenteeism in the Coalmining Industry, Involuntary absenteeism in the Royal Ordnance Factories, Memorandum by the Ministry of Supply, 3 October 1949. The *Daily Mail* suggested the figure was as high as £1.25 million: 'Faked sickness probe by minister', *Daily Mail*, 15 August 1949, p. 2.
[25]   Select Committee on Estimates, *Seventh Report from the Select Committee on Estimates (HC 200 (1947–48))* (London: HMSO, 1948); Select Committee on Estimates, *Fifth Report from the Select Committee on Estimates (HC 141 (1948–49))* (London: HMSO, 1949).
[26]   TNA: T 217/52, Stanley Lees to Mr Blaker, 3 April 1950.
[27]   TNA: CAB 128/15/40, CM(49)40, 2 June 1949.
[28]   See Chapter 3 and Claud Schuster, *Report of the Departmental Committee on Sickness Benefit Claims Under the National Insurance Act (Cd. 7687)* (London: HMSO, 1914).

recover from illness. Officials noted this in their reports to the Ministry, even commenting that there was some anecdotal evidence from management that workers seemed more motivated or fitter when they returned.[29] However, and despite having no estimate of the likely cost before sickness benefit was introduced, the government considered the scale of the growth in sickness claims was excessive. The investigation was charged with measuring the level of absence, explaining it, and finding ways to counteract it.[30] The Joint Co-ordinating Committee for Government Industrial Establishments (JCC), which included representatives from the Ministry of Supply, Treasury, armed forces, and the trades unions, produced its own report in 1950. But to get a more 'scientific' response to the matter, it turned to the Medical Research Council and medical sociologist R. B. Buzzard. Together with a junior colleague, W. J. Shaw, he produced an interim and final report in 1950 and 1951 which detailed the probable causes of absenteeism and offered some tentative solutions for management.[31] Ironically, the 1951 report was delayed for several months because Buzzard got sick.[32]

Sick notes were part of the problem. Since claims to ROF sick pay and National Insurance sickness benefits required a medical certificate, the large growth in claims could only come from an increase in the number of certificates being issued.[33] The Survey of Sickness showed no spike in the levels of morbidity in the general population, casting doubt on the 'thoroughness' of some doctors' examinations.[34] Indeed, in 1951 nine men in Scotland were dismissed after they were found moonlighting while being signed off.[35] The JCC repeated some of the concerns seen in Chapter 2 about how 'panel' GPs in the new NHS were

---

[29] TNA: T 217/47, Air Force to Lees, 30 March 1949; ibid., War Office to Lees, 12 April 1949.

[30] TNA: T 217/52, Secret—Joint Co-ordinating Committee for Government Industrial Establishments, Report of the Sub-committee on Absence from Work Attributed to Sickness, 2 January 1950.

[31] These reports were circulated among the JCC in TNA: T 217/52, R. B. Buzzard, W. J. Shaw— Investigation of Sick Absence among Government Industrial Workers: Summary of Progress and Immediate Prospects, December 1950 and ibid., R. B. Buzzard and W. J. Shaw, Sick Absence Among Government Industrial Workers, Second Report, 1 November 1951. This was written up for wider academic consumption in R. B. Buzzard and W. J. Shaw, 'An analysis of absence under a scheme of paid sick leave', *British Journal of Industrial Medicine* 9, no. 4 (1952): pp. 282–95.

[32] TNA: T 217/52, Lees to Padmore, 28 May 1951. Buzzard blamed overwork for delays, informing the JCC that he needed an extended holiday. Other retarding factors included the difficulty in gathering reliable data and difficulties in finding good support staff.

[33] The lack of increase in 'uncertified' absence suggested this was the case. TNA: T 217/52, Buzzard and Shaw, Second Report.

[34] JCC were sent figures from the Survey that confirmed this. TNA: T 217/52, Survey of sickness. Comparative rates per 100 persons interviewed, attached to memorandum 15 May 1950. On the Survey itself, see Daisy Payling, '"The people who write to us are the people who don't like us:" Public responses to the Government Social Survey's Survey of Sickness, 1943–1952', *Journal of British Studies* 59 (2020): 315–42.

[35] 'Expulsion of union officials', *The Times*, 11 July 1951, p. 3; 'Appeals to union rejected', *Daily Mail*, 11 July 1951, p. 5. There were reports of similar behaviour in Portsmouth.

incentivized to write notes for workers rather than protect management or the public purse. For its 1950 report:

> The point has been repeatedly made…that all absence is justified because sick leave is not granted except on production of a doctor's certificate. We cannot completely accept this because it seems to us that the diagnosis of the physician in the first place must usually be based upon the patient's own account of his symptoms, so that the neurotic and the dishonest stand to gain an advantage over the others.[36]

The Minister of Education, George Tomlinson, confirmed this prejudice, drawing on the interwar experience of friendly societies.[37] Minister of Health Aneurin Bevan assured Cabinet that 'there was no evidence of any relaxation in the standards of medical certification by general practitioners' in general.[38] However, he did recommend that doctors and the Ministry of National Insurance pay closer attention to certificates written for ROF employees until the absenteeism issue was resolved.[39]

Despite this, sick notes were considered only part of a wider problem. Five main causes were found to be far more important.[40] First, higher and longer entitlements to sick pay meant that workers were able to recover in the way the scheme intended. In other words, before September 1948 there had been *too little* sickness absence and the system was correcting itself. Second, the scheme had been well-advertised, so workers were more aware of their entitlements. Third, some workers were financially better off staying at home. Sick workers did not have to pay National Insurance contributions to maintain their benefit entitlements and could avoiding public transport fares and other costs associated with going to the workplace.[41] 'This advantage varies with individual cases', noted the committee, 'but is rarely less than 5s [£0.25]' and could be anything up to a pound a week.[42] Fourth, some factories appeared to be more vulnerable to sickness, either because of the type of work they did or because their workforce was comparatively older. Fifth, many bosses claimed that there was a perverse incentive for workers to stretch their convalescence. The scheme only paid out for the first two days of

---

[36] TNA: T 217/52, Secret—Joint Co-ordinating Committee for Government Industrial Establishments. Report of the Sub-committee on Absence from Work Attributed to Sickness, 2 January 1950. The Ministry of Supply made similar comments in 1949: TNA: T 217/47, Ministry of Supply to Stanley Lees, 28 April 1949.

[37] TNA: CAB 195/7/45, Notes on proceedings at CM(49)49, 27 July 1949.

[38] TNA: CAB 128/15/40, CM(49)40, 2 June 1949.

[39] TNA: CAB 128/16/6, CM(49)49, 27 July 1949.

[40] TNA: T 217/52, Report of the Sub-committee on Absence from Work Attributed to Sickness.

[41] See discussions on 'cultural inflation' of morbidity and 'moral hazard' in Chapters 1 and 2.

[42] This would be used as the rationale for reforming sickness benefits to make them more easily taxable in the early 1980s. See Chapter 5 and Department of Health and Social Security, *Income during Initial Sickness: A New Strategy (Cmnd 7864)* (London: HMSO, 1980).

sickness if the length of illness was five days or fewer. Thus, while a worker could get some National Insurance compensation for shorter bouts, it was financially advantageous to 'extend' illness to a full week. The Admiralty demonstrated a hypothetical case of a worker earning one pound per day who got sick on a Monday. He or she would be £3 7/6 [£3.375] worse off returning on Friday versus taking the entire week off.[43] The committee found 'little evidence in support' of the idea that this behaviour was widespread and deliberate but did note the bulk of the extra absenteeism came from people claiming sickness for over five days, suggesting that workers were willing and able to take more time off than they had before the scheme was introduced.[44]

Even those who did suspect GPs' 'lax certification' acknowledged that structural factors were more pressing. Tomlinson, for example, prefaced his comments on friendly societies and doctors with 'a scheme which means paying people more when sick than working is bound to break down. That is the thing to tackle.'[45] In these criticisms of the scheme and the behaviour of its beneficiaries, class prejudice was evident. A representative from the Royal Air Force acknowledged that it would be unfair for industrial workers to be denied the form of sick pay given to non-industrials, but:

> Nevertheless, I do not like it....My own observations, spread over many years of public service, lead me to think that pretty full advantage is taken of the 7 days uncertificated sick leave [by white-collar workers], and if the industrials are given this my feeling is that the sickness figures will substantially increase.... I am not optimistic that generosity on our part will bring any reward.[46]

The implication was that while this had to be begrudgingly tolerated of the white-collar workers, it could not be for the blue-collar ones. Perhaps, then, certain classes of people needed to be given different kinds of incentive to present themselves for work. Military Transport drivers, for example, took less sick leave the general workforce. This was attributed to the fact that they received significant bonus pay for each delivery they made; thus, they earned more from coming to work and making deliveries than they could from sick pay (which only replaced their basic wage).[47] On the other hand, this could be an incentive to increase presenteeism, and potentially catastrophic for the household reliant upon bonus

---

[43] Accounting for lost wages, differences in National Insurance benefits and in sick pay. TNA: T 217/47, Admiralty to Lees, 29 April 1949.

[44] TNA: T 217/52, Report of the Sub-committee on Absence from Work Attributed to Sickness.

[45] TNA: CAB 195/7/45, Notes on proceedings at CM(49)49, 27 July 1949.

[46] TNA: T 217/47, Air Force to Lees, 30 March 1949.

[47] TNA: T 217/47, Air Force to Lees, 30 March 1949. See also Buzzard and Shaw, 'An analysis of absence'.

pay to cover the bills if overwork led to longer absence.[48] In any case, the quality of the certification process was not the issue—the key factor was the personal incentive for the worker to seek one.

To try to police the system better, other forms of medical validation were considered. Sick visiting in workers' homes and greater use of works' doctors were suggested. These would assess the worker's needs, encourage convalescence, and determine whether it might be possible, in the short term, to redeploy the employee within the organization to a different task until fully fit. It was not, in itself, designed to stop malingering.[49] There were even suggestions to allow self-certification for short bouts of illness, reducing the load on local doctors and removing the incentives to procure documentation of longer illnesses in order to claim benefits. In theory, workers would therefore return as soon as they felt fit rather than having to go through the process of obtaining First and Final National Insurance certificates for minor ailments.[50]

While JCC approached Buzzard in that the hope of finding a 'scientific' solution, it was disappointed. The report provided no clear plan of action. Even where Buzzard and Shaw had recommendations, they argued that changes would have to be implemented long-term to evaluate their potential effects. This was not useful to an organization that wanted quick, decisive scientific advice. Overall, the report simply told JCC what it already knew. Sickness was relative, subjective, and affected by countless structural and personal factors. The ROFs had already worked this out for themselves during the war. An inquiry into women workers showed that married women took more sick leave. Overall, this was partly because they had more caring duties and life commitments; but the specific reasons for each individual case were varied and unpredictable.[51] Even when the ROFs attempted to find a 'correct' level of absenteeism (they decided on four per cent because this was the level of absenteeism seen in other departments and among non-industrial ROF employees), this was based on estimates and guesswork.

---

[48] On the relationship to these sorts of pay structures to the 'gig economy', presenteeism, and ill health, see Chapter 8.

[49] TNA: T 217/47, Treasury Medical Service, Meeting 25 November 1948; ibid., Ministry of Supply to Lees, 28 April 1949. For more on industrial medicine and works doctors see Vicky Long, *The Rise and Fall of the Healthy Factory: The Politics of Industrial Health in Britain, 1914–60* (Basingstoke: Palgrave Macmillan, 2010).

[50] At this time, workers still required a note from their doctor certifying they had recovered from sickness (see Chapter 2). Self-certification was rejected, but these arguments would return during negotiations over the GPs' contract in the 1960s and introduction of Statutory Sick Pay in the 1980s (see Chapter 5).

[51] S. Wyatt, R. Marriott, and D. E. R. Hughes, *A Study of Absenteeism among Women* (London: HMSO, 1943); 'Women workers' lost time', *The Times*, 31 August 1943, p. 2; 'Young wives take the most days off', *Daily Mail*, 31 August 1943, p. 3. On gendered approaches to incapacity, see Chapter 4 and esp. Julie Gulland, *Gender, Work and Social Control: A Century of Disability Benefits* (London: Palgrave Macmillan, 2019).

It also required a staff-wide mean average and could not account for variations in individual factories due to the work they did or their workforce demographics.[52]

ROF management therefore decided not to focus on medical matters. It was not the sick note per se that had caused the problem—though, clearly, certification was not doing enough to help solve it. Instead, the problem was reframed as a behavioural one with focus on the worker. Some bureaucratic changes were made, such as revising some procedural anomalies which could provide a financial incentive for a worker to remain on sick pay rather than returning to work. But the main target was to treat absenteeism like a public health issue; one that, like raising vaccination rates or addressing the risks of smoking, could be remedied through persuasion and propaganda.[53] Notices were placed in break rooms warning workers that 'the future of the scheme depends on you'.[54] Further, Jack Jones, a junior minister at the Ministry of Supply, conducted a tour of ROFs in 1949 at the suggestion of the Ministry and Cabinet.[55] These visits attracted the attention of the press and had a mixed reception from the unions.[56] The union side of the JCC also opposed public statements that implied the government would have to rescind the sick pay scheme if absenteeism remained high (while reminding management that such threats might have the perverse effect of encouraging people to claim their sick pay 'while the going was good').[57] Despite this, it was clear to union officials that they would have to support management to an extent. The levels of absenteeism had become politically embarrassing and reflected poorly on the staff in the public eye. Thus, the unions co-signed a declaration that sick schemes and sick notes ought to be used 'responsibly'.[58] On the day Jack Jones visited Darwen, A. Pearson of the Transport and General Workers Union told workers to report those colleagues whom they suspected were malingering.[59] He further told Union members that the ROFs were being used by some private-sector businesses as an example of why they could not

---

[52] TNA: T 217/52, Report of the Sub-committee on Absence from Work Attributed to Sickness.

[53] Virginia Berridge, *Marketing Health* (Oxford: Oxford University Press, 2007); Alex Mold et al., *Placing the Public in Public Health in Postwar Britain* (London: Palgrave Macmillan, 2019); Hannah J. Elizabeth, Gareth Millward, and Alex Mold, '"Injections-While-You-Dance": Press advertisements and poster promotion of the polio vaccine to British publics, 1956–1962', *Cultural and Social History* 16, no. 3 (2019): pp. 315–36.

[54] TNA: T 217/52, Poster, 1949.

[55] TNA: CAB 128/16/6, C.M. (49) 40th Conclusions (27 July 1949).

[56] See, for example: 'Faked sickness probe by Minister', *Daily Mail*, 15 August 1949, p. 2; 'Arms workers warned: Health scheme in danger', *Daily Mail*, 16 August 1949, p. 1; 'Sickness among R.O.F. workers', *Manchester Guardian*, 16 August 1949, p. 4; 'Abuse of sick pay scheme', *Manchester Guardian*, 20 August 1949, p. 4; 'Sickness at ordnance factories', *The Times*, 15 August 1949, p. 2; 'Tour of ordnance factories', *The Times*, 16 August 1949, p. 2.

[57] TNA: T 217/52, Stanley Lees to Mr Blaker, 3 April 1950.

[58] TNA: T 217/52, Poster, 1949.

[59] 'Union say: Report the dodgers', *Daily Mail*, 18 August 1949, p. 3.

implement a full sick pay scheme.[60] A *Daily Mail* editorial went a stage further, arguing that this was an inevitable result of nationalization:

> Odd, isn't it, that such appeals have to be made only where the State takes over? We do not hear them coming from the steel, cement and sugar industries to name three scheduled for nationalisation. They are not necessary. The workers there have the old spirit. No one wants to restore the bad features of the old days; but unless the good ones are kept alive Britain's recovery will be difficult indeed.[61]

Thankfully for the Ministry of Supply, absenteeism in the ROFs returned to levels more comparable to other industries by the early 1950s, making the need for dramatic intervention less politically urgent and keeping the sector out of the public eye.[62] Whether because of these 'educational' interventions, or merely coincidental, government, management, and the unions seemed content to maintain the new status quo.

National Coal Board

The same could not be said for the National Coal Board (NCB). Absenteeism was part of a long-running problem for coalmining that had taken on a new political dimension. After the 'Vesting Day' of 1 January 1947, coalmining became a nationalized industry. While coal production had come under state control during the War to ensure supplies, most mines remained in private hands. From 1947, the Ministry of Fuel and Power now owned and ran the industry through the Board.[63] Nationalization, coupled with extant figures on output and labour usage during the War, made absenteeism visible in ways that were not necessarily matched in other industries. Crucially, these statistics were not just visible to government authorities and medical sociologists; they were regularly published in economic reports and highlighted by the media.

A lot was riding on coal. The government's economic plans required high enough production and exports to manage Britain's balance of payments and repay the sizable wartime debt to the United States. Furthermore, many industries were reliant upon coal power—and, significantly for public opinion in the new government, domestic use of coal for heating was politically sensitive. When

[60] 'End abuse of sick pay scheme', *Manchester Guardian*, 18 August 1949, p. 6.
[61] 'The old spirit', *Daily Mail*, 20 August 1949, p. 1.
[62] TNA: T 217/52, Buzzard and Shaw, Second Report; ibid., Letter to Chancellor (undated, probably November or December 1951).
[63] Israel Berkovitch, *Coal on the Switchback: The Coal Industry Since Nationalisation* (London: Routledge, 2017); Vicky Long and Victoria Brown, 'Conceptualizing work-related mental distress in the British coalfields (c. 1900–1950)', *Palgrave Communications* 4, no. 1 (2018): pp. 1–10.

production fell below targets, opponents were able to use the NCB's readily-available high (compared to other industries) and rising (compared to the prewar privatized mines) absenteeism figures to attack the government, mine management, miners, and the concept of nationalization itself. Indeed, the criticism of absent miners in the 1946/47 coal shortage was so intense that the National Union of Miners was able to convince the government to launch an inquiry into the written press's partisan coverage.[64]

The stakes were therefore much higher in coal than they were in the ROFs. Cabinet and the Ministry of Fuel and Power took the matter seriously, dedicating time and financial resource. At face value, it seemed that sick notes were part of the problem. Minister of Fuel and Power Philip Noel-Baker informed the House of Commons that around 59 per cent of absenteeism in 1950 was marked as sick leave.[65] Coalmining was notoriously taxing on the bodies of those it employed at the face and required labourers to be in good physical condition for them to be productive.[66] Higher levels of medical absence were therefore expected, either through injury or a lack of fitness that might not be as incapacitating in other industries. However, the government and mine managers doubted that all of the medical excuses provided by miners were genuine—or, at the very least, they doubted that injuries and ailments were serious enough to warrant the levels of 'involuntary' absenteeism presented in the figures. As the Ministry of Fuel and Power put it in 1949:

It might be from a strictly medical point of view and so far as the general well-being of the workers is concerned, this increase in absence from work is justifiable. There was no doubt that the old system operated harshly and some increase in absence was to be expected as the result of the new scheme. It might be too that by giving greater attention to the well-being of the worker today, a dividend will be received in years to come in the shape of a stronger and healthier labour force. The question must be faced, however, whether at the present stage of the nation's affairs, increases in absenteeism of the extent that were being experienced in the coal industry can be afforded. It was not only the cost

---

[64] *Cmd. 7700*, pp. 112–13. The inquiry found that the *Daily Mail* and *Daily Express* (right-wing, tabloid-format) were heavily critical, the *Daily Telegraph* and *Daily Graphic* (right-wing, broadsheet) even more so; but that each did also report when production improved in the late 1940s. The *Daily Worker* (hard left) reported absenteeism only to argue that it was being instrumentalized by the right to attack nationalization.

[65] Philip Noel-Baker, 'Coal shortage', *Hansard [Commons]*, 1 February 1951,vol. 483, cc. 1092–199, at col. 1100. Noel-Barker stated that seven per cent of the 11.95 per cent absenteeism rate in 1950 was due to sickness.

[66] Kirsti Bohata et al., *Disability in Industrial Britain* (Manchester: Manchester University Press, 2020); Arthur McIvor, 'Body talk: Oral history methodology in the study of occupational health and disability in twentieth century British coalmining', trans. Arthur McIvor, *Santé et Travail à la Mine: XIXe–XXIe Siècle*, edited by J. Rainhorn (Rennes: Presses Universitaires du Septentrion, 2014), pp. 238–61.

of the benefits themselves, serious as that might be; it was the loss of coal arising from this increased absenteeism which was the most serious aspect of the matter.[67]

There was a long history of official doubt over miners' incapacity, as recounted vividly in Bohata, Jones, Mantin, and Thompson's exploration of disability in the industry.[68] 1950s' officials, too, were wary. Management and doctors often repeated that absenteeism was particularly bad in coalmining regions and that miners were regular attendees at the GPs' surgery asking for medical certificates. A 'Mining General Practitioner' from Yorkshire wrote to the *Manchester Guardian*:

> I am reasonably sure that coal production could easily and quickly be raised...by using the fit, trained miners, very often face-workers, who every day clutter my waiting rooms to ask for 'Bonus Shift Notes' and insurance sick benefit certificates with specious excuses, difficult to refute or reject clinically, but obvious for what they are to the trained eye.[69]

At face value, then, more-stringent certification might cure the absenteeism problem. But there were significant barriers to putting this into practice. For one thing, doctors were unlikely to comply.[70] As another *Guardian* correspondent put it, the doctor's 'job is to look after the sick, not to act as a sort of policeman searching for malingerers for the benefit of the finances of the National Coal Board'.[71] Better sick pay and industrial injuries protection within the mines and from the state had produced similar incentives as in the ROFs. One 'miners' leader' was quoted at a delegate conference saying: 'it takes...the hell of a good doctor to cure a minor injury when a man is getting over £6 a week while he is away from the pit'.[72]

Just as the ROFs had chosen to focus on behaviour and education, there were deep cultural practices around work (and not working) that would need to be overcome. Various customs allowed miners to declare themselves 'sick' without the need for a note—and while the explicit 'excuse' might be considered medical, they were bound up in the institutional framework around mine employment

---

[67] TNA: COAL 26/170, Cabinet, Committee on Involuntary Absenteeism in the Coalmining Industry, Memorandum by Ministry of Fuel and Power, 7 September 1949.

[68] Bohata et al., *Disability in Industrial Britain*, esp. pp. 1–17, 105–39. The semi-autobiographical novel *The Citadel* by A. J. Cronin (originally published 1937) contains a key scene where the lead character begins work in a mining town and spends most of his first day examining miners for sick notes. A. J. Cronin, *The Citadel* (Basingstoke: Bello, 2013).

[69] 'Mining General Practitioner', letter in *Manchester Guardian*, 25 July 1954, p. 4.

[70] On doctors' reluctance to play 'gatekeeper', see esp. Chapters 2 and 5. Deborah A. Stone, 'Physicians as gatekeepers', *Public Policy* 27 (1979): pp. 227–54.

[71] A. R. Murray, letter in *Manchester Guardian*, 16 July 1954, p. 6.

[72] TNA: COAL 26/170, Cabinet, Committee on Involuntary Absenteeism in the Coalmining Industry, Memorandum by Ministry of Fuel and Power, 7 September 1949.

and wider economic incentives. For instance, there were reports in northern England that faceworkers would work up to their quotas and then claim to be sick, exhausted, or injured in order to end a shift early and still retain a full day's pay and their bonuses.[73] There was some speculation that miners might also be holding back production through absenteeism to avoid bonus pay forcing them into a higher income tax band.[74]

Still, there remained the physical toll that mining took from those it employed. Miners themselves attributed working conditions to the rates of both sickness and 'voluntary' absenteeism. Two Yorkshire miners wrote to the *Manchester Guardian* to argue that 'of course there is absenteeism' but given the conditions of the mines 'the wonder is, it is not higher'. They continued, 'the vast majority of miners turn up day in day out to do the real "donkey work" of the economy'.[75] Another from the same county noted the double standards with white-collar workers. Miners in 1948 were entitled to a total of 13 days' holiday, while 'at Christmas alone Civil Servants are to stop work at noon on the Friday until the following *Wednesday* morning, and, on making enquiries, [he found] that thousands of Civil Servants are entitled to 36 working days off every year....Why the difference?'[76]

Further research confirmed that any answers to the absenteeism crisis would not lie in sick notes. In 1949, Cabinet ordered an investigation into coalmining along similar lines to the one directed at the ROFs. It found that variance in sickness rates with previous years could be explained through administrative changes and seasonal fluctuations in infectious disease.[77] The injury rate had also increased, but the vast majority of these claims were found to be genuine.[78] Yet the political sensitivity of absenteeism ensured that debates continued through-out the 1950s, leading to the internal publication of a series of reviews by the NCB and Medical Research Council into absence rates in 1956.[79] These coincided with

[73] 'Proper poorly', *Daily Mail*, 14 October 1957. In an attempt to cajole miners to work a full week, the NCB had begun paying a bonus to anyone who worked five days in a week; but this would still be paid if a miner was signed off sick.

[74] A Durham Miners' Official categorically denied this rumour, while a representative of the Yorkshire Deputies and Overmen's Association supported it. TNA: COAL 26/170, *Yorkshire Post* cutting, damaged and undated, probably late summer 1949. The Cabinet inquiry later dismissed it as a likely factor in absenteeism rates. TNA: COAL 26/170, Cabinet, Committee on Involuntary Absenteeism in the Coalmining Industry, Effect of P.A.Y.E. on Absence from Work in Coalmines, memorandum by Sir Geoffrey Vickers, 5 October 1948.

[75] J. H. Freeman and A. Woodhall, miners at South Kirkby Colliery, letter to *Manchester Guardian*, 11 October 1955, p. 6.

[76] Emphasis original.'Coal-face Worker, Doncaster', letter to *Daily Mail*, 16 November 1948, p. 2.

[77] TNA: COAL 26/170, Cabinet, Committee on Involuntary Absenteeism in the Coalmining Industry, Results of Enquiry into Absences Following Accidents, memorandum by the Ministry of National Insurance (incorporating data furnished by the National Coal Board), 16 September 1949.

[78] TNA: CAB 129/41/12, Minister of Fuel and Power, 'Report of the Lidbury Committee on Involuntary Absenteeism' (11 July 1950).

[79] TNA: COAL 31/69, R. B. Buzzard, Attendance Investigation. The Scope, General Methods and Development of the Research, December 1956. Later published as R. B. Buzzard and F. D. K. Liddell, *Coalminers' Attendance at Work* (London: National Coal Board, 1963). See also TNA: COAL 74/3539, Reports on Absenteeism by Mr W. H. Sales, 1951.

new sick pay demands by the unions for surface workers.[80] Following his ROF study, Buzzard was invited to head the Medical Research Council investigation, although the NCB were unhappy with his conclusions. Again, Buzzard's findings showed that absenteeism was complex, relative, subjective, and it was difficult to present clear, workable, generalizable solutions. The Board was so unhappy that even though his report was circulated internally in 1956, it did not publish until 1963, including a foreword expressing its disappointment.[81] Some had predicted this. The Labour Relations Department, for example, questioned whether more investigation was needed into a problem that was already well known. Absenteeism 'would not be cured by a scientific enquiry', its representative said to the NCB's personnel committee in January 1952, 'a cure could only be guaranteed by the full and proper use of the established machinery for consultation and conciliation'.[82]

Despite these many competing factors in absenteeism, some in the NCB continued to criticize sick notes and 'the health services'; not because free health care gave miners the opportunity to 'swing the lead' but because it removed oversight from the mines' own doctors.[83] The new National Insurance system used the same form of certification for Industrial Injuries Benefit as for Sickness Benefit. This meant that rather than making a claim under the pre-1948 Workmen's Compensation Acts (where the employer had the right to request its own investigation and medical examination), all that was needed was a sick note from the claimant's GP. The machinery for policing these sick notes shifted to the National Insurance administration, which did not have the same capabilities for sick visiting or specialized knowledge of mining.[84] The Ministry of Fuel and Power, drawing on older criticisms of 'panel' GPs informed Cabinet:

> Compensation is paid by the State on the strength of a medical certificate given by the men's own...doctors [who] have no responsibility to the coal industry; they have a financial interest in retaining the patients on their panel and may naturally have difficulty in granting or refusing a continuance of a certificate for a few days if a man maintains he is unfit. It was widely felt in the coalfields that medical supervision was not as close as under the old system and that this went

[80] These reached a head in 1958. See for example: 'Coal chief and pit stay-away', *Daily Mail*, 9 January 1958, p. 7; policy discussions in TNA: COAL 74/6928.

[81] Berkovitch, *Coal on the Switchback*; Buzzard and Liddell, *Coalminers' Attendance at Work*.

[82] Iestyn Williams in TNA: COAL 31/69, Extract from the minutes of the 13th meeting of the Personnel Committee held on 21 January 1952.

[83] TNA: CAB 129/35/12, Ministry of Fuel and Power, 'Effect of new sickness and injury benefits upon absenteeism in coal mines' (31 May 1949), para 6.

[84] TNA: CAB 129/41/11, CP(5)161, 7 July 1950, para 22; TNA: COAL 26/171, Cabinet, Committee on Involuntary Absenteeism in the Coalmining Industry, Advantages which an absent man derives by submitting a medical certificate to the management, Memorandum by Sir Geoffrey Vickers, 3 November 1949.

a long way to account for benefit being paid more frequently and for longer periods than in the past.[85]

Fuel and Power suggested that the Ministry of Health could do more to ensure medical certificates were tightened and that the Ministry of National Insurance could be more active in re-examining patients.[86] Neither approach appeared to make much headway. The Ministry of Health was used to being asked to tighten certificates, as had been seen with the ROFs, and had become adept at batting such requests away. As for the Ministry of National Insurance, it did not have the same capacity for home visiting and re-examination that the Approved Societies had done before the war.[87] Besides, since the bulk of sickness was accounted for by short-term spells, such examinations would be largely fruitless.[88] NCB had echoed the Ministries of Health and National Insurance to the Cabinet investigation, earning rebuke from the Ministry of Fuel and Power for not backing their 'own' department. This serves as a reminder that there was no singular 'government' view of absenteeism or of sick notes—even within the auspices of a single ministry.

Metropolitan Police

Like the coal mines, police forces had long-running absenteeism data to show change over time in the rates of sickness. Officers were also subjected to fitness tests and had to meet certain physical standards. This made large forces, such as the Metropolitan Police (the Met), ideal sites for research, especially with the rise of 'social medicine' after the war.[89] The physical requirements for (mostly male) police officers meant there was a relatively consistent population to study across time, with fitness, sickness, and accident reporting detailed enough to provide reliable, comparable, and generalizable data for social scientists. When absenteeism increased significantly after the war, this made the police an even more intriguing research subject as a potential source of answers for other industries' problems.

The Met itself did not seem unduly perturbed by absenteeism in the 1950s. There were no high-profile examples of the 'blue flu'—using co-ordinated sick leave in lieu of strike action—that afflicted Stockholm in the 1950s and other

---

[85] TNA: COAL 26/170, Cabinet, Committee on Involuntary Absenteeism in the Coalmining Industry, Memorandum by Ministry of Fuel and Power, 7 September 1949.

[86] TNA: CAB 129/41/11, CP(50)161, 7 July 1950; TNA: CAB 129/41/12, CP(50)162, 11 July 1950.

[87] See Chapter 2 and Gulland, *Gender, Work and Social Control*.

[88] TNA: COAL 26/170, Cabinet, Committee on Involuntary Absenteeism in the Coalmining Industry, Minutes of a Meeting of the Committee, 16 September 1949; Cabinet, Committee on Involuntary Absenteeism in the Coalmining Industry, Memorandum by Ministry of Fuel and Power, 7 September 1949.

[89] Virginia Berridge, 'Jerry Morris', *International Journal of Epidemiology* 30, no. 5 (2001): pp. 1141–5.

police forces across the second half of the twentieth century.[90] In fact, the limited correspondence on the subject in The National Archives suggests that, unlike the ROFs, NCB, and Post Office, it found research an inconvenient annoyance.[91] When a *Daily Express* report on sickness rates among police officers required an official response, one civil servant said that the article was broadly correct, but that the Met had not invited the Medical Research Council to investigate absenteeism: 'on the contrary, we have been doing our best to put them off, as their constant requests for assistance in medical investigations have been a nuisance and have caused us a lot of extra work'.[92]

But while sick notes were not a major political worry for the Met, publicity given to medical absenteeism in the police force does expose wider concerns with changing demographics and a sense of 'decline' in postwar Britain.[93] These issues are explored in greater detail in Chapter 4, but the Met's responses to criticisms of its absence figures show that workforces in the 1950s were understood to be qualitatively and quantitatively different to the prewar generation. In turn, management was convinced that these developments were responsible for greater sickness absence and were outside its control. Healthy men left the force during the war, replaced with less-able-bodied and less-experienced recruits. For those who returned or remained, the age of retirement had been raised (with officers now required to work for 30 years before claiming their pension, not 24 as previously). Since 1944, full sick pay had been offered, producing similar effects on absenteeism as the NCB and ROF schemes. The police also seemed to be convinced that lowering the minimum height requirement for new recruits meant that forces were now employing shorter men who were, because of their diminutive stature, more prone to illness.[94] This was, apparently, so common-sensical that it required no further explanation.[95]

---

[90] On later 'strikes' see: '1,000 policemen go sick', *Manchester Guardian*, 24 June 1955, p. 13; Michael Leapman, 'New York nervous as police go on strike', *The Times*, 16 January 1971, p. 1. 'Crime wave as police report sick in Sweden', *The Times*, 21 October 1985, p. 5; Audrey Magee, '80% of Irish police go sick in protest at salary offer', *The Times*, 2 May 1998, p. 2.

[91] TNA: MEPO 2/8424, S. J. Hobson to Chief Medical Officer, 11 September 1952. For published research, see: E. R. Bransby, 'Comparison of the rates of sick absence of Metropolitan Policemen before and after the War', *Monthly Bulletin of the Ministry of Health and the Public Laboratory Service* 8 (1949): pp. 31–6; E. R. Bransby and D. Thomson, 'Sick absence in the Metropolitan Police, especially that due to respiratory infections', *Monthly Bulletin of the Ministry of Health and the Public Laboratory Service* 12 (1953): pp. 32–42.

[92] TNA: MEPO 2/8484, Met response to *Daily Express*, internal memorandum, undated. See also: 'Post war health of police', *Police Review*, 25 March 1949, pp. 1–2; Chapman Pincher, 'Why should a P.C. take 10 days to get over that common cold?', *Daily Express*, 6 March 1953.

[93] See Chapter 1 and Jim Tomlinson, 'De-industrialization: Strengths and weaknesses as a key concept for understanding post-war British history', *Urban History* 47, no. 2 (2020): pp. 199–219 for a critique of this concept.

[94] 'Post war health of police'.

[95] There was, however, a long-standing association of shortness with malnutrition or 'bad breeding', particularly in eugenicist population studies in the interwar period. See: Roderick Floud, Kenneth W. Wachter, and Annabel Gregory, *Height, Health, and History: Nutritional Status in the United Kingdom, 1750–1980* (Cambridge: University Press, 1990).

'Shortism' aside, the Met was not the only publicly funded organization to note these trends. It, the ROFs, NCB, and Post Office, all accepted that their workforces were very different to the ones they had managed in the 1930s. Thus, even if certification practices could be tightened there would still be new sickness challenges among their staff. When coupled with anxieties about national productivity, these changes became even more politically charged. The declining birth rate after the initial post-First World War 'baby boom' meant there was a shortage of the traditional target for industrial and manual workers: young, white men.[96] Those born immediately after 1945 would not leave compulsory schooling until the 1960s and people were retiring later, creating an older workforce more prone to sick leave.[97] Deaths and injuries sustained by working-age men during the two world wars produced a greater reliance on disabled, female, and migrant labour.[98] Despite Buzzard's focus on male workers in his reports on the ROFs and the mines, it was widely acknowledged that women took more sick leave. A key reason for this was that women had more domestic and caring duties, and therefore often had to take more time off, especially when ill.[99] Indeed, this was a sticking point in a dispute between male bus conductors and London Transport in 1950. The men argued that hiring too many women would lead to absenteeism (putting more strain on the men) and the lower pay offered to women would hamper the men's claims to higher wages.[100]

The NCB had further problems. In coalmining towns and villages, 'young men will not enter what appears to be an unattractive industry offering a heavier than

---

[96] Susan L. Carruthers, '"Manning the factories": Propaganda and policy on the employment of women, 1939–1947', *History* 75, no. 244 (1990): pp. 232–56.

[97] 'Post war health of police'; TNA: T 217/52, Secret—Joint Co-ordinating Committee for Government Industrial Establishments, Report of the Sub-committee on Absence from Work Attributed to Sickness, 2 January 1950. P. M. Thane, 'The debate on the declining birth-rate in Britain: The "menace" of an ageing population, 1920s–1950s', *Continuity & Change* 5, no. 2 (1990): pp. 238–305. See also Gorsky et al.'s account of how an ageing population explains changing sick claim trends in the interwar period in Gorsky et al., 'The "cultural inflation of morbidity"'.

[98] Anxieties over the failures of rehabilitative services in the First World War led to the Disabled Persons (Employment) Act 1944 and the creation of Remploy for sheltered employment. Helen Bolderson, *Social Security, Disability and Rehabilitation* (London: Jessica Kingsley, 1991); Julie Anderson, *War, Disability and Rehabilitation in Britain: 'Soul of a Nation'* (Manchester: Manchester University Press, 2011); Jameel Hampton, *Disability and the Welfare State in Britain: Changes in Perception and Policy 1948-1979* (Bristol: Policy Press, 2016). As will be discussed in Chapter 4, although the employment of women was not a new phenomenon, the scale and political meaning of such employment was significant. Sarah Horrell, 'The household and the labour market', in *Work and Pay in 20th Century Britain*, edited by Nicholas Crafts, Ian Gazeley, and Andrew Newell (Oxford: Oxford University Press, 2007), pp. 117–41. On migration, see Chapter 4 and Satnam Virdee, *Racism, Class and the Racialized Outsider* (Basingstoke: Palgrave Macmillan, 2014).

[99] R. B. Buzzard, 'Attendance and absence in industry: The nature of the evidence', *The British Journal of Sociology* 5, no. 3 (1954): pp. 238–52; Wyatt, Marriott, and Hughes, *A Study of Absenteeism among Women*. On the labour of women at work and in the home see Jane Lewis, 'Gender and the development of welfare regimes', *Journal of European Social Policy* 2, no. 2 (1992): pp. 159–73; Claire Langhamer, 'Feelings, women and work in the long 1950s', *Women's History Review* 26, no. 1 (2017): pp. 77–92; Gulland, *Gender, Work and Social Control*.

[100] Roland Hurman, 'Busmen are winning', *Daily Mail*, 24 March 1950, p. 2.

average accident rate unless some really attractive carrot is offered to them'.[101] Full employment had given people more options to earn a decent wage in jobs that were less dangerous, physically demanding, and unpleasant. Attorney General Sir Hartley Shawcross even suggested in 1949 that the lack of fear of unemployment risked creating 'slackness'.[102] E. M. Nicholson of the Lord President's Office took these arguments a step further when discussing absenteeism in the ROFs. Sick leave, he argued, was an inevitable product of the welfare state.

> Since 1930 we have switched over...to a labour saving and full employment economy in which there is now no social excuse left for any able-bodied, or even partially disabled adult to get out of doing more or less a full year's work at some occupation ....As a result we have about 22 ½ million gainfully occupied people in employment, but if one considers the numbers of the mentally diseased, mentally defective, neurotic and other mental or emotionally handicapped persons, it seems difficult to avoid the conclusion that out present policy is forcing into full-time employment a lot of people who cannot take it, and is also...forcing into a routine type of employment people who are temperamentally better fitted for more spasmodic activity, and are therefore also misfits in existing conditions.[103]

This eugenicist approach to the labour 'stock' suggested that, regardless of monitoring procedures, there would always be a rump within the population unable or unwilling to work full time, despite the needs and expectations of the general economy. Stricter sick notes were not going to change that.

Post Office

Unlike the Met, the Post Office did take an active role in researching its issues with absenteeism. It was unique in these case studies because the staff side of its Whitley Council—comprising representatives from trades unions and workers—actively requested reports on absenteeism so that the data could be used to improve staff health and overall productivity.[104] The Post Office (or Royal Mail) was one of the oldest continuously operating institutions in the world. Indeed, one of the reasons why its postwar increase in absenteeism was visible to the government and management was that statistics on sickness among workers had

---

[101] A. G. Flint, letter to *Manchester Guardian*, 22 September 1947, p. 4.
[102] 'Work', *Daily Mail*, 4 April 1949, p. 3.
[103] TNA: T 217/52, E. M. Nicholson to Sir Frederick Bartlett, 11 May 1950.
[104] The Whitley councils of staff and management worked together to deal with staffing issues within civil service departments. MRC: MSS 89P/196, Note of an informal meeting with representatives of the Staff Side of the Post Office Departmental Whitley Council held on 31 October 1949, to discuss the incidence of sick rates in the Post Office.

been kept since at least 1892, and it had maintained its own medical service since 1854.[105] It also employed thousands of people across the United Kingdom in various roles. Like the Met, some of these were performed outside in all weathers, others were more clerical.

Since Post Office employees were treated as 'civil servants' they had not received a new sick pay scheme in the late 1940s, but the introduction of the health services and changing demographics appeared to have played a part in rising absenteeism. The overall scale of the problem was presented in stark terms. The difference in sick leave between 1938 and 1952 was the equivalent to 5,400 full-time staff, or £2 million per annum. Many of the older men and women recruited in the War remained in post and, for those staff returning, they tended to work longer before retirement. Furthermore, it was known that 'women generally have more sick leave than men' and that younger recruits took a disproportionate amount of leave when accounting for lower levels of morbidity relative to older age groups.[106] It was also clear that there were regional and occupational variations. Management and unions accepted that this might be solved through general education and reminding young employees of their duties rather than attributing it to malingering or abuse.[107]

The Post Office's Medical Officer, Cecil Roberts, acknowledged that structural factors might lead to increased absenteeism, even if the individual worker still bore some responsibility. In an article for the *Monthly Bulletin of the Ministry of Health* he noted that:

If a man is happy at a job, has a team spirit with his mates, a good sense of service to his department and the community, he works off many of his ailments and is usually none the worse for it in health or happiness. On the other hand, if he loathes the sight of a dingy office; doesn't get on with his mates; hates his overseer's face; misguidedly lacks a sense of service to his department and the community, or just can't adjust himself to the essential disciplines in a public service, he escapes into sick absence at the slightest provocation.[108]

The Post Office's approach to absenteeism appeared more sympathetic towards the workers than the NCB or ROFs (and less apathetic than the Metropolitan

---

[105] Cecil Roberts, 'Post Office medical services and morbidity statistics', *Monthly Bulletin of the Ministry of Health and the Public Laboratory Service* 7 (1948): pp. 184–201.

[106] MRC: MSS 89P/197, The Sick Leave Situation, attached to memorandum dated 20 October 1953.

[107] MRC: MSS 89P/196, Note of a meeting with representatives of the Staff Side of the Post Office Departmental Whitley Council held on the 29th August, 1952, to discuss the incidence of sick rates in the Post Office.

[108] Roberts, 'Post Office', p. 186. Roberts' article was a defence of—at times, a eulogy for—the Post Office's Medical Service, which was about to be closed. With the advent of the NHS, there was no need for a full medical service. Roberts' role would eventually be absorbed by the Treasury, allowing him to continue working on Post Office medical matters but not within his own demesne.

Police). There were fewer direct demands on the Post Office for greater efficiency. There were some. For instance, Edwin Wells led an almost-one-man crusade under the auspices of the Postal Reform League to get the Post Office to reduce waste and absenteeism so that there could be a return of the penny post.[109] However the Royal Mail did not have the ROF's financial problems or the politically-charged output targets of the coalmines. Similarly, the history of Post Office employment is instructive.[110] There was a greater proportion of clerical jobs within the organization. These 'white-collar' or 'middle-class' workers enjoyed a greater level of trust from management than their working-class ROF and NCB counterparts. The existence of the medical service, full sick pay, and other benefits before the War meant that there was a welfare relationship between management and workers that did not necessarily exist in other companies. It also meant that National Insurance did not provide much greater incentive to remain absent than before 1939.[111] Indeed, there was even call for a significant wage rise from some trade unionists who argued the welfare state effectively meant a pay cut given the relative loss of benefits compared to the general population.[112]

As with the other cases studies, investigation showed that sick notes were not the major factor that they might have appeared at face value. While 'sometimes doctors are blamed' for the increase in absenteeism the Post Office found it important to stress that 'this is not altogether fair, for it is up to the patient, when he is not seriously ill, to tell his doctor when he feels he can return to work'.[113] In a list of suggestions raised by local Whitley committees, medical certificates did not appear as one of the proposals.[114] There was general acceptance that sick notes alone would not be able to police absenteeism and that the solution would have to be to improve 'discipline and morale'.[115] The exception to this general picture was over one-day absences. These typically did not require a doctor's note, and there was evidence that in some cases this had been abused. The most high-profile example of this came when several telephonists—or 'hello girls' as the *Daily Mail* described them—were dismissed in Manchester and Liverpool.[116] Most of the

---

[109]   See, for example, Letter from Edwin Wells, Secretary and founder of the Postal Reform League, *The Times*, 13 August 1952, p. 5; 'Obituary', *Manchester Guardian*, 2 July 1954, p. 7; 'Life was a struggle to restore 1d post', *Daily Mail*, 2 July 1954, p. 5.

[110]   Martin J. Daunton, *Royal Mail: The Post Office since 1840* (London: Athlone Press, 1985).

[111]   The core sick pay provision for white-collar civil servants had changed little from the 1920s. See Raymond E. Priestley, *Royal Commission on the Civil Service 1953–55. Report (Cmd. 9613)* (London: HMSO, 1955), pp. 64–6.

[112]   'Post Office workers seek wage increase', *Manchester Guardian*, 17 June 1948, p. 3.

[113]   MRC: MSS 89P/197, The Sick Leave Situation, attached to memorandum dated 20 October 1953.

[114]   MRC: MSS 89P/197, Sick Absence—Suggestions by Local Whitley Committees for Improving the Position, attached to memorandum dated 12 January 1955.

[115]   'Green Ink' letter to *Manchester Guardian*, 1 March 1954, p. 4.

[116]   Three of those dismissed, however, were men. 'Hello girls are sacked after taking too much leave', *Daily Mail*, 16 February 1954, p. 3.

workers were part-time but had taken several one-day absences alongside longer periods of illness.[117] The local unions appealed, withdrawing from any further discussions on how to reduce absenteeism. The National Guild of Telephonists questioned why their sector of the Post Office appeared to have been singled out ahead of other occupations.[118] But even if the two sides in this dispute had been able to point to a sick note—or lack thereof—as proof one way or the other of the degree of incapacity, would notes for such a small period of time be worth the administrative hassle for worker or bureaucrat?[119]

The political question for the Post Office, however, was over how absenteeism would affect the organization's reputation. Both bosses and workers noted that civil servants had developed a reputation for 'tea-drinking and form filling...[taking] a day off whenever they feel like it'.[120] For management, Post Office staff had a duty to reduce absenteeism as part of their responsibilities to local communities and the wider state:

> As Civil Servants we have to be careful that the privileges we receive under government employment are not criticised by the rest of the community as being too expensive. Our sick pay arrangements are probably better than most...in outside industry....We should keep down our expenses in terms of manpower as well as the money cost of the extra staff and the relatively high costs for overtime.[121]

The Post Office offered to be a site of scientific enquiry for sickness absence. It felt the organization had responsibilities as a public service, as well as the means and geographic spread to make any data generalizable for political authorities.[122] The Deputy General of the Union of Post Office Workers agreed during the telephonist dispute that there was no 'right' to excessive numbers of sick days.[123] Yet the exact balance between the rights to sick leave, the duty towards the organization and the nation, the need to avoid presenteeism, and the expectations that could be placed on an ageing and increasingly female workforce was difficult to define objectively.

Of course, there was one area of absenteeism that remained perplexing. Captain Lawrence Orr asked deputy Postmaster General David Gammans MP 'when the allowance payable for the maintenance of cats...was last raised'. Cats

---

[117] 'Check of telephonists' records', *The Times*, 1 March 1954, p. 3; 'Too many off sick', *Manchester Guardian*, 15 February 1954, p. 1.

[118] 'Telephonists "not tea-drinkers"', *Manchester Guardian*, 2 March 1954, p. 2.

[119] On the problems of short-term certification and 'ipse dixit' notes, see Chapters 2 and 5.

[120] National organizer for the National Guild of Telephonists quoted in 'Telephonists "not tea-drinkers"', *Manchester Guardian*, 2 March 1954, p. 2.

[121] MRC: MSS 89P/197, The Sick Leave Situation, attached to memorandum dated 20 October 1953.

[122] MRC: MSS 89P/196, K. Hind to F. T. Dixon, 14 November 1950.

[123] 'Postal union reply to critics', *Manchester Guardian*, 26 February 1954, p. 8.

had been used historically in Post Offices to catch mice nibbling on envelopes and raise the morale among staff. Gammans lamented:

> There is, I am afraid, a certain amount of industrial chaos in the Post Office cat world. Allowances vary in different places, possibly according to the alleged efficiency of the animals and other factors. It has proved impossible to organise any scheme for payment by results or output bonus. These servants of the State are, however, frequently unreliable, capricious in their duties and liable to prolonged absenteeism....There are no Post Office cats in Northern Ireland. Except for the cats at Post Office Headquarters who got the special allowance a few years ago, presumably for prestige reasons, there has been a general wage freeze since July, 1918, but there have been no complaints![124]

The joke—aside from the absurdity of discussing such a trivial matter in the House of Commons—certainly fit the debates about nationalized industries at the time. Pay and conditions were often linked to absenteeism, as seen particularly with the NCB. At least, unlike with human bus drivers in 1950, Gammans was able to confirm that male and female cats enjoyed equal pay.

Conclusion

In these examples, the sick note was representative of a problem, but not necessarily the cause of it. 'Lax certification' from doctors and the eagerness of workers to procure sick notes seemed synonymous with absenteeism. In scratching the surface, however, authorities came to see a much more complex web of industrial relations and economic incentives baked into state and employer sick pay schemes. Sick notes and absenteeism were rhetorically linked, the first thing to be raised whenever there was talk about needing to do something to improve attendance—but this was not an adequate base for any form of effective policy. One could not police sick notes more strictly and maintain morale among the workforce. One could not insult the professional integrity of GPs and expect them to provide a free medical gatekeeping service. As Buzzard wrote in his report that was subsequently maligned by the NCB, 'the opinions held about absence...were not only contradictory but were often expressed in strongly emotional terms'. It did not really matter, then, whether the population was 'really' getting sicker—only how statistical data around sickness and work were generated and interpreted.

---

[124] 'Cats (Maintenance Allowances)', *Hansard [Commons]*, 18 March 1953, vol. 513 cc. 4–5. See also '#MuseumCats Day: "Industrial chaos in the Post Office cat world"', The British Postal Museum and Archive Blog, 30 July 2014, accessed 16 July 2019, https://postalheritage.wordpress.com/2014/07/30/museumcats-day-industrial-chaos-in-the-post-office-cat-world; 'Enough to make OHMS cats laugh', *Daily Mail*, 19 March 1953, p. 2.

Besides, sick notes were not going to be an adequate way of determining that 'real' level of morbidity.

But this rhetorical conflation proves useful for exploring the meaning and implementation of the welfare state. Investigating sick notes inevitably leads down a path to absenteeism and the interconnected areas of economic, employment, health, and social security policy. The story quickly shifts to a series of anxieties around the future viability of the welfare state. It exposes narratives of decline that pervade the chapters of this book: decline in the economic power of a country struggling to rebuild after the war, but also in the moral fibre of the labour necessary for that reconstruction. Absenteeism, like decline, was always relative.[125] In the cases here, that relativity was mainly to the past, a past that was qualitatively and (selectively) quantitatively 'better'. In turn, this brought attention on how work and the population that performed that work had changed since the 1930s. Medical certification policy is a window onto these issues, but what we uncover has far wider implications than simply the interaction between National Insurance benefit claimant and his or her GP.

Crucially, even though discussion moves quickly onto these deeper concerns, in each of the case studies presented here the sick note never disappears. Despite the 'scientific' investigations that showed medical certification to be a minor factor in the rise of involuntary absenteeism, officials, politicians, doctors, and workers all brought it up as a central part of the process of securing leave from work. An observable part of the bureaucracy that was supposed to curb malingering, sick notes might not have caused the absenteeism problem but there was consternation that they could not do more to help tackle it. Once again, we see how the sick note survived the 1950s just as it did the 1940s. It was not a perfect solution, and its failings were very visible—but even a cursory investigation into absenteeism showed that there were much more pressing issues to tackle before replacing medical certification with something else.

---

[125] Jim Tomlinson, 'De-industrialization'.

4

Chauvinists and Breadwinners in the 'Classic Welfare State'

Despite the teething troubles with the British Medical Association and the nation-alized industries, the previous chapters have shown that the British welfare state had successfully integrated sick notes into the system. Liberal state institutions and Approved Societies before the war had been replaced by social democratic structures, but the sick note had been able to adapt. The 'classic welfare state' period, as Anne Digby has described the era between the end of the Second World War and the oil crisis of the 1970s, had fully embraced the sick note.[1] Even employers (both as private welfare providers via occupational sick pay schemes and as policers of absenteeism) had been able to integrate medical certification into everyday personnel decisions. Thus far, however, this book has largely relied upon source materials that tell us about the dominant images of workers and claimants in the welfare state. The picture is much more complicated once we consider people who fell outside this imagined 'ordinary' worker.

The National Insurance sick note and National Insurance system discussed in the previous two chapters were designed for 'heads of households' with stable employment and full insurance contribution records. Such people—usually men—could access the system with relative ease when sick. There might be debates about the 'real' extent of incapacity, absenteeism, and the role of the doc-tor, but the general question of eligibility for benefit fell mainly on the burden of medical proof. When we examine the archive of the sickness system more closely, however, it becomes evident that claims from the very poor, non-British born claimants, and married women were treated rather differently. These were not policy 'problems' of legitimate sickness—the issue was whether such groups were legally or morally entitled to support at all.

Even if liberal and social democratic regimes could incorporate the sick note, this chapter moves beyond these traditional political and economic 'regimes' to consider other modes of power in the postwar welfare state. Notably, it builds upon the growing literature on European 'welfare chauvinism'—the idea that national welfare states exist to serve native populations and not those coded as

---

[1] Anne Digby, *British Welfare Policy: Workhouse to Workfare* (London: Faber, 1989); Jameel Hampton, *Disability and the Welfare State in Britain: Changes in Perception and Policy 1948–1979* (Bristol: Policy Press, 2016). On welfare state periodization see Chapter 1.

immigrants—and the 'breadwinner model' of welfare—that posits that the British welfare state was erected to maintain 'traditional' gender roles.[2] The everyday operation of sickness policy has left an archival trail that can be read 'against the grain' to uncover how wider prejudices and structural discrimination manifested in the design and operation of welfare state policy. This chapter shows that while medical certification could be adapted to meet the needs of chauvinists and those keen to protect conservative 'family values', in practice other forms of gatekeeping meant that the sick note rarely stood as the main difference between accessing welfare services and not.

Focusing on the 'classic welfare state' period, the three sections that follow build upon each other to show how these processes played out. First, it is important to understand the Beveridgean welfare state's position on the poorest in society. As discussed in Chapter 2, National Assistance (from 1968, Supplementary Benefit) was designed to provide a subsistence income to those whose household earnings and assets fell below the poverty line. Many payments were conditional upon sickness and relied upon medical evidence indistinguishable from the National Insurance sick note. However, because the system was designed for those without recourse to National Insurance benefits, it is here that we see claims from people most disadvantaged in a capitalist society built on waged labour. Therefore, only considering the story of National Insurance sick notes *in relation to National Insurance* erases a range of experiences in postwar Britain. Investigating National Assistance shows that the utility of sick notes got stretched by concerns over other eligibility criteria for claimants with complex financial and social needs. At the same time, the cases that did involve sick notes show the nuances and inconsistencies in sickness-related benefits that give us a richer picture of how the welfare state operated day-to-day. National Assistance therefore makes visible those cases—indeed, those people—that were not in mind when the system was established. It helps illuminate how the British state determined who was entitled to support and, in turn, who qualified for full citizenship in this new era of 'social rights'.[3]

In the second and third sections, two of these marginalized groups are considered in more detail. Though by no means exhaustive, they are useful ways to explore the structural inequalities in the welfare state. The second section

[2] Jane Lewis, 'Gender and the development of welfare regimes', *Journal of European Social Policy* 2, no. 2 (1992): pp. 159–73; Jeroen van der Waal, Willem de Koster, and Wim van Oorschot, 'Three worlds of welfare chauvinism? How welfare regimes affect support for distributing welfare to immigrants in Europe', *Journal of Comparative Policy Analysis: Research and Practice* 15, no. 2 (2013): pp. 164–81. On the use of 'welfare regimes' or logics as hermeneutic devices, see Chapter 1, esp.: Gøsta Esping-Andersen, *The Three Worlds of Welfare Capitalism* (Cambridge: Polity, 1990); Keesvan Kersbergen and Barbara Vis, *Comparative Welfare State Politics: Development, Opportunities, and Reform* (Cambridge University Press, 2014), esp. pp. 53–77.
[3] See Chapters 1 and 2 and T. H. Marshall, *Citizenship and Social Class, and Other Essays* (Cambridge: Cambridge University Press, 1950).

considered the position of newly arrived migrants from Commonwealth countries. The discourse around immigration and the welfare state rarely confronted sickness certification directly. In using medical certification policy as the starting point, however, the trail through the archive shows how 'problems' regarding migrant claimants were racialized and categorized by certain sections the media, government departments, front-line staff and the public. 'Welfare chauvinism', often examined in Europe as a more-recent phenomenon, was clearly evident in Britain as soon as the welfare state was established.[4] As a result, problems in the sickness system that involved people born outside the UK were treated as migration issues first and foremost. For example, even when there was reason to consider sick notes a major security risk following the exposure of a fraud gang run by Indian criminals, the government continued to focus on administrative responses to migrant claimants rather than taking action with the system itself.

The third section then details the categorization of women in the 'breadwinner' welfare state model.[5] Married women were disadvantaged in a system designed to uphold a particular vision of the nuclear family. However, as with debates on migration, sickness benefits were complicated by changing patterns of employment and demographic shifts. More women were entering and remaining in paid work. Maternity claims were not as simple as originally thought, while the growing demand for gender equality in social security led to contradictory responses to new sickness benefits for 'housewives'. Gendered attitudes towards paid and domestic labour also placed greater responsibility on women to care for sick relatives; but while the state acknowledged the need to provide support, it was unclear whether such payments—and the sick notes used as a gateway to them—should be given to the carer or the cared-for. In total, these three sections show the prejudices baked into the original design of the sickness welfare system and how they quickly buckled under contact with claimants' lived experience.

Poverty

As discussed in Chapter 2, when the Victorian Poor Laws were revoked on 5 July 1948 three key institutions emerged to take their place: National Health, National Insurance, and National Assistance.[6] Designed as a stop gap for those few who would not have adequate insurance records in a prosperous nation with full employment, the medical certification needs of the National Assistance Board

---

[4] The term is attributed to Jørgen Goul Andersen and Tor Bjørklund, 'Structural change and new cleavages: The progress parties in Denmark and Norway', *Acta Sociologica* 33, no. 3 (1990): pp. 195–217. On recent analyses, see: Waal, Koster, and Oorschot, 'Three worlds of welfare chauvinism?'; Marko Grdešć, 'Neoliberalism and welfare chauvinism in Germany': An examination of survey evidence', *German Politics & Society* 37, no. 2 (2019): pp. 1–22.
[5] Lewis, 'Gender and the Development of Welfare Regimes'.   [6] See Chapter 2.

(NAB) were an afterthought. This has two significant implications for the history of sick notes and what they tell us about the wider welfare state. First, it shows that designers had assumed that NAB would largely run itself along similar lines to National Insurance (despite the fact that NAB dealt with the most insecure section of British society, a group that disproportionately included women, older people, people with chronic health conditions, and those born outside the British Isles). This leads to the second implication: that sick notes and the sickness welfare system in general was designed for British-born, able-bodied, regularly employed 'breadwinners'.[7]

Digging through the archive to find the few mentions of sick notes in NAB policy is illuminating. Despite there being no such thing as a 'NAB sicknote', National Insurance Med 1s (or statements from doctors which functionally served the same purpose) were regularly processed by the NAB. Three types fall into this category.[8] First, claimants with medical conditions were exempt from the requirement that National Assistance would only be provided to claimants registered for work at the local Labour Exchange. Unemployed sick people, therefore, had to 'prove' that they were sick in the same way as employed sick people. Second, claimants that required a special diet were entitled to additional allowances. Although there was no direct equivalent in National Insurance, the standard and type of proof required was very similar to a traditional sick note. Third, NAB dealt with claimants who were not themselves sick but were the best person available to look after a family member who was. These were often referred to as 'housekeeper' cases.[9] After successful campaigns by poverty lobby organizations in the 1960s and 1970s, several non-contributory benefits (i.e., benefits payable regardless of National Insurance status) were also made available outside of National Assistance and required similar 'sick note' evidence.[10] The difficulty here was that the sick note was not technically for the claimant—it was for the person being cared for. Issues around confidentiality abounded, as did the question of whether a doctor should be writing sick notes for someone other than the claimant (especially if the cared-for person was not on that doctor's list). A combination of these cases will recur throughout this section and the rest of the chapter.

---

[7] On 'breadwinners' see below and Lewis, 'Gender and the Development of Welfare Regimes'.

[8] As noted in the NAB's first annual report. However, one group will not be discussed. Certificates required for the 'special' rate of National Assistance provided for 'blind' and 'tuberculous' claimants were more akin to medical reports than National Insurance sick notes. National Assistance Board, *Report of the National Assistance Board for the Year Ended 31st December 1948 (Cmd. 7767)* (London: HMSO, August 1949), p. 11.

[9] The National Archives (hereafter TNA): AST 7/1494, T. E. Nodder to A. G. Beard, 22 October 1959; A. G. Beard, internal NAB memorandum, 16 June 1960.

[10] Hampton, *Disability and the Welfare State in Britain*; Gareth Millward, 'Social security policy and the early disability movement – expertise, disability and the government, 1965–1977', *Twentieth Century British History* 26, no. 2 (2015): pp. 274–97.

In September 1956, the NAB Controller in Scotland wrote to headquarters in London with a problem. Since 1948, a woman had looked after her elderly father. She wanted an additional payment for a special diet because she had been ill following 'the after-effects of an attack of coronary thrombosis'. A local Councillor had correctly advised her that this was common practice. However, her doctor disagreed that her symptoms required a change of diet. When asked by the NAB to provide a report, he refused, arguing that NAB reports did not come under the provisions required of NHS doctors. When the local NAB queried this with the Scottish Office, it found that the doctor was completely correct. NAB wrote to the Ministry of Health to discuss the possibility of including their requirements in the NHS regulations in summer 1956 but was told this was unlikely to happen because of the 1949 Safford Report.[11]

NAB had never heard of it. When Safford was being assembled, nobody had thought to include NAB or ask for its recommendations despite the lengthy evidence requested from, and supplied by, the Ministry of National Insurance and 26 other departments.[12] This was typical of the ad hoc way in which NAB's regulations were formed. As another example, local offices could sometimes require a medical report on the suitability of a claimant to undertake occupational rehabilitation. The agreed fee paid to GPs was 10s 6d [£0.525]. How had this figure been found?

> It is not clear .... As far as Mr. Jackson [a civil servant] can recollect, there was no analogy in mind in 1951: and the papers only show that Dr. Gould [a BMA representative] thought that the examination would be much less searching of than that of, say, a fireman, for which the fee then was 25s [£1.25].[13]

Although infrequent, further irregularities continued to arrive at headquarters through the 1950s. A sick widow in Newcastle had applied for an additional payment. Although she worked infrequently and received Widows' Pension, she did not have enough contributions for National Insurance sickness benefit. Her doctor provided a note, but charged her 1s 6d [£0.075], which she then attempted to claim back from National Assistance. The local Board eventually convinced the doctor not to charge in the future, but the case suggested that such incidents were becoming more common.[14] An enquiry into selected regional offices further

---

[11] TNA: AST 7/1494, H. M. Roffey [Ministry of Health] to F. M. Collins [NAB], 30 June 1956. For more on the report, see Chapter 2.

[12] TNA: PIN 7/368, Ministry of Health and Department of Health for Scotland, 'Report of the Inter-Departmental Committee on Medical Certificates', 1949.

[13] TNA: AST 7/1494, Medical Arrangements made by the Board outside the National Health Service, late 1959.

[14] TNA AST 7/1494, Regional Controller, Northern to Headquarters, 19 December 1957; W. Peel [Area Officer, Newcastle (North) to Regional Controller, Northern, 10 January 1958. Fees usually ranged from one to two shillings [£0.05–£0.10].

revealed doctors had charged: 'a married man who stated he was obliged to stay off work on account of his wife's illness, as he was unable to arrange for anyone to care for his four children'; 'a single woman without title to Sickness Benefit, who stated she had given up her employment on her Doctor's orders'; 'a single woman who claimed she was required at home full time to care for her sick and aged parents';[15] 'a need for the full time services of a daughter';[16] a woman with 'neurosis' whose sickness benefit had been rejected and needed NAB while her appeal went through;[17] and a husband needing 'to look after wife confined'.[18]

Given that financial hardship was a precondition of applying for National Assistance, these cases posed a problem for the NAB, claimants, and doctors.[19] The BMA noted:

> The difficulty at present arises in that the doctors are reluctant to charge persons known to be on national assistance for obvious reasons. Nevertheless, we have received many complaints…from doctors who feel that they should not be expected to supply such certificates as a charitable donation.[20]

Though NAB acknowledged that 'people on assistance are very rarely charged', the volume of claims and the acute financial needs of its claimants meant this was a hole in the regulations that had to be patched.[21] The Ministry of Health supported NAB on the basis that, had they been considered by Safford, the basic sick notes for inability to work and special diet would have been approved as essentially the same as those provided though National Insurance.[22] The simplest bureaucratic procedure was not to make a 'NAB sick note' but to officially allow Med 1s and Med 2s to be used for NAB purposes (the de facto position in many cases).[23] Still, in keeping with what now appeared to be a NAB tradition, the Board and the Ministry of Health chose to keep the ad hoc arrangements for 'housekeeper' cases believing that drawing more attention to the problem was more hassle than letting the matter go unnoticed.[24]

---

[15] All these cases from week commencing 23 November 1959. List is not exhaustive. TNA: AST 7/1494, Area Officer, Carlisle to Headquarters, 30 November 1959.

[16] TNA: AST 7/1494, Area Officer, Grimsby to Headquarters, 1 December 1959.

[17] TNA: AST 7/1494, Area Officer, London (North) to Headquarters, 2 December 1959.

[18] TNA: AST 7/1494, Area Officer, Nottingham (East) to Headquarters, 30 November 1959.

[19] TNA: AST 7/1494, Walter Hedgcock [Assistant Secretary, BMA] to The Secretary of NAB, 11 February 1957; Hedgcock to Secretary, 20 May 1957.

[20] TNA: AST 7/1494, J. D. J. Harvard [Assistant Secretary, BMA] to A. G. Beard, 11 June 1959.

[21] TNA: AST 7/1494, A. G. Beard to H. M. Roffey [Ministry of Health], 3 July 1959.

[22] TNA: AST 7/1494, T. E. Nodder to A. G. Beard, 3 September 1959.

[23] A short note from a doctor would be enough for a special diet. The National Assistance Act was also added explicitly to the regulations. See: TNA: AST 7/1494, Fifth Schedule to the General Medical Service Regulations, 1956. On decision to allow National Insurance sick notes to be sued see: ibid., T. E. Nodder to A. G. Beard, 3 September 1959; A. G. Beard to T. E. Nodder, 9 October 1959; TNA: AST 7/1494, A. G. Beard, internal NAB memorandum, 16 June 1960.

[24] TNA: AST 7/1494, T. E. Nodder to A. G. Beard, 14 October 1960. Technically, the note would be free if the claimant and cared-for person had the same GP, but a doctor could charge if the two were

In some ways, flexibility in policy was a strength. The same room for manoeuvre in regulations that allowed doctors to charge for medical certificates also allowed NAB officers to make discretionary decisions about the acute and chronic needs of the cases that came before them.[25] Once again, the sick note could adapt to circumstances and survive changes in the welfare state's operation. However, there was a difference between flexibility and a lack of specificity born of neglect. The National Assistance Act received Royal Assent less than two months before the Appointed Day, with regulations on how to determine eligibility coming two weeks after the Act. This gave the Board little time to implement everything, and such 'muddling through' continued.[26] Internal contradictions in policy and in practice led to NAB's restructure as the Supplementary Benefits Commission in 1966.[27] Significant, too, was the willingness of the Ministry of National Insurance, NAB, Ministry of Health, and BMA to support the 'muddling'. It showed that National Assistance claimants could be seen as part of the 'deserving poor' and worthy of, as the BMA assistant secretary put it in his 1959 letter, 'a charitable donation'[28]—but certain cases could slip through the cracks of a system dependent upon good will rather than concrete regulation. The poorest were not a priority.

It is those 'cracks' to which the chapter will now turn. Fringe cases expose the nuances of sickness policy, while the wider context of their existence shows how the prejudices of designers were baked into the design and operation of the welfare state. If the needs of the most disadvantaged and most at risk of poverty were an afterthought, then the same was also true of those who did not fit 'breadwinner' and 'chauvinist' models. As Mike Savage, Florence Sutcliffe-Braithwaite, and others have shown, Britain had a 'pervasive discourse of "ordinariness"', particularly around class.[29] So, how did the welfare state deal with groups who were decidedly not 'ordinary'?

---

registered with different practices. NAB believed this would happen very rarely, and since doctors had fully agreed with the principle of writing NAB sick notes it was best not to create more confusion. See also: TNA: AST 36/348, S. Muldoon to E. O. F. Stocker, 23 February 1970; TNA: AST 36/349, Supplementary Benefits Commission Headquarters to Regional Office, London (North), 23 September 1976.

[25] M. Kelly, 'Theories of Justice and Street-Level Discretion', *Journal of Public Administration Research and Theory: J-PART* 4, no. 2 (1994): pp. 119–40.

[26] Cmd. 7767.

[27] David Vernon Donnison, *The Politics of Poverty* (Oxford: Robertson, 1982); Carol Walker, *Managing Poverty: The Limits of Social Assistance* (London: Routledge, 1993); Rodney Lowe, *The Welfare State in Britain since 1945* (Basingstoke: Palgrave Macmillan, 2005).

[28] TNA: AST 7/1494, Harvard to Beard, 11 June 1959.

[29] Florence Sutcliffe-Braithwaite, *Class, Politics, and the Decline of Deference in England, 1968–2000* (Oxford: Oxford University Press, 2018), p. 5. See also: John Lawrence, 'Class, "affluence" and the study of everyday life in Britain, c. 1930–64', *Cultural and Social History* 10, no. 2 (2013): pp. 273–99; Mike Savage, 'Working-class identities in the 1960s: Revisiting the affluent worker study', *Sociology* 39, no. 5 (2005): pp. 929–46; Claire Langhamer, ' "Who the hell are ordinary people?" Ordinariness as a category of his historical analysis', *Transactions of the Royal Historical Society* 28 (2018): pp. 175–95.

Migration

Non-UK born migrants were one such group who were not considered 'ordinary'. Resistance to outsiders was reflected in the design of the postwar welfare state as well as in the discriminatory way in which rules were applied by politicians and street-level bureaucrats. As David Feldman shows, one cannot understand resistance to migrants' use of National Assistance without considering older stances towards attitudes to poor people migrating within the British Isles. Rate payers resented 'outsiders' drawing on local funds, often 'deporting' them back to their parish of origin.[30] This 'nativism' has been noted in welfare systems across Europe and North America, but 1948 highlighted the *national* aspects of the welfare system.[31] These tensions became more acute, especially from conservative critics, as the volume of incomers rose from the late 1940s.[32] Anybody from the Commonwealth was considered a British citizen, and therefore entitled to enter and settle in Britain and use the newly established welfare state. These rights were restricted after successive immigration acts from the 1960s onwards, including the Commonwealth Immigration Acts of 1962 and 1968.[33]

While this section examines a bureaucratic understanding and management of a group labelled 'immigrants', this focus obviously cannot be separated from the contemporary history of race and racism in Britain. Criticisms of welfare spending and eligibility for people not born in Britain were imbued with racist language and attitudes, while the regulations around sickness benefits and other forms of welfare also perpetuated structural discrimination. Even when migrant groups could be coded as 'white', it is important to consider Satnam Virdee's work which has shown how Jewish and Irish 'outsiders' were consistently racialized and othered using many of the same tropes applied to non-white people.[34] At the same time, the material circumstances that drove new arrivals to claim their entitlements to support were not necessarily identical to those of the many settled diasporic communities in Britain by the end of the Second World War.[35] Moreover, recent work on 'welfare chauvinism' in twenty-first-century Europe has drawn attention to the fact that while there are clear overlaps with racism and racist attitudes, the focus on 'citizenship' is present in otherwise-progressive-

---

[30] David Feldman, 'Migrants, immigrants and welfare from the Old Poor Law to the welfare state', *Transactions of the Royal Historical Society* 13 (2003): pp. 79–104.

[31] Hans-Georg Betz, 'Facets of nativism: a heuristic exploration', *Patterns of Prejudice* 53, no. 2 (2019): pp. 111–35.

[32] On the way these issues intersected with sick notes in the 'public sector', see Chapter 3.

[33] Nick Kimber, 'Race and equality', in *Unequal Britain: Equalities in Britain since 1945*, edited by Pat Thane (Oxford: Oxford University Press, 2010), pp. 29–51.

[34] Satnam Virdee, *Racism, Class and the Racialized Outsider* (Basingstoke: Palgrave Macmillan, 2014).

[35] Notably, but not limited to, the many diasporic communities in port cities such as Cardiff and Liverpool, or the refugee communities of French Huguenots and Eastern European Jews. See: Kimber, 'Race and equality'.

leaning individuals and organizations.[36] The following should not, therefore, be read as a comprehensive analysis of 'race'. Rather, it is an analysis (using select cases) of how the welfare state managed a bureaucratic category of 'immigrant' within its social security departments and how this interacted with wider cultural attitudes towards people coded as immigrants.

Bias against non-UK born migrants was based in cultural attitudes rather than empirical evidence. Even though 'coloured' immigrants claimed 55 per cent less from the NAB than the nationwide average, the perception of increased demands from Commonwealth citizens forced social security authorities to consider the issue of immigration from the earliest days of the new system.[37] New arrivals were more likely to need accommodation and support while they sought work; and, in poorer communities, were more likely to lose their jobs before building entitlements to National Insurance benefits. Discrimination in hiring and firing practices from employers and trades unions dominated by white men compounded this.[38] The public debate was framed by xenophobic concerns spread by the press and conservative critics of immigration and poverty-relief. For example, an article in the *Daily Mail* in 1949 described Britain as a 'fairyland' for one Nigerian convicted of assault in Liverpool, lamenting the fact that (even though he arrived as a stowaway) he was a British subject, 'could not be sent home' and was 'entitled to national assistance while out of work.'[39] As *The Times* noted in 1968, myths became established around immigrants' personal hygiene, rates of tuberculosis, and effects on house prices.[40] Thus, a key, lasting prejudice was that people came to Britain primarily to claim benefits.

These attitudes are reflected in the NAB's archive. 'As far as I know the majority of them are penniless and are kept until they find work at the expense of the British tax payer', wrote one man from Leeds in 1954. 'It seems strange that Winston Churchill says that England is overpopulated and that it is a good thing for Englishmen to emigrate to the Dominions and yet their places are being filled with Negroes.'[41] Instead, argued a Londoner, the money spent on 'Africans and West Indians etc.' should be used to increase the old age pension. 'It is about time the British tax payer thought about keeping his own breed—not everyone elses

---

[36] Andersen and Bjørklund, 'Structural change and new cleavages'; Waal, Koster, and Oorschot, 'Three worlds of welfare chauvinism?'

[37] Jack Halpern, 'The facts on coloured immigrants', *The Times*, 28 April 1968, p. 6.

[38] Virdee, *Racism, Class and the Racialized Outsider*. See also testimony from migrants, such as: Nisar Ahmad, 'Disintegration...', letter to *The Sunday Times*, 7 May 1967, p. 12; Jerry Okoro, 'Coloured jobless blame prejudice', *The Times*, 21 February 1972, p. 4.

[39] 'Moma finds fairyland', *Daily Mail*, 9 November 1949, p. 5.

[40] Brian Priestley, 'Race myths keep colour issue smouldering', *The Times*, 16 April 1968, p. 6. See also: 'Fake! Race-hate letter is trick to win election says candidate', *Daily Mail*, 10 May 1962, p. 11; '190,000 coloured people in Britain', *The Times*, 8 May 1958, p. 7; 'Renewed call for changes in immigration law', *The Times*, 28 August 1958, p. 4.

[41] TNA: AST 7/1211, [HAC] to Osbert Peake MP, 27 April 1954. The letters in these paragraphs are not exhaustive. TNA: AST 7/1211 contains letters of a similar tone from 1949 to 1961.

[sic]. All this nonsense about the coloureds being British subjects—trash!'[42] These letters showed racist attitudes towards Commonwealth immigrants could be expressed in relation to 'National' Insurance and Assistance. The welfare state was, in these terms, established for Britain to redistribute risk and resources amongst Britons, which required a definition of who was—and was not—British.[43] In the main, this form of xenophobia focused on unemployment and the idea that immigrants came to Britain intending to be economically inactive, or that the social security system encouraged 'too much' immigration before immigrants could be gainfully employed. Some focused on the groups of Britons who did not qualify for support. For example, the man from London argued 'I am a disabled ex-serviceman from the 1939-45 war and I'm not eligible for assistance so I can't see how a fit but lazy n——who prefers not to work can be.'[44]

'Fit but lazy' was key. In searching the archive for sickness-related welfare and migration, attention quickly turns to unemployment. In part this was because sickness-related payments from the NAB offered no substantial increase to what could be claimed as an unemployed person.[45] A crude pilot survey was conducted in 1968 on Supplementary Benefit offices in Bradford and Birmingham regarding the number of 'coloured' claimants. The generalizability of the results was limited, in part because of the small sample size but also because offices did not differentiate their claims by race or country of origin. Still, the DHSS accepted them as accurate enough to get a rough idea of what was going on. The report suggested that the amount of 'coloured' sick claimants was comparable to the number of 'coloured' unemployed claimants. More tellingly, however, these claims were on average much shorter than by the population as a whole. Most white claimants had been receiving money for over a year from Supplementary Benefit, while 'coloured' claims were much more likely to be under three months.[46]

In fact, sick immigrants could literally be removed.[47] While infrequent, NAB could provide funds to secure return passage for sick immigrants for whom it was unlikely they would ever find work. In a press briefing, the Minister of Social Security Judith Hart presented some case histories of people who had applied for

[42] TNA: AST 7/1211, [GR] to NAB, 21 April 1954. Some formatting added. The original letter was handwritten in all capitals.

[43] Virdee, *Racism, Class and the Racialized Outsider*; Kimber, 'Race and equality'. Note, too, the difference between the *National* Assistance Board and the old Poor Law regime administered at the level of local authorities. Clifford Williamson, ' "To remove the stigma of the Poor Law": The "comprehensive" ideal and patient access to the municipal hospital service in the city of Glasgow, 1918–1939', *History* 99, no. 334 (2014): pp. 73–99; Feldman, 'Migrants'.

[44] Censoring mine. TNA: AST 7/1211, [GR] to NAB, 21 July 1954. Follow up letter to previous. Some formatting added. The original letter was handwritten in all capitals.

[45] Except for blindness and tuberculosis. Some discretionary grants might have been available, but these did not appear to concern nativists correspondents to the NAB.

[46] TNA: BN 72/1, Supplementary Benefits—Coloured Claimants, attached to memorandum 18 March 1969.

[47] On other health and port controls, see: Roberta E. Bivins, *Contagious Communities: Medicine, Migration, and the NHS in Post-War Britain* (Oxford: Oxford University Press, 2015).

grants to be repatriated. Of the five examples, three had their passage paid. Of those, two received grants because they had sick notes that showed they had developed mental health conditions and wished to return home.[48] In another case, a widow and her two sons were repatriated to Mauritius because she and the children were diagnosed with schizophrenia. The local office appeared indignant that, despite buying her luggage, packing it, and arranging her trains, she still complained that they had 'omit[ted] to pack the family collection of gramophone records'.[49]

Instead of malingerers, then, the focus remained on the 'workshy black men'[50] who used National Assistance, an attitude reflected by staff within the welfare system. Such attitudes, however, are crucial to understanding why controversies around sickness benefits and migrants focused on the migrants themselves rather than sick notes or potential failures in the system. The discretion allowed to street-level bureaucrats, which was a potential strength in tailoring the social security system's response to acute need, also gave room for the prejudices in society to be magnified and barriers to be put in place.[51] In public, the NAB (and its replacement from 1966, the Supplementary Benefits Commission (SBC)) presented an air of tolerance. Indeed:

> Individual officers say they have little idea of the proportion of coloured applicants who come to the counter. But they do notice one thing: large numbers of white people refused assistance mutter something along the lines of: 'The blacks are getting it – why can't I?' Similarly, many black men refused complain: 'I'd get it if I was white.'[52]

When the SBC dug below the surface, however, it was not difficult to see that prejudices were replicated in the staff drawn from British society. With tensions stoked by Enoch Powell's 'Rivers of Blood' speech in April 1968, Secretary of State Richard Crossman asked the social security side of the DHSS to investigate how its offices handled cases involving 'coloured immigrants'.[53] The reports make for grim reading.[54] Consistently, SBC staff repeated similar stereotypes. People from

[48]   TNA: BN 72/1, Ministry of Social Security press briefing, 4 May 1968.
[49]   TNA: BN 72/1, 'Illustrative accounts of repatriation', 2 May 1968.
[50]   'The last hand-out', *Sunday Times*, 7 August 1966, p. 9.
[51]   Michael Lipsky, *Street-Level Bureaucracy: Dilemmas of the Individual in Public Services* (New York: Russell Sage Foundation, 1980); Kelly, 'Theories of justice'; Nissim Cohen, 'How culture affects street-level bureaucrats' bending the rules in the context of informal payments for health care: The Israeli case', *The American Review of Public Administration* 48, no. 2 (2018): pp. 175–87.
[52]   'The last hand-out'.
[53]   TNA: BN 72/1, Richard Crossman to Judith Hart, 15 May 1968.
[54]   The following comes from various reports filed in TNA: PIN 37/13. Most undated, but from around May to June 1968.

West Indian backgrounds were described as hard-working, but prone to cohabit-ing with their sexual partners and not declaring it.[55] People from South Asian backgrounds were also considered hard-working, but were regularly accused of 'hiding' information about their property or jewellery, thus appearing to have fewer assets for the means test. Where there was a question of irregularities, this was often not attributed to deliberate fraud but misunderstanding of the rules.[56] The relative 'praise' given to groups for their willingness to find employment, however, changed according to how familiar offices were with the groups they had pigeonholed. West Indians were, according to the Bradford West office, too ready to give up work for 'unacceptable reasons'.[57] Here and in Leeds, where similar atti-tudes were expressed, South Asian immigration was more common. In Brixton, where the reverse was true, West Indians were commended for their willingness to find and maintain work.[58] The office in Smethwick—which by its manager's own admission had been the focus of immigration-related attention after the infamous Smethwick parliamentary election campaign in 1964—noted that it had relatively few problems in its offices, primarily because staff had years of experi-ence of dealing with now-settled communities.[59]

Staff resented having to talk to claimants where English was not their first lan-guage, arguing that it was impossible to know if the family member or friend of the claimant was properly conveying 'the true facts' of the case.[60] Some were described as 'devious and sinister',[61] others accused of criminal activity (despite acknowledgement from investigators that the evidence from the case files did not back these stories up).[62] Meanwhile, outright hostility could be extended to fellow SBC workers. In Leeds, two officers refused to play in an intra-office bowls com-petition because 'coloured' staff would be taking part.[63] The staff there also argued that they did not want 'a coloured person as a colleague', believing that white claimants would refuse to be seen, potentially leading to violence.[64] Attitudes in headquarters could be just as bleak. Parts of the DHSS resisted providing leaflets

---

[55] Accusations of 'promiscuity' were also common. See esp.: TNA: PIN 37/13, Visit to Leeds North Area Office.
[56] A good example is the description of cohabitation: TNA: AST 37/13, Visit to Derby South Area Office. These stereotypes were repeated in DHSS evidence submitted to the Fisher Report: TNA: BN 60/32.
[57] TNA: AST 37/13, Visit to Bradford West Area Office. See also ibid., Leeds North Area Office.
[58] TNA: AST 37/13, Visit to Brixton Area Office.
[59] TNA: AST 37/13, Visit to Smethwick Area Office. A similar report comes in ibid., Visit to Moss Side Area Office.
[60] TNA: AST 37/13, Visit to Bristol Central Area Office.   [61] Ibid.
[62] TNA: PIN 37/13, Visit to Leeds North Area Office.   [63] Ibid.
[64] Ibid. In Bradford, it was felt younger staff would be OK with it, but that white claimants could still pose a problem. TNA: PIN 37/13, The Immigrant in Bradford. In Brixton, Irish claimants were thought to be particularly hostile to 'coloured staff'. Ibid., Visit to Brixton Area Office.

in other languages—with the 'embarrassing exception' of Welsh—although this opposition was quickly lifted.[65]

There were signs of resistance to this racism in the SBC accounts, but it appeared so rarely that it was worthy of special reference in a report from Brixton. A woman had threatened to report management to headquarters if they enacted a local policy to limit the amount of rent allowance given to 'coloured single men'.[66] Perhaps more striking were attitudes that, while attempting to be progressive, reinforced notions of 'the good immigrant' and welfare chauvinism about expected behaviours from outsiders.[67] An officer from the Wandsworth Council for Community Relations exposed such class and racial prejudices about the growing numbers of Asian immigrants from Kenya. These people were 'most valuable' because they were 'able, intelligent and often highly cultured'. 'Kenyan Asians' had the power to overcome prejudice, according to the officer. 'One air hostess heard we were handing out national assistance to these people as they stepped into the airport. She stormed off the plane to complain, but quickly found there was nothing to complain about.'[68]

This is vital context to understanding the wider chauvinist concerns about welfare 'abuse' in the 1960s and 1970s. These reached a head in 1972 when the Fisher Report was commissioned by the Conservative Heath government to investigate social security fraud.[69] It did not find systematic abuse from claimants coming to Britain from elsewhere in the world, even though it had specifically investigated the matter due to the widespread belief that this was so.[70] The Commission worried about the increased number of short-term claims, but blame was placed upon 'younger claimants' without reference to ethnicity.[71] It found even fewer irregularities with sick notes. Fisher and the DHSS stressed the need to continue certification while being mindful about opposition from doctors and demands from the BMA for sick note reforms.[72] The only 'myth' for which it was able to find any evidence concerned Irish claimants in the construction industry, where a

[65] One civil servant argued Irish and Asian languages were not precise or concise enough to explain social security regulations clearly. TNA: PIN 35/413, H. S. McPherson, 'Fisher and the Tower of Babel', 28 December 1972.

[66] TNA: AST 37/13, Visit to Brixton Area Office.

[67] Madeline Yuan-yin Hsu, The Good Immigrants: How the Yellow Peril Became the Model Minority (Princeton: Princeton University Press, 2017). See also Nikesh Shukla (ed.), The Good Immigrant (London: Unbound, 2016).

[68] Ronald Faux, 'Reality and ideal in immigration colour question', The Times, 2 March 1968, p. 8.

[69] Such views were echoed by MPs. See: 'Hush-up on fraud, MP says', The Times, 15 June 1970, p. 1. The Conservatives had pledged to 'take firm action to deal with abuse of the social security system' in their manifesto: Conservative Party, A Better Tomorrow (London: Conservative Party, 1970).

[70] Henry Fisher, Report of the Committee on Abuse of Social Security Benefits (Cmnd 5228) (London: HMSO, 1972), pp. 57–9.

[71] Ibid., pp. 229–30.

[72] For example, TNA: BN 60/25, L. Errington to Parliamentary Secretary (Social Security) and Secretary of State, 10 January 1973. For the specifics of how the BMA and DHSS negotiations preceded on this question, see Chapter 5.

minority were known to 'sign on' as unemployed or sick in one National Insurance office and then work in another town 'cash in hand'. In doing so, the worker could claim benefit on top of their wages, and his or her National Insurance contributions would continue to accrue.[73] This was framed as an Irish problem, despite clear evidence that British workers could pull this trick too. In Middlesbrough in May 1971, eight men were convicted of working while claiming by pretending to be sick and then working shifts at a nearby refinery that was paying higher wages.[74]

Irish claimants did, however, present a specific bureaucratic headache for National Insurance authorities. These issues were well known to officers, particularly in Northern Ireland, but were difficult to police. Irish citizens had the right to work and draw benefit in the United Kingdom, and there were full reciprocal arrangements for social security between the two nations.[75] Crossing the land border into Northern Ireland or catching ferries to Great Britain was relatively easy, meaning that permanent immigration as well as seasonal working or commuting were common behaviours, particularly in times of high unemployment in the Republic of Ireland. There was some concern that this problem would increase after the United Kingdom joined the European Economic Community.[76] Nevertheless, fears of abuse were based largely on the 'feeling' of National Insurance offices in Northern Ireland and charities in the UK rather than hard data.[77] It is difficult not to see these attitudes outside the context of long-term prejudices against Irish workers and poor Irish citizens on the mainland. Certain British communities had long resented migration from Ireland, which was associated with driving down wages and reducing the quality of the areas of cities in which they lived.[78] Given that Fisher argued no special measures were required other than general tightening of regulations to prevent abuse from all communities, singling out Irish 'outsiders' was administratively unnecessary—yet public and voluntary sector organizations felt the need to do so.

Even when sickness could be tied directly to an issue involving the movement of people to and from Britain and the Commonwealth, authorities' conclusions focused on how to police migrant flows. This is best exemplified in a remarkable account of an organized crime group led by an Indian man. This story is worth repeating in full—and not just because it is a salacious account that exposed the limits of the Ministry's gatekeeping procedures. It shows that sick notes were never neutral arbiters of medical fact. Moreover, once an issue could be coded as

---

[73] *Cmnd 5228*, p. 58. On the problems of short-term claims in general, see Chapter 5.

[74] TNA: PIN 35/390, Press cutting, *Middlesbrough Evening Gazette*, 19 May 1971.

[75] This was for historical reasons going back to the pre-war National Insurance system and the transition to the Irish Free State. For examples of how this agreement affected sickness claims in the 1960s, see the file: TNA: PIN 57/26.

[76] *Cmnd 5228*, p. 59.

[77] TNA: BN 60/32, 'Note of a meeting on 16 April 1973, The Fisher Report and the Irish'; ibid., E. T. Randall, Meeting with the Secretary of State, 12 April 1973.

[78] Virdee, *Racism, Class and the Racialized Outsider*; Feldman, 'Migrants'.

an 'immigrant problem', questions about real or feigned illness became less pressing than those about how to administer, survey and discipline people who had
not been born in Britain.

Ranjit Singh—alias Santokh Singh Sihota—was the only man convicted of a
series of frauds perpetrated between 1963 and 1965. In total, he was charged with
obtaining £5,197 8s [£5,197.40], around £2,500 of which concerned sickness
benefit. The precise details of how he operated are sketchy. Singh gave conflicting
reports about his accomplices, often providing the names of men who lived in
India and were difficult to trace. Authorities were convinced that he could not
have acted alone but could not secure evidence that would have allowed further
convictions. The investigation was not aided by the fact that many of the witnesses 'were most reluctant to give any information' because they were convinced
that Singh or his 'friends' would murder them.[79] As one civil servant put it: 'quite
powerful forces are ranged against us'.[80]

The sickness benefit frauds all followed a similar pattern.[81] Singh entered a
National Insurance office armed with the names and National Insurance numbers
of men who had worked in Britain but had returned to India. Combined with a
fake sick note, he would claim sickness benefit on their behalf, having the payments sent to various properties where he knew they would not be intercepted. In
the end, the police were able to tie him to crimes around Luton, Kettering,
Huddersfield, Leicester, Birmingham, and Coventry.

The early sick notes appear to have been for genuine illnesses filled for the
wrong person. Reports from Huddersfield suggested that the group had found
members of the Indian diaspora with back trouble or other conditions, persuad-
ing them to get signed notes from their doctors. The gang would take the note
and ensure the details matched the National Insurance numbers and names of the
individuals they knew had returned to India. However, at some point around
early 1965 a pad of blank sick notes was stolen. Authorities believed that the
group was able to copy the pad and forge a new set with a different doctor's
stamp—giving the fraudsters unlimited access to genuine-looking counterfeits
that could barely be spotted on close inspection. It was only in October 1965
when a clerk in Smethwick noticed that the stamp on one form looked like it had
been altered that the authorities discovered the modus operandi, two years after
the first frauds had been committed.

---

[79] The case from the Ministry's perspective is recounted in TNA: PIN 42/62, especially: Inspector
SIS, Midlands Regional Office, 'Police investigation of fraudulent Indian sickness benefit claims', 28
January 1966.

[80] TNA: PIN 42/62, I. J. Bayliss to R. W. C. Cocksedge, 13 December 1965.

[81] The local Black Country and Birmingham press covered this in some detail. Press cuttings in
TNA: PIN 42/62 include: 'Fictitious names given as cover up', Birmingham Evening Mail, 29 December
1965; 'Sent for trial on £2,850 fraud charges', Birmingham Post, 30 December 1965; 'Wholesale frauds
on Ministry story', Smethwick Telephone and Warley Courier, 23 December 1965; 'Ministry fraud net-
ted £2,584 – police', Express & Star, 20 December 1965. The 'gang' also obtained goods on hire purchase with fake credentials, stole Post Office orders and committed unemployment benefit fraud.

Singh told the police that a gentleman called the 'Doctor' had masterminded the plan, sending the forms from a secret counterfeit press based in India via a Birmingham travel agent. The police were never able to substantiate the claims, but Singh did have impressive knowledge of how GPs wrote sick notes and how the National Insurance offices processed them. Claims were never made for longer than a month, which would have triggered follow-up investigations. In the Huddersfield cases, Singh got 'Final' certificates from doctors fairly easily as the note was only needed to show that the claimant was fit for work and GPs rarely bothered to check the patient's identity. The authorities believed that Singh's wife might have been a doctor at one time, which would explain this level of expertise.

After Smethwick detected the forgeries, the net began to close in. More counterfeits appeared in Handsworth, and a man matching Singh's description was also seen in Ladywood.[82] Staff in neighbouring West Bromwich had considered Singh suspicious months earlier in May. They tried to keep Singh distracted and telephoned Birmingham CID. However, West Bromwich was in Staffordshire, outside their main jurisdiction, so they did not consider it a worthwhile drive. Singh got spooked and left before an arrest could be made.[83] It was not until November that another office was able to apprehend him. In Handsworth (conveniently in the same county as Birmingham), staff closed the post box on the side of the building, forcing all claimants to come to the desk. They waited for Singh to appear and, when he did, he was arrested. In searching his car, the police found a list of National Insurance numbers and addresses, a benefit envelope, forged medical certificates, and other forms. Somewhat ironically, there was also a *genuine* sick note for Singh himself. Police raided a house in Leicester which was legally in the name of one of Singh's associates but which they were able to show belonged to Singh, in part due to the testimony of the paper boy who delivered the *Daily Telegraph* there each morning. The house had been cleared of any evidence, but the legal owner gave enough false evidence at the trial that prosecutors were seriously considering charging him with perjury and suspected his wider involvement in the enterprise.

Singh's crimes were detected through the National Insurance system. They could not have existed through National Assistance because the means-testing and qualification criteria would not have allowed claims solely on the production of a sick note and a National Insurance number. It also required a level of expertise about how the system worked from the point of view of the claimant, National Insurance officers, and the GP. If any of the people associated with the National Insurance numbers returned to Britain and made a genuine claim, the disparity would alert the authorities immediately. One civil servant noted that 'Singh had a

[82] Smethwick, Handsworth, and Ladywood are all districts to the west of Birmingham city centre, no more than six kilometres from each other.
[83] TNA: PIN 42/62, Bayliss to Cocksedge. West Bromwich was in Staffordshire; Birmingham in Warwickshire.

good run for his money, but he had to go to great lengths to keep it up and [the custodial sentence] is likely to be discouraging for his associates. I hope we shall not be over nervous about the risk of repetition.'[84]

This explains, in part, why neither the government nor the general press used the incident to indict certain immigrant groups as malingerers or frauds. Indeed, none of the major national newspapers even ran the story. This remained a crime understood as specific, localized, and out of the ordinary. On the other hand, while the case looks exceptional, the operational documents expose many of the same attitudes towards immigration and social security exhibited elsewhere. The Ministry of Pensions and National Insurance scrambled to work out how its security had been breached so readily and what could be done to prevent it happening again. Some of their solutions were technical. The new 'Med 3' sick note forms due to enter circulation in 1966 offered a defence by printing part of the text in red ink, making them much more difficult to photocopy or forge.[85] Others, however, leaned on the same chauvinist tropes expressed elsewhere. On at least two occasions, the Ministry issued nationwide edicts to scrutinize all sickness-related claims coming from claimants with 'Indian or Pakistani' names. (Pakistanis were included because one of Singh's frauds used a Muslim name.) Some officials wanted further scrutiny for longer periods but were persuaded that this would disproportionately affect regions with higher levels of immigration and there simply was not the labour power to forensically analyse every claim.[86]

Still, when an Irish man was arrested in Bristol for stealing a pad of sick notes from a doctor in an outreach centre, the Ministry asked the police to question him about any possible involvement with Indian gangs. It was immediately evident that the man had long-standing mental health problems, a history of alcohol dependency, and had been in and out of NAB accommodation and prison for years. His only possible connection to wide-scale fraud was that one of his spells outside institutions was spent in the West Midlands while Singh's operation was active. It is difficult to consider any reason why the Ministry would have been suspicious other than his nationality. For example, they did not appear to be concerned that all Welsh men were potential fraudsters after a 37 year old man with a common English surname was convicted of stealing benefit postal drafts in Newport in December 1965.[87] Nor were pubgoers considered suspect when a Gravesend man claimed he had bought a pad of blank notes from a gentleman in his local hostelry in 1956.[88] Yet they were suspicious of a Pakistani boilerman

[84] TNA: PIN 42/62, T. C. Stephens, internal memorandum, 3 January 1966.

[85] TNA: PIN 42/62, Bayliss to Cocksedge. On the Med 3 and changes with previous forms, see Chapter 5.

[86] TNA: PIN 42/62, Mr Smith, Inspector SIS, Fradulent Claims to Sickness Benefit by Indians, 29 November 1965.

[87] TNA: PIN 42/62, newspaper cutting 'Newport man obtained cash wrongly', *South Wales Weekly Argus*, 23 December 1965.

[88] TNA: PIN 35/100, C. M. Regan [MPNI] to W. Turner [Ministry of Health], 5 June 1961.

who had acted as an interpreter in court and became interested in understanding the law around social security claims. Officials couched this in administrative terms, noting the difficulty of policing identity and post-Commonwealth Immigration Bill entitlements because 'Pakistanis never have birth certificates' or other documentation.[89] Nevertheless, it fed into wider suspicions about South Asians speaking in languages other than English as a way to 'hide' information and game the system. Even more bizarrely, one notices a much more aggressive attitude towards a confused Irish thief or an enthusiastic working-class Pakistani than towards a Derbyshire printing company which had been commissioned to produce medical certificates and used superfluous rolls of blank Med 3s as wrapping paper for their other deliveries.[90] This presented a much more obvious and easily exploited security breach than the complex operation involving counterfeit presses and clandestine packages routed through travel agents.

The Singh case and the others outlined here show that even when sick notes were part of the relationship between authorities and immigrant claimants, they were understood as a separate category. These were always 'outsiders' who did not fit the model of the 'ordinary' British-born worker entitled to support when sick by right. Instead, out-of-work immigrants, regardless of medical reasons, were suspicious because they were unemployed and not from 'this parish'.[91] Even when there was an outright attack on the sickness system, those involved were categorized differently to UK-born fraudsters.

Women

These cultural prejudices were integral to the welfare state's design and operation as processes of welfare chauvinism looked to exclude migrants. Yet, women were in a slightly different position. Prejudice had a material impact on whether women could access support—but it was never the intention that they be excluded entirely. Instead, a range of different qualification criteria and benefits existed to provide welfare in specific circumstances based on the claimant's relationship to her husband. Attempting to apply the same sick note logic to such benefits as the general National Insurance sickness benefit system for 'breadwinners', however, was fraught with difficulties. Tracing these anomalies through the archive not only exposes similar discriminatory processes as seen with migrants, it also shows

---

[89] TNA: PIN 42/62, E. Hoskins [High Wycombe National Insurance Office] to M. Thorns [London South Regional Office], 26 October 1965. Those who entered the country before the passing of the Commonwealth Immigration Act 1962 were treated as full citizens. As the late 2010s 'Windrush Scandal' shows, this was not always easy to prove. Wendy Williams, *Windrush Lessons Learned Review (HC 93 (2019–20))* (London: TSO, March 2020).

[90] Some of this wrapping paper, as well as details of the investigation, is stored in TNA: PIN 35/100. See also: ibid., Bemrose & Sons Ltd to Her Majesty's Stationery Office, 15 May 1967.

[91] Feldman, 'Migrants'.

that determining sickness was only one of many criteria imposed to determine moral and legal desert.

Britain's 'breadwinner' welfare state regime reflected majority public attitudes in the 1940s.[92] Documentary evidence, Mass Observation testimony and oral history research show that for many Britons the war had strengthened a desire to 'return' to 'traditional' gendered roles of the masculine 'breadwinner' and the feminine 'housewife', with these attitudes being more strongly expressed among the working classes.[93] As Stephen Brooke reminds us, the Beveridge Report itself 'was, in gender terms, an ode to the pre-war world'.[94] This structure had significant implications for both employment and social security. As more married women—and mothers—entered and remained in paid employment, these gender norms were challenged, increasing the visibility of gendered disputes in employment policy. Despite the growing importance of wives' earnings to household incomes, such wages continued to be understood as 'extras' in contrast to the 'meaningful' wage of the husband (regardless of its relative or absolute monetary value).[95] Even as women's paid employment became more common and 'socially acceptable', its status remained below men's paid work and women's domestic work in what Laura King calls the 'hierarchy of value' of labour.[96] But these challenges did not suddenly appear in the Women's Liberation movement of the 1960s.[97] Debates around the use of sick notes show that the increased presence and agency of women in paid work also meant more women claiming employment-related social security. When they did so, it became clear that the sickness system was inadequately set up to meet women's needs or moral entitlements.

Just as the bureaucratic category of 'immigrant' cannot be considered a comprehensive analogue of race, so too this section cannot consider 'women' as a corollary for 'gender'. A key example of this is the way *married* women were administratively separated from single women and men. Gender cannot be ignored, as the same patriarchal power structures that affected other groups of women help explain the specific ways in which married women were discriminated against. For instance, Pat Thane and Tanya Evans have detailed the problems

---

[92] Lewis, 'Gender and the development of welfare regimes'.

[93] Whether or not those ideals ever really existed is another matter. See: Stephen Brooke, 'Gender and working class identity in Britain during the 1950s', *Journal of Social History* 34, no. 4 (2001): pp. 773–95; Laura King, 'How men valued women's work: Labour in and outside the home in post-war Britain', *Contemporary European History* 28, no. 4 (2019): pp. 454–68; Susan L. Carruthers, '"Manning the factories": Propaganda and policy on the employment of women, 1939–1947', *History* 75, no. 244 (1990): pp. 232–56; Helen McCarthy, 'Women, marriage and paid work in post-war Britain', *Women's History Review* 26, no. 1 (2017): pp. 46–61.

[94] Brooke, 'Gender and working class identity', p. 777.

[95] Dolly Smith Wilson, 'A new look at the affluent worker: The good working mother in post-war Britain', *Twentieth Century British History* 17, no. 2 (2006): pp. 206–29.

[96] King, 'How men valued women's work'.

[97] King, 'How men valued women's work'; Helen McCarthy, 'Social science and married women's employment in post-war Britain', *Past & Present* 233, no. 1 (2016): pp. 269–305.

faced by single mothers within the welfare state, including the moral panics around their ability to parent, provide for their household and threat to 'family values'.[98] Yet, these debates did not explicitly revolve around sickness; rather, they played on other welfare state anxieties about unemployment, sexual morality, and the creation or maintenance of the 'underclass'.[99] With married women and sickness-related welfare, examples emerge from the archive of claimants, citizens, and authorities wrestling with how the family unit's lived experiences of paid and domestic work clashed with Beveridgean 'breadwinner' assumptions. Age, class, and race were confounding factors, as we have already seen and will continue to see in this book.

Women's position regarding sickness benefits in 1948 was complicated. Single women were entitled to the same rate as men (26s [£1.30] per week). However, the rate for married women was much lower (16s [£0.80] per week).[100] Married women automatically paid a lower rate of National Insurance contributions to compensate, in part, for lower benefit entitlements. The justification was that women would be mostly dependent upon their husband's income and, in old age, his pension. Despite this, a married woman could opt to pay the higher rate of National Insurance to secure a pension in her own right as well as a higher rate of maternity grant and a maternity benefit. Regardless of whether she paid the lower or higher rate of contributions, she was only entitled to the lower rate of sickness benefit. This was an ongoing debate in the first decades of the postwar welfare state. *The Times*, *Guardian*, and *Daily Mail* regularly published advice in their women's and finance sections on the pros and cons of paying the higher rate of National Insurance, often noting that this imperfect trade off was only possible if the household could afford to lose the extra chunk of the wife's pay packet.[101] The Labour Party spoke about equalization in parliament and campaign material from the mid-1960s, but, despite a campaigning research paper published towards the end of Harold Wilson's first period as Prime Minister, it was not until 1977 that all women entering employment, regardless of marriage status, paid the same rate—and received the same benefits—as men.[102] Even then, just as with the equalization in pension age in the 1990s, this was seen by some women's groups

[98] Pat Thane and Tanya Evans, *Sinners? Scroungers? Saints?: Unmarried Motherhood in Twentieth-Century England* (Oxford: Oxford University Press, 2012).

[99] John Welshman, *Underclass: A History of the Excluded, 1880–2000* (London: Hambledon Continuum, 2007).

[100] 'Benefits (statistics)', *House of Commons Official Report (Hansard)*, 9 March 1948, vol. 448, col. 128W.

[101] Examples include: Pauline Young, 'Women must pay', *The Times*, 2 December 1979, p. iv; Dryden Gilling-Smith, 'The five million wisest wives', *Daily Mail*, 30 December 1970, p. 16; Halldora Blair, 'A wife's choice: To pay or not to pay', *The Times*, 25 September 1971, p. 19; Dryden Gilling-Smith, 'Should a wife pay?', *Daily Mail*, 9 May 1973, p. 20; Joanna Slaughter, 'Women who pay in full', *Guardian*, 18 March 1979, p. 24.

[102] Labour Party, *Towards Equality: Women and Social Security* (London: Labour Party, 1969); Social Security Pensions Act 1975; 'Women's low-insurance option ends', *The Times*, 11 May 1977, p. 2.

as discriminatory. It increased the financial contributions of women workers but did not consider the health needs or the additional domestic duties that continued to be placed on women.[103] Breadwinner models, whether inadvertent or not, were thus internalized by authorities from a range of political traditions.[104]

Of course, to categorize in this way one must define marriage. This was not a trivial task, nor was the policing of a woman's relationship to her 'husband' confined to social security. Jordanna Bailkin has detailed how the British state had to wrestle with the legal and moral implications of polygamy and the imposition of Western family values on colonial law since at least the 1880s.[105] By the late 1940s, a woman's right to reside in the UK could depend upon her marital status; as could her entitlement to any war pensions or National Insurance contributions built by her husband during and after the war. Bailkin notes that approaches to polygamy or the legality of non-Christian, non-British marriages could be vastly different according to government department or even policies within each department. Her work on the social security system focuses primarily on widows' and old age pensions. However, sickness benefits expose these contradictions too.

The logic of the breadwinner model meant that exemptions had to be provided if the 'breadwinner' was not able to perform 'his' duties. Separated wives could therefore claim the higher rate of benefit if they could show that their husbands were not supporting them financially. One woman in 1954 had been found to have married twice—once in 1934 to 'Thomas' and again in 1952 to 'Harold'.[106] She claimed sickness benefit at the single women's rate in 1951 and 1952, but on marrying Harold declared a change in status and moved down to the married rate. When the authorities found that the marriage to Thomas was never dissolved, the question arose as to whether she should always have received the lower rate. As she could not get financial support from Thomas and because the marriage to Harold was void, she ended up qualifying for the single woman's rate even after 'marrying' Harold. The only question for National Insurance was whether Thomas—her legal husband—could support her. The issue of cohabitation, a major factor in National Assistance cases, never arose.[107] Indeed, even when women wanted to be paid at a lower rate in recognition of their relationship with their partner, National Insurance refused to do so. A woman in Coventry in 1951 had been living for years with a man and had changed her name to his, though they had never actually married. She wanted to be paid at the married rate, despite the loss of income, so that her employer would not find out that she

---

[103] Hugh Pemberton, 'WASPI's is (mostly) a campaign for inequality', *The Political Quarterly* 88, no. 3 (2017): pp. 510–16.

[104] Ben Jackson, 'Free markets and feminism: The neo-liberal defence of the male breadwinner model in Britain, c. 1980–1997', *Women's History Review* 28, no. 2 (2019): pp. 297–316.

[105] Jordanna Bailkin, *The Afterlife of Empire* (Berkeley: University of California Press, 2012).

[106] Names have been changed. Original report: TNA: PIN 35/92, H. Davis to R. S. Harris, 3 July 1954.

[107] Ibid.

was unmarried when her occupational sick pay scheme made up the difference between her sickness benefit and her regular wage.[108] Despite a request from her MP, the Ministry of National Insurance argued that it was illegal to 'underpay' her.[109]

For National Assistance claims, on the other hand, cohabitation and a woman's financial relationship with her partner were more pressing. Any support a married woman received from the husband, no matter how inconsistent, could put her income at risk.[110] Bizarrely, it was possible for a husband to support his wife without her knowledge, making her an unwitting recipient of overpayments. In 1951 in Birkenhead, the NAB attempted to recover £57 4s 4d [£57.217] from a woman who had received the single woman's rate of sickness benefit. Despite being separated from her husband since 1944 and having no contact with him, he had been paying the NAB £2 10s [£2.50] a week to cover some of the costs of her benefits. He instructed the Board not to tell the wife or any other authorities because he did not want her to know where he was living or anything about his financial circumstances. National Insurance paid her the married woman's rate because neither they nor she knew anything about it. It was only when the husband died that National Insurance were informed. Despite no attempt to deceive or any reasonable knowledge of what had happened, NAB recovered £13 from the wife and planned to extract more.[111]

Authorities had assumed that this scenario would be uncommon.[112] Only two other cases of this type were considered by headquarters' policy division in the NAB's first decade, one in Scotland in 1949 and another in England in 1954.[113] Still, given that there were an estimated 700,000 claims between 1948 and 1953 from married women applying for the single woman's rate, qualification criteria and the definition of 'financial support' were consistent issues with which NAB and National Insurance had to wrestle.[114] As family breakdown and divorce became more common and easier to apply for after the 1969 Divorce Reform Act, the boundaries between being a 'married' or a 'single' woman became more blurred.[115]

---

[108] On how occupational sick pay interacted with National Insurance entitlements see Chapters 2 and 5.

[109] TNA: PIN 35/23, D. H. Fulcher to Smith, 27 March 1951; Edith Summerskill to Elaine Burton MP, [n.d.] March 1951. The employer would have found out about the woman's living arrangements as many occupational sick pay schemes 'topped up' National Insurance benefits to cover an employee's regular wage. This system is explored in more detail in Chapter 5.

[110] TNA: PIN 35/91, Claim for Sickness Benefit, Decision of the Commissioner [C.S.6/61], 23 August 1961.

[111] TNA: PIN 35/91, Re: overpayment of sickness benefit to Mrs. [MN], 15 July 1958; N. Salisbury, Regional Controller, North Western to Headquarters, 24 June 1958; A. Gibbons, MPNI Report to Regional Office of Overpayments Exceeding £50, 17 June 1958; and surrounding documents.

[112] TNA: PIN 35/91, R. E. Higginson to R. M. Arnott, 3 August 1954.

[113] TNA: PIN 35/91, Claim for Sickness Benefit, Decision of the Commissioner, 20 December 1949; R. M. Arnott to R. E. Higginson, 18 August 1954.

[114] TNA: PIN 35/91, R. S. Harris to Waldron, [n.d.] May 1953.

[115] On the issues surrounding annulment, separation and divorce, see: TNA: PIN 35/135; National Insurance Advisory Committee, *Report of the National Insurance Advisory Committee on the Question of Contribution Conditions and Credit Provisions (Cmd. 9854)* (London: HMSO, 1956), p. 62; Fergus Morton, *Royal Commission on Marriage and Divorce (Cmd. 9678)* (London: HMSO, 1956).

If it was difficult to police the boundaries of 'marriage', greater complications came from the changing behaviour of 'married' women. Recent scholarly interest in the history of working women in Britain has illuminated the profound political and social implications of the increase in the number of married women in paid employment. Married women had worked before 1948—and not just in periods of total war when labour was scarce.[116] But from the late 1940s onwards, three compounding factors led to significant growth in the proportion of married women in paid work. First, the number of women entering employment increased generally. Second, women did not, as had been traditional, resign on getting married. Instead, they tended to remain in employment until they had their first child. And third, women had fewer children, younger, and in a shorter space of time. This meant that when women returned to work after their youngest had come of school age, they spent more time over the course of their lives in paid employment. Dolly Wilson has demonstrated that 42.6 per cent of all women were in work in 1971, as opposed to 34.7 percent and 34.2 per cent in 1951 and 1931 respectively. More significantly, 51.3 per cent of married women were in work in 1971, versus 21.7 per cent and 10 per cent in 1951 and 1931.[117] Another factor that made these statistical shifts possible was the greater availability of part-time work and shift patterns after the war, partially due to the needs of industry in postwar reconstruction and partially due to demand from women who wanted to, rather than solely felt the financial need to, work.[118] The labour shortage in the 1940s and 1950s could not be satisfied entirely by men or from new workers from the Commonwealth, leading the government to encourage married women with older children to take up these opportunities for paid employment.[119] All of this disrupted the assumptions of National Insurance. The system was built largely for the regularly full-time employed British man. The part-time worker whose insurance status could fluctuate according to her relationship with her 'breadwinner' created problems.

National Insurance offices early on appreciated that they would have to pay closer attention to diagnoses on sick notes such as 'climacteric', 'menorrhagia', 'abortion', and 'menopause'. Sick visiting was recommended for all claims after two, three, or four weeks (depending on the illness category); but for these gynae-cological diagnoses specific rules were put in place to deal with the sensitivity and potential need for specialist examination.[120] It is not clear in the memoranda whose modesty these rules were designed to protect: the claimant's or the investi-

---

[116] Carruthers, '"Manning the factories"'.

[117] Wilson, 'A new look at the affluent worker'.

[118] Ibid.; McCarthy, 'Women, marriage and paid work';Laura Paterson, '"I didn't feel like my own person": Paid work in women's narratives of self and working motherhood, 1950–1980', *Contemporary British History* 33, no. 3 (2019): pp. 405–26.

[119] Carruthers, '"Manning the factories"'.

[120] TNA: PIN 135/746, Ministry of National Insurance, Sickness and Injury Benefit, Control of Claims, April 1952.

gating officers'. Regardless, more women in work meant more claims, and not just because of the aggregate number of people in paid employment. As discussed in Chapter 3, the statistical returns showed that women were more likely than men to take sick leave and for longer periods, with married women more prone to sickness than single women.[121] The reasons for this were debated. Partly, it was argued, married women in paid employment were likely to be older, since they were more likely to be absent from work while they (and their children) were younger. Partly, it was acknowledged that their increased caring responsibilities for elderly relatives or children meant that they needed more time off that could either be classified as sickness (i.e. they were genuinely mildly ill, but had to choose between caring or paid work) or their double work load meant they were more likely to be run down.[122]

The social security archives show how these questions affected the development of policy from an early point, with medical certification a critical—if not the only—part of this process. Perhaps nowhere was this more obvious that around pregnancy and maternity. Maternity grant was a lump sum payable on the husband's insurance (at a lower rate) or on the wife's if she had full contributions (at a higher rate). Maternity benefit, paid weekly for the first 26 weeks after birth, was payable only to a woman with full contributions. This reflected the idea that taking time off to have children was the 'normal' state of being for a woman who would not be working anyway, and therefore would not affect the core income for the household. These benefits were paid according to the circumstances of the woman's 'confinement'.[123] Even if pregnancy was not considered a 'sickness' in itself, the medical implications of birth and recovery meant that women were considered incapable of paid work.

The definition of confinement created numerous grey areas even for those following the rules to the letter. As Bailkin notes with regard to polygamy, the definition of certain terms in law could vary according to the department writing them and the policy being enacted.[124] In the original 1948 National Insurance regulations, 'confinement' was 'labour resulting in the issue of a living child'.[125]

---

[121] In 1965, a Ministry briefing document for the minister outlined that men took 2.1 weeks off per year, versus 2.2 weeks for single women and 3.1 for married women. PIN 35/91, '"Women in industry". Minister's briefing', 4 May [1965]. See also discussions about rising absenteeism and demographic changes, including the feminization of the workforce in Chapter 3.

[122] Pemberton, 'WASPI's is (mostly) a campaign for inequality'.

[123] The certificates for this purpose were so functionally similar to sick notes that they were governed by the same regulations. See: National Insurance Advisory Committee, *National Insurance (Maternity Benefit) Regulations 1948: Report (HC 147 (1947–48))* (London: HMSO, 1948); National Insurance Advisory Committee, *Maternity Benefits (Cmd. 8446)* (London: HMSO, 1952), p. 40; National Insurance Advisory Committee, *National Insurance (Medical Certification) Amendment Regulations 1966. Report of the National Insurance Advisory Committee (Cmnd 2875)* (London: HMSO, 1966).

[124] Bailkin, *The Afterlife of Empire*.

[125] TNA: PIN 52/6, F. M. Collins to G. M. Kemp Jones, 24 May 1951.

'Issue' had no basis in medical practice or science. It was a term used by social security authorities to refer to the completion of labour, but could refer to anything from the moment the baby left the birth canal, through the cutting of the umbilical cord, to the passing of the afterbirth. Given the way the regulations were written, that could have major implications for paying of benefit. If the child died before 'confinement' was completed, technically this would not be the 'issue of a living child' and so full benefit would not be payable. This contradicted the definition of 'birth' from the General Register Office. If the child survived for any length of time outside the womb it would have to be registered for a birth and a death certificate rather than being classed as a still birth. Even more shockingly, strict interpretation of 'confinement' could leave women who experienced complicated or traumatic births in legal limbo. In one case in Leeds a woman had to undergo an emergency hysterectomy while pregnant. The child survived for about an hour before dying. The Deputy Chief Medical Officer to the Ministry of National Insurance advised against paying maternity benefit on the grounds that a hysterectomy was not 'labour'. He then recommended that the definition of confinement was refined so that such cases would qualify in the future.[126] To make these definitions easier to manage, as well as to provide a degree of justice for claimants, the National Insurance Advisory Committee advised in 1952 that it would be better to pay maternity grant in two halves: the first at confinement and the second two weeks later, provided both the mother and the baby survived.[127] In this way, women received some financial benefit for the birth itself—generally considered to be a medically acceptable reason to miss work—without having to ask invasive questions about the way it was conducted or the potentially devastating outcomes.

One key prejudice reinforced by these kinds of regulations was the position of women's incomes in the 'hierarchy of value'. The relevance of this hierarchy becomes even more apparent when we consider how and when the social security authorities recognized the financial value of domestic work. 'Housekeeper' cases in National Assistance are a good example. NAB adopted the shorthand 'housekeeper' for claimants who were considered unable to work because they were required at home full time to look after a relative.[128] 'Require', 'home', 'full time', and 'relative' were all contestable terms which will be left for now. For sick notes, however, we see a fundamentally different form of certification. In the other situations hitherto described, claimants provided their own evidence of incapacity. Here, the sick note was technically a report on the person being cared for. Thus, the primary obstacle for claimants was often not whether their relative was 'really' sick; it was whether or not the claimant was the one with the duty to provide that

---

[126] TNA: PIN 52/6, F. M. Collins to Parr, 24 August 1955; East and West Ridings Region to Chief Insurance Officer, August 1955.
[127] *Cmd. 8446*, p. 14.
[128] See especially the policy memoranda in TNA: AST 36/348 and AST 36/349.

care. Given that caring duties fell disproportionately on women, this affected judgements on such cases, whether the woman was the one caring or the one being cared for.

A married woman's entitlements to support were restricted, especially if she was caring for her husband. This was, according to Beveridgean logic, entirely natural. As with sickness benefit, the loss of earnings for the wife was simply a loss of 'extras'. These benefits were not designed to pay a wage to wife, who was performing her 'duties'. A subsistence income would therefore come from the husband's entitlements to National Assistance or National Insurance benefits such as sickness, industrial injuries, and, after 1971, invalidity benefits. Yet, in many cases, women were outside the purview of National Insurance. The National Council for the Single Woman and Her Dependents repeatedly made the case for women who had to give up work to care for relatives after its foundation in 1965.[129] These claimants were disproportionately middle-aged unmarried daughters caring for parents. Unlike wives or widows, they could not claim specific benefits on their husbands' insurance.[130] An article in the *Guardian* in 1970 summed up the situation succinctly: 'single daughters are often the breadwinners for the family. A drop in their income means the whole family faces poverty.'[131]

The disparity in treatment by social security authorities was emphasized further by the position of a husband who was the carer for his wife. In 1972, a case came to the DHSS's attention of a man who had been charged £0.25 every time he needed a sick note for his wife to claim supplementary benefit.[132] While the Department worked out how to compensate the husband, the underlying entitlement to benefit remained clear. A payment was necessary because the family was losing the income of its breadwinner on the one hand and the provision of domestic duties on the other. Even if the domestic work itself was not given a financial value, it became pertinent if the loss of such work affected the ability of the breadwinner to earn the household's core income. This position was moral as well as legal. In 1973 a doctor attempted to circumvent the regulations to allow his patient to claim sickness benefit in a timely manner, though he felt the need to inform the DHSS about what he had done. He had written a sick note for a husband even though he knew the real reason he was unable to work was because the wife was unable to look after the household or their young children. She was, by the GP's estimation, 'an incompetent alcoholic who has made suicidal attempts' but, despite the doctor's advice, the parents were not willing to put their children in care.[133] The idea that the husband, as the breadwinner, was entitled to support

[129] Alice Hall and Hannah Tweed, 'Curating care: Creativity, women's work, and the Carers UK Archive', *Journal of Contemporary Archive Studies* 6 (2019).
[130] May Abbott, 'Single and silent', *Guardian*, 4 January 1963, p. 6.
[131] 'Hardships that face single women with dependents', *Guardian*, 14 July 1970, p. 7.
[132] TNA: AST 36/348, E. J. Dowling, Senior Medical Officer to G. Morgan, 25 September 1972.
[133] TNA: AST 36/349, K. A. E. Spence to E. J. Dowling, 19 November 1973.

was not in question. A sick note was enough to allow the husband access—the wife, however, was excluded from this system.

The expansion of disability-related benefits in the 1970s did not resolve these inequalities.[134] When Attendance Allowance became available in 1971 to cover the extra costs associated with long-term care, payments were made to the disabled claimant rather than the person providing the 'attendance'. While avoiding the moral dilemma of who received the sick note, it did not pay at a high enough rate to cover for the lost earnings of the person providing the care—often a woman—or the likely decrease in the household income if the claimant was the 'breadwinner'. But it was never designed to.[135] This role was supposedly played by Invalidity Benefit, which was payable to a married woman only if she had a complete contribution record.[136] More complicated was Invalid Care Allowance. This was paid to the carer based on the benefits claimed by the person being cared for; but it was *not* available to married women on the basis that a wife was not a breadwinner. It was designed primarily for unmarried daughters caring for older relatives, although it was technically available to both men and women.[137] A long legal campaign using equalities legislation in the United Kingdom and European Economic Community saw these regulations changed in the 1980s and a significant increase in the number of claimants as a result.[138]

These contradictions are best exemplified by Housewife's Non-contributory Invalidity Pension. The very existence of this benefit showed how the welfare state struggled to resolve the moral claims from women for adequate support with the perceived need to maintain the principles of National Insurance and the breadwinner model. HNCIP was introduced in 1977 for women between 16 and 60 years old, resident in the UK, 'married' or 'living with a man as his wife', and '*continuously* incapable of [her] normal household duties for at least 28 weeks; and *continuously* incapable of paid work for at least 28 weeks'.[139] The final two criteria were measured with a 'household duties test'.

The 'household duties' test amounted to a report from the claimant's GP about her ability to perform certain tasks. The list is instructive. Broken into four categories—'shopping', 'meals', 'washing and ironing', and 'cleaning'—it asked whether the claimant was 'able to do it all', 'most of it', 'a little of it', or 'not able to do it at all'. Very quickly it became clear that married women had varying degrees of skill and need. One tribunal case from 1981 highlighted by Jackie Gulland in

[134] Hampton, *Disability and the Welfare State in Britain*.
[135] Millward, 'Social security policy and the early disability movement'.
[136] TNA: PIN 35/92, V. Southon to Watts, 10 July 1972.
[137] See the negotiations between DHSS and Treasury on releasing funds for the allowance, especially TNA: T 277/4045, J. A. Atkinson to P. R. Baldwin, 19 June 1974.
[138] Hall and Tweed, 'Curating care'.
[139] Emphasis original. TNA: PIN 15/4481, DHSS Leaflet NI 214, NCIP for Married Women, June 1977, pp. 1–2. Copy also consulted in Peter Townsend Collection, University of Essex (hereafter PTC): 78.19.

her work on gendered discrimination within disability benefits policy perfectly demonstrates this. A 59-year-old woman 'of Indian origin' was initially denied HNCIP because it was found that she could perform enough of her 'household duties'. On appeal, however, the Commissioner granted her the benefit on the basis that her 'duties' were much more intensive than would have been expected of a white British family. The cooking was considered more complex as were her laundry requirement (including the careful washing of saris). Moreover, as an older mother in her cultural setting she had more duties towards the care of her children, their partners and her grandchildren.[140] There was no sense from the record that the claimant was any more 'sick' than had been written on her sick note. The question of eligibility centred on the definition of 'normal' household duties.

A woman from Leicester in 1978 was also denied benefit because it was determined that she could perform many of the tasks on the 'duties test' list. However, her living situation and the circumstances of her injury suggested that these tasks would be very difficult to perform. 'Janice'[141] had cut her hand and suffered nerve damage breaking a window to get into her own house to rescue her children from her husband who had locked her out. Her testimony from her appeal outlines her moral entitlement to help, both as a mother and as a disabled person.

> I would like to work. but I carnt. Thats why I put in for this benefit at the moment I am homeless....I put my hand thow a window to save my children as my husband had been drinking. its not the first time hes hurry my children. he is now in prison and we are left with nothing No Home no furnicher. he sold that....but What can I do thats why I put in for this pension. So I could find some where of my owne. I am disabled.[142]

The commissioner upheld the original decision to deny benefit. The presence of Janice's social worker suggests that she was getting some support from the local authority, but we do not have any records to tell us whether this support was adequate, nor what happened to her and her children after this. In any event, the sick note was not the issue here. Neither Janice nor the authorities disputed her incapacity for paid work, though this was only half of the medical qualifying criteria. The only question was whether Janice could perform her 'duties', which evidently did not take into account the dangerous husband, her living conditions in her brother's home (which was without electricity) nor, crucially, her inability to do *paid* work. The 'hierarchy of value' did not just extend to the financial

---

[140] Jackie Gulland, 'Conditionality in social security: lessons from the household duties test', *Journal of Social Security Law* 26, no. 2 (2019): pp. 62–78.

[141] Not her real name.

[142] TNA: PIN 19/514/4. The tribunal transcribed a letter from Janice onto a form, reproducing the typographical errors. Letter received by the local tribunal on 4 October 1978.

compensation for work, but also to the supposed physical and mental difficulty of doing it.

Janice was also affected by changes in the qualification rules which were rewritten soon after the benefit was introduced. Campaigners drew attention to the unfairness of subjecting married women to the duties test. The Disablement Income Group (DIG), which had been formed by two women who self-identified as housewives, led the charge. The need to prove inability for both paid and domestic work appeared self-evidently contradictory. Surely inability to do one meant inability to do the other; and why did married women have to go through this, but not single women or men?[143] This inequality was made even stricter after a tribunal decision in September 1978 which had been supported by groups such as DIG and the Disability Alliance's 'Equal Rights for Disabled Women Campaign'. The commissioner in the case emphasized the regulations should focus on what a woman could not do rather than what she could. Essentially, this was a benefit to provide for lost capacity in the home, and should not be denied on the basis that a woman could do many of the items on the duties list if she could not perform other core tasks. This interpretation could have led to the tripling of the HNCIP budget, according to the DHSS.[144] Again, neither the actual severity of the person's medical condition nor its impact upon the ability of the woman to work were in question. Within four days, the DHSS imposed new wording into the regulations to reassert the stricter standard for qualification it had originally envisaged.[145] The inequality of treatment between married women and other claimants, combined with the severity of the test, meant that campaigners were successfully able to leverage sex equality legislation to force the government into reform. As we will see in Chapter 6, the DHSS's answer was not to revise the way it provided support for loss of domestic work, but to scrap the benefit altogether and fold it into a new one.

Conclusion

The sickness system was built for a perceived 'ordinary' claimant. An otherwise healthy, regularly employed, British-born man could claim National Insurance benefit for short periods using a sick note and his National Insurance contributions status. As we have seen in previous chapters, there were individual cases that garnered suspicion and the overall population could come under scrutiny if total absenteeism rose too much. Still, when we look deeper at sick note policy it

---

[143] See for example the Disability Alliance complaints in a meeting with the disability minister Alf Morris. 'Better deal for the handicapped in prospect', *The Times*, 19 July 1978, p. 2; and their policy discussions in PTC: 77.02, Minutes of DA's steering committee, 18 October 1978.

[144] TNA: PIN 35/495, B1, Reference of the HNCIP question to NIAC, pp. 6–8.

[145] PTC: 77.02, Minutes of DA's Steering Committee, 18 October 1978.

is obvious which demographics were—and were not—in mind when the Beveridgean welfare state was created in the 1940s. It was generally assumed that British men would qualify for benefit. The sick note determined whether they were eligible specifically for sickness-related welfare. For migrants and women, however, there were far more hoops to jump through just to prove moral and legal desert. The sick note is discussed far less because the legitimacy of the medical complaint was of much lower importance for determining access.

This is vital for understanding the design and implementation of the British welfare state, especially as shifts in employment patterns, demographics and equality politics clashed with the assumptions made in 1948. By tracing sick note policy, we see these tensions manifested in the 'classic welfare state' era. The system struggled to deal with cases that fell outside the 'ordinary', and the volume of such cases was only to increase as the twentieth century went on. It was going to be harder to treat all migrant cases as if they were manifestations of different versions of 'unemployment' or a modified form of border control. Women were not going to revert to the 'default' of performing full-time domestic labour when they married a breadwinning man. Even as reactionary and conservative forces attempted to push back against immigration and changing gender roles in domestic and paid employment, it was becoming legally and socially less acceptable to engage in overt discrimination on these grounds.[146] Sick note policy exposes that these challenges did not appear in the 1960s. Instead, they were problematic from the Appointed Day. Moreover, the system was slow to respond because its administration was not designed to quickly adapt. Sick notes might not have worked for migrants and women, but there was no great rush to get rid of them. In part because this would require significant resources to create a viable alternative—in part because this was a very minor 'failure' in a system that was never designed to cater to their needs.

As the relationship between employment, social security and health continued to evolve, however, changes were eventually required. The next chapter shows that the system had become too inefficient for business, government, and the medical profession. The way sick notes were used by claimants, employers, and various other institutions had put too much strain on GPs surgeries, while political shifts across the postwar period had led some to question whether the private sector could take on the functions that had been placed on the state in the 1940s.

---

[146] Not, of course, that this did not still happen. Virdee, *Racism, Class and the Racialized Outsider*; Bivins, *Contagious Communities*; McCarthy, 'Women, marriage and paid work'; Paterson, ' "I didn't feel like my own person" '.

5

Privatization?

The Sick Note into the 1980s

'Many were sceptical when British workers were put on trust to sign their own short-term sick notes' wrote the *Daily Mail* in July 1983. 'Surely, they said, the number of absentees would increase sharply? Now, just a year after the scheme's introduction, the British worker has been vindicated.'[1]

The introduction of self-certification in 1982 acknowledged what had been articulated for decades: sick notes were inherently flawed. Allowing workers to 'take a week off on your honour' removed the unnecessary bureaucratic hurdle for patients to see the doctor, for the doctor to write the note, and for employers and the state to process the paperwork.[2] Given the complaints seen in previous chapters, one might wonder why it took so long. Indeed, it did not happen overnight. The Ministries that would eventually become the Department of Health and Social Security (DHSS)[3] progressively reduced the certification demands on doctors and claimants from the mid-1960s. These concessions—largely the result of lobbying from the British Medical Association (BMA) and brought to a head by moments of tension between the health ministries and general practitioners—accepted that short term certification created more bureaucratic waste than it was worth for the small gains in reducing inappropriate claims. At the same time, the businesses that had come to rely upon the National Insurance certification system for policing their own absenteeism and maintaining staff discipline were cautious. They were less willing to give sick notes up; and nobody was willing to throw them out altogether.

The early 1980s are a turning point for the story of sick notes. Self-certification was a major break from past practice, yet it was only possible because the DHSS radically restructured sickness benefit. From 1983, employers would administer a new Statutory Sick Pay (SSP) to employees for the first eight weeks rather than National Insurance offices. While some of the cost would be reimbursed from the

---

[1] Michael Jeffries, 'Now the sceptics look sick', *Daily Mail*, 1 July 1983, p. 6.
[2] John Stevenson, 'Take a week off on your honour', *Daily Mail*, 25 April 1981, p. 10.
[3] The social security ministries went through many changes between 1948 and 1968 when the DHSS was created. For simplicity, this chapter will refer to 'social security' as a catch-all for the Ministry of National Insurance, the Ministry of Pensions and National Insurance and the Ministry of Social Security. See also Chapter 1.

government, the DHSS was no longer directly responsible for paying short-term sickness benefit. Thus, it had no need for short-term sick notes. Furthermore, demand would be reduced because free notes would be harder to come by. In theory, employers would no longer be able 'to grasp at any piece of paper which they can accept as explaining an absence from work as "involuntary" and so relive themselves of any obligation to check on absenteeism'.[4]

This chapter is therefore about two interconnected trends. On the one hand, successful (albeit incremental) BMA lobbying had weakened the defences of those determined to force patients to seek short-term certificates and to force doctors to write them. To understand how and why this happened, the chapter first examines the various arguments the BMA and others made against sick notes up to 1980 alongside contemporary attitudes from employers and employees. The chapter then considers the two major disputes between the BMA and DHSS that led to significant reform of sick note regulations: one that coincided with the 1966 GPs' contract; and another that took place during reforms to the NHS and threatened strike action in the mid-1970s. These changes led to the reduction in the number of forms GPs were required to complete as well as downgrading the status of the sick note from a 'certificate' to a 'statement' of the doctor's opinion about the ability of the patient to work.

On the other hand, the evolution of employment practices and the election of Margaret Thatcher in 1979 meant that it was possible—practically and politically—to effectively 'privatize' sickness benefit. While there was some degree of financial compensation in its early running, the early 1980s' sick pay reforms were part of a deliberate incremental plan to eventually make all short-term sickness benefit administered and paid in full by employers. The chapter ends by discussing how and why the DHSS decided to shift the responsibility for administering short-term sickness to employers while still retaining its role in providing for longer-term sickness and disability. By the 1980s, the majority of employers now provided some form of occupational sick pay, and the success of Pay As You Earn (PAYE) income tax had shown that payroll could deal with the administration of such functions. Even though this was only designed as a supplement to (rather than a replacement of) the basic rate of National Insurance sickness benefit, Secretary of State for Social Services Patrick Jenkin and others at the DHSS argued that it was now unnecessary to duplicate bureaucracy by having the state process sickness benefit payments as well as employers. These reforms would even incentivize businesses to crack down on absenteeism once they appreciated the additional costs of sickness. Still, not all businesses were convinced. The insurance principle had spread the risk of sickness across the

---

[4] The National Archives (hereafter TNA): PIN 35/150, 'Medical Certificates for National Insurance Purposes' attached to memorandum Hellon to Swift, 23 March 1965.

population, but it had also collectivized the risks to businesses which had different rates of morbidity and industrial accidents. Representatives from the Confederation of British Industry (CBI) and Trades Union Congress (TUC) were worried that the relationship between employers and employees could be significantly altered by the removal of the automatic application of 'adjudication machinery...which is independent of both claimant and employer'.[5] The sick note, then, had become much more than just a passport to benefit—it was inextricably tied into the relationship between employers, employees, and the state.

Combined, we see how sick notes were always a tool of the bureaucracies that demanded them. The changing position of medical certification in the welfare state was driven by practical concerns about how to administer sickness-related benefits as well as reflecting wider changes in public attitudes towards work, welfare, and how the state ought to be managed. Questions about how far the state ought to collectivize its response to sickness could not be separated from wider political and economic concerns about the long-term viability and suitability of the welfare state. As James Vernon's research on Heathrow Airport has shown the seeds of neoliberal policy existed long before the election of Margaret Thatcher (and social democratic trends continued long after), the policy debates leading to SSP expose how sickness certification was able to adapt to the needs of different welfare state logics.[6]

The Limitations of Sick Notes

The arguments against sick notes were well-rehearsed by 1982, especially among doctors. As seen so far in this volume, many of the problems experienced in the prewar National Health Insurance system carried over into the Beveridgean welfare state. Tighter certification was not an answer to absenteeism, and the entire network of employment, insurance, and healthcare was built around a 'breadwinner' nuclear family ideal that no longer (if ever) applied to large parts of the working population.

It is, however, worth repeating some of these complaints again, especially over short-term certification. (Longer-term certification will be discussed in more detail in Chapter 6.) Short-term certificates constituted the bulk of sick notes for doctors and administrators.[7] Complaints also explain why doctors pushed for self-certification for short periods of illness and why the state and businesses could be convinced that this was a workable solution to the BMA's problems.

---

[5] The Modern Records Centre (hereafter MRC): MSS 200/C/3/EMP/5/21, Trades Union Congress, 'Government Green Paper: "Income During Initial Sickness"', 30 September 1980, p. 11.

[6] James Vernon, 'Heathrow and the making of neoliberal Britain', *Past & Present* (2021).

[7] Department of Health and Social Security, *Income during Initial Sickness: A New Strategy (Cmnd 7864)* (London: HMSO, 1980). See also the discussion of absenteeism statistics in Chapter 3.

While these complaints recurred throughout the postwar period, the significance for policy change within the British welfare state is in *when* doctors were able to successfully present these grievances and press their collective bargaining power.

The main source of consternation for BMA members was the sheer volume of paperwork generated by the National Insurance system. A culture had developed around sick notes, exponentially fuelled by demand from businesses, the state, and workers. 'Sickness' had been established as a legitimate reason for absence, and 'sickness' had become defined de facto as absence from work *certified by a sick note*. Thus, the sick note was sickness—and without a sick note, there was no sickness. Before even considering National Insurance benefit entitlement, certification was essential for employers' absenteeism management and for workers to protect themselves against charges of 'voluntary absenteeism'. As a BBC interviewer put it on *World at One* in 1974, 'the act of going along to your doctor and getting a sickness note is a traditional part of the British way of life'.[8]

Doctors were annoyed enough at the requirement in their terms of service to write certificates for National Insurance. However, they believed that this was being exploited as much by businesses as it was by work-shy patients. The pseudonymous 'Scrutator' of *Medical News* wrote in his or her sketch:

> The real bugbear, I am afraid, is the employer. Insidiously, this gross abuse of our services has been allowed to creep in until it has now become accepted as quite normal and proper by industry, patients and – alas! – by too many doctors that we must act as unpaid attendance officers....The Saturday night hangover has passed, they need no treatment, but – mark this well! – it is the employer who wants a certificate to keep his books tidy.[9]

Could they, as one civil servant wrote in 1965, 'be prepared to reduce their apparently insatiable demands for "pieces of paper" to cover the odd day's absence from work of their employees'?[10] It seemed not. Even when patients did not qualify for a 'free' sick note, employers were insistent on private ones. Doctors could charge for sick notes for absences less than three days—the standard rate in the 1960s was two shilling [£0.10]—but the volume of demand still clogged waiting rooms. For the reasons explored in Chapter 2, doctors could feel a mix of duty and financial necessity to agree to perform these services, and so refusal was difficult. That

[8] TNA: PIN 35/435/1, transcript of *World at One* interview with R. B. L. Ridge, member of the GMSC and Joint Working Group, 5 April 1974.

[9] TNA: PIN 35/151, Cutting, 'Scrutator', 'Certification gone wrong', *Medical News*, September 1964, pp. 17–19. The author could be George Macpherson who wrote for the *British Medical Journal* under the nom de plume 'Scrutator' from 1970 to 1991 dissecting medico-political news. Richard Smith, 'Farewell Scrutator', *British Medical Journal* 302, no. 6767 (1991): p. 6; Linda Beecham, 'Gordon Macpherson: Editor who bridged the gap between the BMJ and the BMA', *British Medical Journal* 366 (2019).

[10] TNA: PIN 35/150, 'Medical Certificates for National Insurance Purposes', March 1965.

position had been exploited by employers who had come to expect as a right the use of NHS GPs as an absenteeism watchdog. For 'Scrutator':

> Because we have hitherto given our co-operation as a courtesy, it is now being demanded as our bounden duty....One simple way of achieving [a reduction] would be to charge...at least 10s. 6. [£0.525]...Should the employer...reimburse the employee, then I fancy cheaper ways of keeping the books tidy will soon be found.[11]

Besides, as one group of GPs in Tamworth put it: 'The boss knows the workers he can trust and those who are scrimshankers. It is not up to use to arbitrate and decide if a worker is telling the truth.'[12]

The BMA was also frustrated because even if doctors were compelled to write them, sick notes were not scientific 'proof' of capacity for work. Especially in the case of short-term illnesses, most notes were nothing more than 'ipse dixit' confirmation that the patient presented themselves and told the doctor they were sick. In some cases, incapacity for work was so obvious the worker required not 'the service of a doctor, but the attention of a much lower-paid clerk with two eyes, one hand, and two legs'.[13] As a BMA official was recorded saying in an unguarded comment to junior doctors in 1974, sick notes were little more than 'bogus chits'.[14] There was general consensus that long-term sickness could be monitored well through the existing system. These conditions required extended contact with medical authorities and were likely to be diagnosed more formally through tests. For mild illnesses (such as colds) it was impossible for a doctor to say with any scientific certainty what virus was responsible for the patient's symptoms, making the 'diagnosis' useless.[15] Under the 1948 system, if the patient had come back for a 'Final' certificate, could the doctor say that the now-non-existent symptoms were real or debilitating enough to warrant time off work in the first place? In any case, patients rarely sought or required medical treatment.[16] For workers, having to go to the doctor for these certificates was inconvenient and medically unnecessary. For the government, these notes were difficult to police, a source of tension in industrial relations with the BMA, and, potentially, a drain on the NHS. The BMA argued that doctors might be tempted to write prescriptions for patients who needed nothing more than bedrest, a costly

---

[11] TNA: PIN 35/151, 'Scrutator', 'Certification gone wrong'.

[12] Keith Collling, 'The 10/6 sick note', Daily Mail, 17 December 1965, p. 9.

[13] S. S. Lawson, 'Points from letters: Sickness certification', British Medical Journal 4, no. 5675 (1969): p. 114. See also 'Doctor wants sick notes to be abolished', The Times, 14 August 1970, p. 3.

[14] TNA: PIN 35/435/1, Cutting, 'Leap forward on certificates', Pulse, 6 April 1974, p. 1.

[15] On this argument, repeatedly made, see: TNA: PIN 35/435/1, Cutting from General Practitioner, 5 July 1974. See also the debates over 'Repeat short-term claimants' in TNA: PIN 35/229.

[16] TNA: PIN 35/150, 'Medical certificates for National Insurance purposes', March 1965.

side-effect that would not happen if the worker could stay at home and simply telephone in sick.[17]

As annoying as sick notes were to GPs, all this would be a price worth paying if they acted as an effective check on malingering and absenteeism. But short-term certification could not even provide that. A Glaswegian doctor grumbled that the system had not changed substantially since the 1910s and 'astute' citizens had already worked out that, 'with a little ingenuity and perseverance...in the welfare state, one need not work'.[18] Such cynicism about the utility of sick notes—and the moral fibre of patients—extended beyond the medical profession. The *Daily Mail* suggested that the growing generosity of sick pay coupled with easy access to medical certification created ' "legalised" absenteeism'.[19] It was happy to print stories from doctors who admitted that they no longer bothered to fight their belligerent patients and become 'like Horatio on the bridge or Canute stemming the tide'.[20] Good copy was also to be found in what appeared to be comical diagnoses. A man allegedly received a sick note for 'cyesis' (pregnancy). A woman obtained a certificate for prostatitis.[21] Given that people could self-declare or alter the gender they were assigned for National Insurance purposes since the 1950s, such diagnoses were not impossible,[22] but they were improbable enough for the jokes to land in 1970s Britain. The key point—that the certificates were 'not worth the paper they [were] written on'—stood.[23]

Doctors and officials complained about the 'repeat short period claimant' who exploited the quirks in the system. Just as Ranjit Singh in Chapter 4 had been able to time his fraudulent claims so that they ended just before a regional medical officer might investigate the case, so too could enterprising individuals take several short illnesses that would never result in sick visiting or other monitoring procedures. During an investigation, the social security ministries highlighted internally the example of two men who had each claimed 55 separate spells of sickness between 1964 and 1967. Their lack of cooperation with authorities was evidence to National Insurance officers that they were not 'really' suffering from

---

[17] TNA: MH 153/299, BMA, 'Reduction in Certification' report for the Ministry of Health, early 1965. The DHSS also made this argument: TNA: BN 118/46, W. McConnachie to A. Brown, 23 February 1981.

[18] Alex Crawford, 'Certification', *British Medical Journal* 2, no. 5360 (1963): p. 808.

[19] Julian Holland, 'How many of us go sick of the money?', *Daily Mail*, 29 March 1966, p. 8.

[20] 'Sick note sickness', *Daily Mail*, 30 June 1978, p. 19.

[21] John Illman, 'Abusing the sick note system', *Sunday Times* (20 April 1975), p. 13. The author's name is not a pun. See also the later story of 'a man recovering from a mastectomy' in 'The papers', *The Times* (9 July 1982), p. 24.

[22] Adrian, Kane-Galbraith, 'Male breadwinners of "doubtful sex": Trans men and the welfare state, 1945-1969', in *Twentieth Century British Masculinities* (Manchester: Manchester University Press (under review));Mar Hicks, 'Hacking the cis-tem: Transgender citizens and the early digital state', *IEEE Annals of the History of Computing* 4, no. 1 (2019): pp. 20–33.

[23] J. A. Eddington and J. L. A. McVicker, 'The curse of certificates', *British Medical Journal* 2, no. 5402 (1964): p. 192.

chronic health issues and were merely manipulating the system.[24] Employers were similarly annoyed as regularly absent workers made it difficult to plan shift patterns. A Production Superintendent wrote to the Liverpool DHSS office in 1977 about one worker in his early fifties who was coincidentally always sick when his shifts fell on Friday, Saturday, or Sunday. He attached the worker's time sheets as evidence—an anti-sick note, of sorts. Each spell had been legitimized by a medical certificate, but it seemed obvious to management that the man was manipulating the system to avoid his obligations to the company at weekends.[25]

'Convenient' sick notes were not always repeated or long term, however. The act of taking an isolated day or two off for a local event or just to remain idle was sufficiently understood to be the subject of humour. Welsh comic poet Max Boyce's '9-3' from his album *Live at Treorchy*, for example, tells the story of Llanelli Scarlets beating the New Zealand rugby union team in the style of an epic.[26] In his introduction he tells of the camaraderie (even complicity) of functionaries because the game meant so much to the town. The local traffic policeman is shown to still be drunk having celebrated a little too much; while the town's GPs sign everyone off work with 'Scarlet fever'.[27] Authorities in general had been somewhat less amused by these absences across the period, however. There were specific procedures for local offices dealing with an increase in claims 'at times of holiday periods, local sporting events or strikes'.[28] The coincidence of sickness benefit claims with the traditional 'Barnsley feast week' in late August drew investigation. Most factories in the Yorkshire town shut during this period of local holiday, but some workers attempted to claim sick pay anyway. Without doubt, many were genuinely ill and otherwise entitled. Nevertheless, the volume of new claims suggested—on the population level, at least—an increase in malingering.[29] Similarly, an official in the Admiralty warned that giving working-class men more leeway on short-term sickness would only encourage more skiving to watch sport.[30] During the productivity crisis covered in Chapter 2, the government had placed restrictions on greyhound racing, encouraged big horse racing events such as the St Leger Stakes to take place on a weekend, and persuaded the Football League to keep its midweek fixtures to a minimum.[31]

---

[24] TNA: PIN 25/229, N. Hellon to J. P. Cahsman, 13 March 1968.
[25] MRC: MSS 2002/C/3/EMP/5/24, HL Johnson, United Reclaim Limited to The Inspector, DHSS Liverpool, 4 April 1977 (copied to the local CBI branch).
[26] My thanks to Martin Johnes for directing me to this song.
[27] Max Boyce, '9-3', *Live at Treorchy* (EMI, 1974).
[28] TNA: PIN 35/105, Extract from regulations, 1954.
[29] See discussions in TNA: PIN 35/105, esp. Barnsley NIO, Barnsley 'Feast' Week—1955—Seventh Annual Report.
[30] TNA: T 217/47, Admiralty to Lees, 29 April 1949.
[31] TNA: COAL 31/69, file on 'Manpower Absenteeism Mid-week Sport'; TNA: CAB 124/1060–61; 'Saturday for big races', *Daily Mail*, 22 July 1949, p. 6; Daryl Leeworthy, 'A diversion from the new leisure: Greyhound racing, working-class culture, and the politics of unemployment in inter-war South Wales', *Sport in History* 32, no. 1 (2012): pp. 53–73.

The Welsh National Insurance office speculated that the Empire Games in Cardiff might have been responsible for a spike in injury claims relative to previous years in July 1958.[32] Businesses, too, were unhappy. For example, a quirk of the fixture list in 1949 led to FA Cup replays at the two big Birmingham football clubs (Aston Villa and Birmingham City) to be organized for the same Monday afternoon. The general manager of GEC called on the government to step in 'if the [Football Association] haven't got enough sense' to avoid such clashes and would 'remind workers of the "gentleman's agreement"...that workers would not quit their jobs to see mid-week soccer matches'.[33]

Moreover, it was not just the idle that could exploit the system. As seen in previous chapters, miners could moonlight while claiming benefit with genuine sick notes, and there were long-standing prejudices that Irish claimants were claiming sickness in one region while working cash-in-hand in another. In 1971, a high-profile case of eight workers in Middlesbrough drew complaints against the DHSS from two Conservative MPs. The men had claimed sickness from their regular jobs to take short-term, highly paid work at a local oil refinery. The DHSS responded that unless they treated every single claim to sickness benefit as a potential fraud then it would be impossible to eliminate all abuse. Regardless, such a system would be administratively impractical and cripplingly expensive.[34] Given that these claims, from Welsh sporting events to North Yorkshire oil refineries, were accompanied by a sick note, it was clear that medical certification was not a check on short-term wilful absence.

Opportunities for Change

While these complaints about short-term certification were consistent, opportunities for reform were rare. As Mark Drakeford and Ian Butler have argued about political scandals, the mere existence of a problem is not enough to motivate institutions to effect change.[35] The problem needs to be recognized as serious enough to warrant action and there needs to be a politically-acceptable alternative course available.[36] Two such windows opened for the BMA, one in

---

[32] TNA: PIN 35/105, New claim to injury benefit, Wales, 5 August 1958.

[33] The combined capacity of both clubs' stadiums was over 100,000. At this time, teams were not allowed to play under floodlights and so had to play during daylight hours. '250,000 warned: "shun cup-tie"', Daily Mail, 17 January 1949, p. 1.

[34] TNA: PIN 35/390, Paul Dean letters to Oscar Murton MP and John Sutcliffe MP, 5 July and 23 June 1971; A. G. Beard to Mr Errington, 18 June 1971.

[35] Mark Drakeford and Ian Butler, Scandal, Social Policy and Social Welfare, 2nd edn (Bristol: Policy Press, 2006).

[36] This is the 'policy streams' theory of policy making. See: John W. Kingdon and James A. Thurber, Agendas, Alternatives, and Public Policies (Boston: Longman, 2011); Gil Walt, Health Policy: An Introduction to Process and Power (London: Zed Books, 1994).

1966 and the other in 1975. Both led to significant concessions on the type and number of National Insurance sick notes doctors would be compelled to write. Successful lobbying also made it easier for the BMA to press for self-certification in the 1980s.

In March 1965, the BMA published 'A Charter for the Family Doctor Service' to demand changes to working conditions and increased funding for general practice.[37] This became the prelude to negotiations with GPs that would lead to the 1966 GP contract.[38] Doctors' workloads had increased significantly since the introduction of the NHS. In part this was due to advances in medicine that made primary care more complex, while GPs had also taken on an expanded role in preventative medicine, providing more immunizations and prophylactic care for chronic conditions such as diabetes.[39] Another major problem was that the population had expanded while the number of GPs had (proportionately) decreased.[40] The profession needed to become more attractive and ditch, as described in one popular 1950s' novel, the 'common knowledge in medical schools that general practitioners in the National Health Service are all seedy men signing forms in insanitary surgeries until they drop dead at forty from overwork'.[41]

As with the disputes over the National Health Service Acts in Chapter 2, pay was the central issue.[42] Jane Lewis notes, however, that conditions and professional autonomy were important concerns.[43] While the Charter did not demand a significant reformulation of a GPs duties within the NHS, there was one exception: sick notes.

This is by general consent one of the most time-wasting of the family doctor's tasks, particularly in the present era of over-work and shortage of doctors. Employing clinicians, whose services are in such demand, on clerical and

[37] British Medical Association, 'A Charter for the Family Doctor Service', *British Medical Journal* 1, no. 5436 (1965): pp. S89–91.

[38] John Lewis, 'The medical profession and the state: GPs and the GP contract in the 1960s and the 1990s', *Social Policy & Administration* 32, no. 2 (1998): pp. 132–50.

[39] National Insurance Advisory Committee, *National Insurance (Medical Certification) Amendment Regulations 1966. Report of the National Insurance Advisory Committee (Cmnd 2875)* (London: HMSO, 1966); Martin D. Moore, *Managing Diabetes, Managing Medicine: Chronic Disease and Clinical Bureaucracy in Post-War Britain* (Manchester: Manchester University Press, 2019); Gareth Millward, *Vaccinating Britain: Mass Vaccination and the Public since the Second World War* (Manchester: Manchester University Press, 2019).

[40] TNA: PIN 35/151, Medical Certification. Note for the Minister's meeting with representatives of the Trades Union Congress, Confederation of British Industries, British Medical Association, Ministry of Pensions and National Insurance, Ministry of Labour and Scottish Home and Health Department, August 1965. See also *Cmnd. 2875*.

[41] Richard Gordon, *Doctor at Large* (London: Michael Joseph, 1955), p. 8.

[42] Charles Webster, *National Health Service: A Political History*, 2nd revised edn (Oxford: Oxford University Press, 2002); Rudolf Klein, 'The state and the profession: The politics of the double bed', *British Medical Journal* 301, no. 6754 (1990): pp 700–2.

[43] Lewis, 'The medical profession and the state'.

administrative duties of this kind cannot be justified....The first immediate step must be to reduce to a minimum the burden of certification for National Insurance purposes....Our concern is with the benefit to the public which will result from releasing the doctor's time in order to attend to his patient's medical needs.[44]

No sick notes would be possible at all if the family doctors resigned *en masse* (or 'dropped dead at forty'). The Ministry of Health therefore needed a solution that could be passed relatively quickly and would have the blessing of the CBI, TUC, social security ministries, and, above all, the Treasury.[45] The BMA accepted that some sort of certification was probably necessary and that GPs were best placed to provide it.[46] At the same time, the government, at least overtly, did not take GPs' acquiescence for granted. The Ministries were well aware that if doctors pushed their terms of service to the limit the National Insurance system would break down through a lack of certificates and the need to install new gatekeeping procedures.[47] 'It would probably be better than having concessions dragged out of us later on', reasoned one civil servant.[48] And while it would be easy to be cynical about the motivations of doctors focusing on their own pay awards from the Ministry of Health, the social duties of family doctors were repeated regularly. 'We owe [our patients] not only a therapeutic but an administrative service', noted one occupational physician, 'dull though this may be'.[49]

The compromise was to reduce (rather than eliminate) the bureaucracy. It was generally accepted the use of 'First' and 'Final' certificates was unhelpful and created extra clinical work that had no therapeutic benefit. These were merged into a new form, the 'Med 3' (see Figure 5.1). This allowed doctors to sign a 'closed' certificate which would grant patients up to a week off work without the need to return to the surgery if it seemed clear that the incapacity would be short term. An 'open' Med 3 was also possible for up to four weeks for conditions likely to be long term (such as a broken leg with a clear prognosis and no need for reassessment). Should additional certificates be required, or the illness change, Med 3s could be used as 'Intermediate' certificates, while GPs reaffirmed that a four-week note did not mean that a patient could not come to see the doctor for follow-up care.[50] In total, the Ministry of Pensions and National Insurance

[44] British Medical Association, 'A Charter for the Family Doctor Service', p. 90.
[45] TNA: MH 35/151, Secretary to Sir Arnold France, 21 September 1965.
[46] See arguments made in Chapter 2 about the family doctor's duty to patients and TNA: MH 153/299, BMA, 'Reduction in Certification' report for the Ministry of Health, early 1965.
[47] TNA: PIN 35/150, Swift to Deputy Secretary of State, 31 March 1965; Watkins to Swift, 6 April 1965.
[48] TNA: PIN 35/150, Swift to Deputy Secretary of State, 31 March 1965.
[49] K. H. Nickol, 'Certification', *British Medical Journal* 1, no. 5487 (1966): p. 614.
[50] *Cmnd. 2875.*

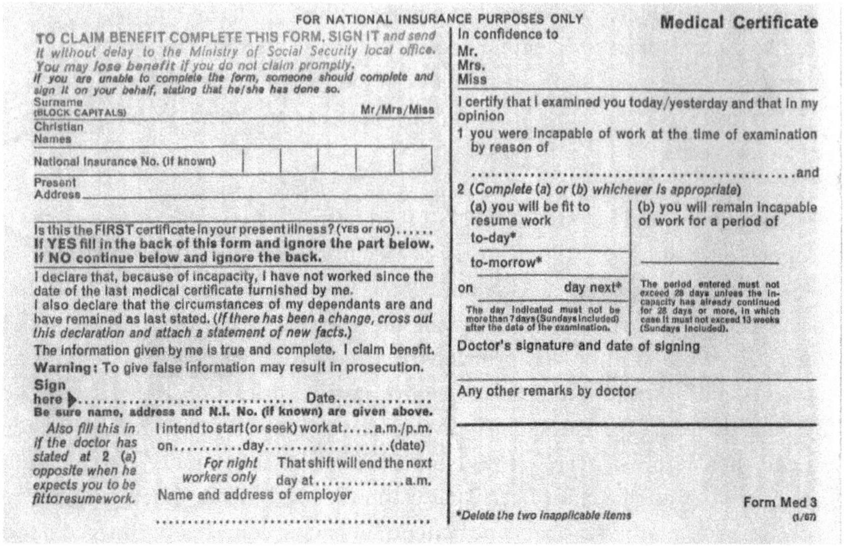

FOR NATIONAL INSURANCE PURPOSES ONLY

Medical Certificate

TO CLAIM BENEFIT COMPLETE THIS FORM, SIGN IT *and send it without delay to the Ministry of Social Security local office.*
You may lose benefit if you do not claim promptly.
If you are unable to complete the form, someone should complete and sign it on your behalf, stating that he/she has done so.

Surname (BLOCK CAPITALS) Mr/Mrs/Miss
Christian Names
National Insurance No. (If known)
Present Address

Is this the FIRST certificate in your present illness? (YES or NO)......
If YES fill in the back of this form and ignore the part below.
If NO continue below and ignore the back.

I declare that, because of incapacity, I have not worked since the date of the last medical certificate furnished by me.
I also declare that the circumstances of my dependants are and have remained as last stated. (*If there has been a change, cross out this declaration and attach a statement of new facts.*)
The information given by me is true and complete. I claim benefit.
Warning: To give false information may result in prosecution.
Sign here ▶.................................. Date...............
Be sure name, address and N.I. No. (if known) are given above.

Also fill this in if the doctor has stated at 2 (a) opposite when he expects you to be fit to resume work.
I intend to start (or seek) work at......a.m./p.m. on...........day....................(date)
For night workers only That shift will end the next day at..............a.m.
Name and address of employer
....

In confidence to
Mr.
Mrs.
Miss

I certify that I examined you today/yesterday and that in my opinion
1 you were incapable of work at the time of examination by reason of
....and
2 (*Complete (a) or (b) whichever is appropriate*)
(a) you will be fit to resume work
to-day*
to-morrow*
on day next*
The day indicated must not be more than 7 days (Sundays included) after the date of the examination.
(b) you will remain incapable of work for a period of
The period entered must not exceed 28 days unless the incapacity has already continued for 28 days or more, in which case it must not exceed 13 weeks (Sundays included).

Doctor's signature and date of signing

Any other remarks by doctor

**Delete the two inapplicable items*

Form Med 3 (1/67)

Figure 5.1 'Form Med 3', First/Final medical certificate used for National Insurance purposes, 1967.
TNA: PIN 35/100.

estimated this could eliminate around 14 million certificates.[51] A survey of the first year of the Med 3's use suggested some gains had been made because workers that had been signed off for a week would return to their jobs immediately, rather than having to go to the doctor for a 'Final' certificate on Monday morning, thus effectively reducing their absence by at least half a day.[52] Further, the Ministry was able to secure a general agreement from the CBI to reduce industry's demands for private certification.[53] While the CBI had misgivings that employees would push their week-long entitlement to the limit, the benefits outweighed the negatives.[54] Besides, was this situation much different to the 'ipse dixit' status quo?[55]

If the new contract in 1966 brought in a '"golden age" of general practice',[56] it was one in which sick notes continued to cause annoyance. An alternative seemed possible when in January 1969 the *British Medical Journal* published two studies of self-certification which sparked an exchange of correspondence in the letters

[51] TNA: PIN 35/150, 'Medical certificates for National Insurance purposes', March 1965.
[52] Ministry of Social Security, *Report of the Ministry of Social Security for the Year 1966 (Cmnd 3338)* (London: HMSO, 1967), p. 95.
[53] TNA: PIN 35/151, Medical Certification. Note for the Minister's meeting... August 1965; TNA: PIN 35/150, 'Medical certificates for National Insurance purposes', March 1965.
[54] 'New medical certificates save time all round', *The Times*, 20 January 1966, p. 5.
[55] 'Open to abuse?', *The Economist*, 29 January 1966, p. 417.
[56] Stephen Gillam, 'The Family Doctor Charter: 50 years on', *British Journal of General Practice* 67, no. 658 (2017): pp. 227–8.

pages.[57] Both drew on a series of complaints from GPs and small experiments with self-certification to show that self-certification would not increase absenteeism appreciably and doctors' time would be saved.[58] While they acknowledged that rates of absenteeism had been rising in the general population, they sought to show that certification was not the cause.[59] Businesses that continued to demand them were, therefore, adding to GPs' already-heavy workload for no tangible gain.[60] As the 1970s arrived, there was renewed pressure to get rid of short-term notes and replace them with self-certification.

GPs threatened to stop writing medical certificates altogether in 1969 in protest at workloads and as part of a larger pay dispute with the DHSS.[61] While this withdrawal of labour did not materialize, there were two periods in 1970 where sick notes were suspended. Early in the year, GPs were not required to write National Insurance medical certificates due to an influenza epidemic.[62] Instead, emergency claim forms allowed patients to self-certificate. In part this was to avoid infection by congregating patients in surgery waiting rooms; but it was also an acknowledgement that doctors themselves were not immune to influenza and that many GPs would themselves be on sick leave. The epidemic was followed by a sick note 'strike' in the summer.[63] (One doctor described this period as 'the happiest in his career'.)[64] The level of absenteeism and the amount paid in benefits during this period actually decreased, though experts predicted this was only because the situation was temporary. Claimants had not had time to work out how to use the National Insurance system without sick notes and the government had been hypervigilant during what amounted to a short-term crisis.[65]

The 1970 epidemic was the first time that the DHSS or its predecessors had suspended certification on such a large scale. Usually, the emergency claim forms were printed in small numbers and held in local National Insurance offices, as it

---

[57] P. J. Taylor, 'Self-certification for brief spells of sickness absence', *British Medical Journal* 1, no. 5637 (1969): pp. 144–7; Stuart Carne, 'Sick absence certification. Analysis of one group practice in 1967', *British Medical Journal* 1, no. 5637 (1969): pp. 147–9.

[58] In particular: John H. Swan, 'The Curse of Certificates', *British Medical Journal* 1, no. 5384 (1964): p. 703; R. P. C. Handfield-Jones, 'Who shall help the doctor? Ancillaries, prescriptions and certificates', *The Lancet* 284, no. 7370 (1964): pp. 1173–4; P. J. Taylor, 'Individual variations in sickness absence', *British Journal of Industrial Medicine* 24, no. 3 (1967): pp. 169–77.

[59] Office of Health Economics, *Work Lost through Sickness* (London: Office of Health Economics, 1965). See also Figure 1.1.

[60] R. E. Dawson, 'Sickness certification', *British Medical Journal* 1, no. 5640 (1969): p. 377; Michael T. Wade, 'Sickness certification', *British Medical Journal* 3, no. 5672 (1969): p. 720.

[61] See especially discussions in June 1969 in Anon, 'Annual Conference of Representatives of Local Medical Committees', *British Medical Journal* 2, no. 5660 (1969): pp. 155–65.

[62] TNA: PIN 35/116, K. J. Wright to N. W. Cossins, 10 February 1970.

[63] 'BMA denounced after threat to the Health Service', *Sunday Times*, 7 June 1970, p. 1; David Wilson, 'Doctors are divided on protest action', *Financial Times*, 8 June 1970, p. 1; John Windsor, 'We will sign again say young doctors', *Daily Mail*, 22 June 1970, p. 7; 'Doctors vote to end sick-note sanctions', *Sunday Times*, 28 June 1970, p. 1.

[64] Anon, 'A.R.M. Round Up', *British Medical Journal* 3, no. 5770 (1971): pp. 319–20.

[65] Anon, 'Self-certification?', *British Medical Journal* 4, no. 5729 (1970): pp. 192–3; Tom Davies, 'Ministry claims doctors split on sick notes', *Sunday Times*, 14 June 1970, p. 4.

was considered that any suspension would be localized and short-lived.[66] The influenza epidemic had demonstrated how vulnerable the system was to a lack of sick notes—but both it and the 'strike' had shown that the world did not collapse when they disappeared. The BMA had been asking for an inquiry on the subject for a while.[67] With the pressure building in the context of wider disputes over pay and conditions between the BMA and DHSS, Secretary of State Richard Crossman agreed in principle to set up a committee. After the 1970 General Election, the new Secretary of State, Sir Keith Joseph, established a Joint Working Group between the DHSS and BMA's General Medical Services Committee (GMSC) to investigate further changes to the certification system. It finally published after repeated delays (primarily to allow the Fisher Report[68] to be concluded and give the Group the opportunity to consider any of its recommendations) on the day of the February 1974 General Election.[69]

The Report's main recommendation—enacted in 1975—was that the 'medical certificate' should be renamed a 'medical statement'. These statements could be used for National Insurance purposes and be seen by the employer, but doctors had no obligation to print a diagnosis. They simply stated whether the doctor recommended that the patient should refrain from work. In principle, this acknowledged that diagnoses and occupational health assessments were not possible from a GP consultation and emphasized the potential 'ipse dixit' nature of most short-term certificates. The new 'statement' forms were also designed to take less time to complete and required less information from the doctor, saving administrative time (though doing nothing to prevent the additional consultations required by the request for the note in the first place).[70]

Even though BMA leadership and DHSS had agreed to this action, the BMA membership had not. It had hoped for much more radical reform. A representative from Leeds stated that the recommendations did 'nothing to deal with the problems', with a Dyfed member declaring the report 'wriggled its way to irrelevant conclusions'.[71] A group from Manchester wrote in the *Guardian* that it was 'the worst of both worlds': statements that did not include a specific diagnosis would be more open to challenge from hostile benefit agencies and employers, while workloads would not be appreciably reduced. The correspondents called for

[66] TNA: PIN 35/116, K. J. Wright to N. W. Cossins, 10 February 1970; N. W. Cossins to all Area Regional Controllers, 7 January 1969.
[67] Since at least mid-1969. Anon, 'Annual Representative Meeting, Aberdeen, 1969', *British Medical Journal* 3, no. 5662 (1969): pp. 9–67.
[68] For more on the Committee and its relationship to sickness benefits see Chapter 4. Henry Fisher, *Report of the Committee on Abuse of Social Security Benefits (Cmnd 5228)* (London: HMSO, 1972).
[69] TNA: PIN 35/435/1, The Report on the Joint Working Group on Medical Certification, February 1974.
[70] Ibid.
[71] Anon, 'Conference of Representatives of L.M.C.s', *British Medical Journal* 3, no. 5922 (1974): pp. 57–63.

self-certification as a better alternative.[72] The Child Poverty Action Group (CPAG) echoed these sentiments, with director Frank Field alleging that 'the people who stand to lose most are the groups most prone to illness, particularly those ailments connected with heavy labour which are difficult to diagnose. Authority...will pass from the family doctor to social security clerks, and an "unspecified" entry on the doctor's statement will almost certainly become a code word to advise them to withhold benefit.'[73]

Still, the concessions held because the justification for some sort of certification within the British work and welfare systems remained. The *Guardian* noted that certificates could be important to a patient's well-being, but 'whatever problems were there before do not disappear because the doctor has signed a sick note. The rent man, the hire purchase commitment, the bills, and the emotional problems remain.'[74] The Principal Medical Officer at the DHSS noted to the social security side of the Department that the British had a unique relationship with general practice:

apparently in keeping with the wishes of the general community, the State, the practitioners and the medical profession as a whole. If it is accepted that general practice should be retained and fostered in the and by the community, it cannot be avoided that the community must turn to general practitioners for their assistance in many spheres where there are advances in social welfare.[75]

The Med 3 statement was, at least for now, a compromise that allowed gatekeeping procedures to remain in place while maintaining cooperation with the medical profession that was necessary for running it.[76]

The report and the plans to implement its recommendations coincided with major NHS reforms that were enacted by the Heath government and executed under Wilson. Strikes in 1975 showed that the medical profession was willing and able to assert its demands.[77] BMA representatives passed a motion to stop writing sick notes from 1976 by 96 votes to 54,[78] and although this 'strike' was averted it

---

[72] Stuart Bailey, Pat Brien, Johnathan Burton, Judith Gray, Ian Jones, Narayan Kutty, Sheila Stainthorp, and Graham Worral (Manchester MPU/ASTMS) letter to *Guardian*, 11 April 1974, p. 16.

[73] 'New doctor's note "could hit the sick"', *Guardian*, 27 February 1976, p. 4. Field had written an editorial defending certificates in 1974: Frank Field, 'Untitled', *Guardian*, 16 May 1974, p. 13.

[74] Roger Beard, 'At the doctor's back', *Guardian*, 30 April 1975, p. 21. See also 'What is it all about?', *The Economist*, 15 June 1974, p. 24. The article drew from similar points made in Office of Health Economics, *The Work of Primary Medical Care* (London: Office of Health Economics, 1974), esp. p. 26.

[75] TNA: PIN 35/435/1, M. R. Hayes, Principal Medical Officer DHSS M1 to E. B. McGinnis, 17 July 1974.

[76] Ibid.

[77] Jack Saunders, 'Emotions, social practices and the changing composition of class, race and gender in the National Health Service, 1970–79: "Lively discussion ensued"', *History Workshop Journal*, 88 (2019), 204–28.

[78] Anon, 'Conference of Representatives of L.M.C.s', p. 58.

caused political headaches for the Department and the Association.[79] Even if 1975 did not secure the kind of change BMA members had hoped for, it emboldened them to push harder the next time an opportunity for change came about. The premise of 'certification' had already been undermined. With reforms to the social security system under the new Thatcher government, the DHSS's opposition to self-certification for short periods of sickness would become much less fierce.

Statutory Sick Pay

The introduction of self-certification for illnesses under a week came in July 1982, with SSP coming online in the following April. Both were created from the Thatcher government's 1980 Green Paper *Income During Initial Sickness* and subsequent consultation process.[80] The latter garnered responses from the CBI, BMA, TUC, and numerous other individual businesses and voluntary organizations.[81] Proposed by Patrick Jenkin and completed by his successor, Norman Fowler, the plans for SSP underwent revision between the Green Paper and final implementation but the core principles remained. Employers, not National Insurance offices, would be responsible for administering sick pay for employees for the first eight weeks of sickness in a financial year. This would also make sickness benefits taxable since they could be paid through the PAYE taxation system in the regular pay packet, reducing the probability that a worker could end up with more net pay being sick than being at work. Employers would be compensated primarily through a rebate on their National Insurance contributions. Traditional sickness benefit would remain for insured claimants who were unemployed or needed support for longer than eight weeks, while Invalidity Benefit provided for longer-term incapacity after one year.[82]

The plan amounted to the privatization of short-term sickness benefits. As the Green Paper made clear, the Conservative government was committed to the principle that 'the State should, wherever possible, disengage itself from activities which firms and individuals can perform perfectly well for themselves'.[83] This marked an important shift in the political dynamics around sick notes. If the government withdrew from directly paying and policing short-term incapacity, it

---

[79] See the extended correspondence during 1974 in TNA: PIN 35/435/1, esp. E. B. McGinnis, Certification for National Insurance Purposes—Publicity in Favour of Retention, 2 July 1974.

[80] *Cmnd 7864.*

[81] For the CBI's correspondence with its members and other organizations in its response to the Green Paper, see MRC: MSS 200/C/3/EMP/5/17–23. For the DHSS's internal discussions, see TNA: BN 118/1–40.

[82] For uninsured claimants, entitlements to Supplementary Benefit remained. On these proposals, see *Cmnd 7864.*

[83] Ibid., p. 2.

no longer had such strong interests in maintaining the existing medical statement system.

Moreover, it is significant in the history of the administration and relative weight of responsibility for 'welfare' in the British 'welfare state'. Histories around privatization usually concentrate on the sale of large nationalized industries, such as British Rail or British Telecom. In doing so, the focus remains on the second Thatcher administration from 1983 onwards when the major denationalizations took place. Recent studies have noted smaller-scale changes in the 1979–83 years to show that privatization was always part of the Thatcher project, albeit a more cautious and politically sensitive one in the first term.[84] In this sense, recent work on neoliberalism and its emergence in British social policy is instructive.[85] James Vernon's work on Heathrow has shown how 'there was no dramatic moment of rupture' when fully-formed neoliberal ideas took hold in Britain.[86] Even if historians can identify certain governments as neoliberal or adherents to market liberalism in social security, the incremental changes to sickness certification policy show liberal, social democratic, and neoliberal elements of policy articulated at different times in different relationships between the various constituencies in the welfare state.[87] As covered in Chapter 6, SSP, like other welfare state reforms, did not become a monolithic enterprise overnight, with state oversight and funding remaining significant throughout the 1980s even as responsibility for its administration moved ever further onto employers.[88] It also did not suddenly arrive in 1979. Jenkin and Geoffrey Howe had been working on plans to reform sickness benefits for years and saw success in this area as key to implementing the New Right economic and social politics espoused by figures such as Thatcher and (former Secretary of State at the DHSS) Sir Keith Joseph.[89] Moreover, the Labour government had also been forced to reduce its planned

---

[84] Mark Billings and John Wilson, '"Breaking new ground": The National Enterprise Board, Ferranti, and Britain's prehistory of privatization', *Enterprise & Society* 20, no. 4 (2019): pp. 907–38; Jacob Ward, 'Financing the information age: London TeleCity, the legacy of IT-82, and the selling of British Telecom', *Twentieth Century British History* 30, no. 3 (2019): pp. 424–46; Lewis Charles Smith, 'Marketing modernity: Business and family in British Rail's "Age of the Train" campaign, 1979–84', *The Journal of Transport History* 40, no. 3 (2019): pp. 363–94; Jacob Ward, 'Computer models and Thatcherist futures: From monopolies to markets in British Telecommunications', *Technology & Culture* 61, no. 3 (2020): pp. 843–70.

[85] On health, see: Moore, *Managing Diabetes*, esp. pp. 160–1.   [86] Vernon, 'Heathrow', p. 34.

[87] Avner Offer, 'The market turn: From social democracy to market liberalism', *Economic History Review* 70, no. 4 (2017): pp. 1051–71; Peter Sloman, 'Redistribution in an age of neoliberalism: Market economics, "poverty knowledge", and the growth of working-age benefits in Britain, c. 1979–2010', *Political Studies* 67, no. 3 (2019): pp. 732–51.

[88] Colin Hay, 'Whatever happened to Thatcherism?', *Political Studies Review* 5, no. 2 (2007): pp. 183–201.

[89] See MRC: MSS 200/C/3/EMP/5/19, Notes on a meeting with Sir Kenneth Stowe, 2 September 1981. On 'Thatcherites' in opposition: Moore, *Managing Diabetes*, pp. 160–1; Robert Saunders, '"Crisis? What crisis?" Thatcherism and the seventies', in *Making Thatcher's Britain*, edited by Ben Jackson and Robert Saunders (Cambridge: Cambridge University Press, 2012), pp. 25–42.

expenditure on the welfare state due to the oil crisis and the conditions of an International Monetary Fund loan in 1976. There was a sense, regardless of the analysis of the causes of the problems, that something must be done—a political narrative that served opponents of the Beveridgean welfare state and Keynesian economics well.[90]

Sickness benefits provided an opportunity to see these principles of state retrenchment and privatization manifested in welfare state governance. SSP was sold as more efficient because it eliminated the duplicated bureaucracy of both National Insurance and the employer's own absenteeism procedures. Until this point, the National Insurance benefit had been the 'base' of sick pay. Workers would claim their state entitlements, and then employers who had their own schemes would 'top up' this amount to equal the claimant's regular wage. SSP responded to the changing needs of the state—the government noted that in 1948 national sick pay was necessary since so few employers provided any coverage, whereas in 1980 around 80 per cent had their own schemes. Why, then, could employers not pay the 'base' amount themselves and remove the costly state bureaucracy? SSP allowed sick pay to be taxed (only the 'top up' was eligible for taxation), reducing economic incentives to remain off work and emphasizing the need for benefit claimants to exercise personal responsibility.[91] While the state would remain as a regulator to ensure a statutory minimum level of coverage, 'good' employers were not prevented from providing higher levels of benefit to their employees to encourage recruitment and retention.[92] Perhaps just as importantly, it allowed a degree of continuity. For most workers, little would materially change in the process of getting sick pay and leave—and it would not seriously undermine any chauvinist, breadwinner model, or Conservative approaches to welfare.[93]

The BMA, realizing that SSP would not be a National Insurance benefit, argued that doctors would not be required to write medical statements for it under the NHS terms of service. The Association put pressure on the DHSS and businesses to accept self-certification for incapacity lasting six days or less, threatening to unilaterally refuse to sign any short-term certificates if no agreement could be

[90] Rodney Lowe, *The Welfare State in Britain since 1945* (Basingstoke: Palgrave Macmillan, 2005), p. 6; Hay, 'Whatever happened to Thatcherism?'; Colin Hay, 'Chronicles of a death foretold: The Winter of Discontent and construction of crisis of British Keynesianism', *Parliamentary Affairs* 63 (2010): pp. 446–70.

[91] The argument was that net pay after taxation was higher when claiming sickness benefit because the state benefit could not be taxed. On the rhetoric around 'scroungers' see Chapters 6 and 7 and Stuart Hall, 'The great moving right show', *The Politics of Thatcherism*, edited by Stuart Hall and Martin Jacques (London: Lawrence & Wishart, 1983), pp. 19–39.

[92] See especially the introductory paragraphs to *Cmnd 7864*, pp. 1–3.

[93] See Chapter 4 on these models of welfare. On Conservative adherence to breadwinner welfare after 1979, see: Ben Jackson, 'Free markets and feminism: The neo-liberal defence of the male breadwinner model in Britain, c. 1980–1997', *Women's History Review* 28, no. 2 (2019): pp. 297–316.

reached.[94] The health side of the DHSS required good relations with its doctors in the NHS, and the social security side had less incentive under SSP to cling to physician-signed notes. For Jenkin in 1981, the benefits were clear. The BMA would be placated, there would be less strain on the NHS, and workers would be more likely to return to work when they felt ready rather than waiting out the full week of the medical certificate.[95]

While there was split opinion among CBI members about the principle of self-certification and whether it would lead to greater absenteeism, most (albeit reluctantly) accepted the inevitability that the DHSS would bow to the BMA's demands.[96] Changes to the notes would be difficult to absorb, but if adequate access to tribunal apparatus and second opinions from doctors remained available, the system would not collapse. Besides, there seemed to be comforting news from Europe. A sick note 'strike' in Belgium resulted in a temporary system of self-certification. Absenteeism dropped because workers had returned to their jobs once they felt ready to do so rather than waiting out the full week of the certificate.[97] Unlike in the 1960s and 1970s where self-certification had been rejected based on the absenteeism rates in Sweden, it seemed this evidence was enough to help convince the CBI to give the system a go.[98] The greater consternation came from the DHSS's decision to rollout self-certification a year before SSP. The CBI made clear its concern that the DHSS appeared to be making policy solely in the context of National Insurance and industrial relations with the BMA rather than considering the needs of employers.[99] This created further points of contention for the CBI to exert pressure on the government to provide them with a better deal on the terms of SSP, most notably the size of the rebate businesses would receive on their National Insurance contributions. The first draft Bill was even scrapped in this hostile atmosphere. But enough common ground was eventually found to effect the changes, with self-certification beginning in July 1982 and SSP in April 1983.[100]

Employers had always relied upon sick notes, but the changes in SSP made explicit what had hitherto been taken for granted. The DHSS had hoped that passing the responsibility for short-term sickness onto employers would

[94] MRC: MSS 200/C/3/EMP/5/19, CBI, Self-certification: Meeting at DHSS, 24 September 1981.
[95] MRC: MSS 200/C/3/EMP/5/19, CBI, Meeting with Mr Patrick Jenkin...at Preston, 9 September 1981.
[96] The CBI set out this position to the DHSS in a letter: MRC: MSS 200/C/3/EMP/5/19, R. Worsley, Director of Social Affairs, CBI to P. R. Oglesby, DHSS, 2 October 1981.
[97] TNA: BN 118/46, W. McConnachie to A. Brown, 23 February 1981; MRC: MSS 200/C/3/EMP/5/19, Summary of the views expressed by delegates during the July and August 1981 Kininmonth Sick Pay Seminars and the reaction of the DHSS.
[98] TNA: PIN 35/150, Watkins to Swift, 6 April 1965.
[99] MRC: MSS 200/C/3/EMP/5/19, R. Worsley, Director of Social Affairs, CBI to P. R. Oglesby, DHSS, 2 October 1981.
[100] MRC: MSS 200/C/3/EMP/5/18, Leaflet, CBI, 'Why the Government needs to think again on sick pay', January 1981.

incentivize them to better police absenteeism.[101] Yet it also made businesses aware of how they were beneficiaries of collectivized approaches to sickness absence just as much as their employees. When the CBI polled its members on how it should respond to the Green Paper it found that many sectors were fearful.[102] Mining, construction and dock work produced more sickness and injury than white-collar office work. Forcing businesses to pay sickness benefits would disproportionately fall on the shoulders of businesses with higher sickness loads, whether because of occupation, workforce demographics, geography, or whatever else.[103] Different levels of risk produced conflicting responses to the SSP proposals. One smaller company argued that larger businesses might be able to absorb the costs of hiring occupational physicians and other absenteeism management teams, while small employers were less equipped to challenge patients' or doctors' certificates.[104] The personnel department at Imperial Chemical Industries countered this view, arguing the very existence of such policing procedures would lead directly to conflict with trades unions and doctors, creating problems that were hitherto handled by the 'third-party' National Insurance machinery.[105] Others argued small firms would be protected because everyone would know each other and co-workers would automatically police the 'layabout'.[106] Treating all businesses as if they had the same medical certification needs was also problematic once they became responsible for paying sickness benefits. The brewing industry, for example, wanted to know how to deal with 'sick ghosts'.[107] Given the high turnover of staff in the catering and pub trades, it was difficult to know who would have responsibility for managing sickness. Shifts were irregular, and a worker could be employed by multiple businesses in a local area. Which of the employers would be responsible for SSP? How would they share records to determine whether the claimant had used up their allocation? What was to stop someone claiming to be too ill to work at one pub and then doing a shift at the same time in another?[108] The 'ghost' claimant would be an untraceable artefact running through the payrolls of multiple businesses, while also representing a real claimant looking to secure sickness benefit from his or her employer(s).

---

[101] *Cmnd 7864.*   [102] See in particular MRC: MSS 200/C/3/EMP/5/17–21.

[103] MRC: MSS 200/C/3/EMP/5/18, Leaflet, CBI, 'Why the Government needs to think again on sick pay', January 1981.

[104] MRC: MSS 200/C/3/EMP/5/21, Lucas & Co., Knaresborough to CBI, April 1980. See also C. T. Kiching, Company Personnel Manager, Pirelli to R. Worsley, 9 July 1980.

[105] MRC: MSS 200/C/3/EMP/5/21, P. Reilly, Group Personnel Department, Imperial Chemical Industries Limited to R. Worsley, 5 August 1980. The view was backed by MRC: MSS 200/C/3/EMP/5/21, Courtaulds Limited, Coventry to R. Worsley, 10 July 1980.

[106] MRC: MSS 200/C/3/EMP/5/21, A. Cherrill, Refrigeration Spares Ltd., London to Sonia Elkin (CBI), 21 August 1980. See also: Lucas & Co., Knaresborough to CBI, April 1980.

[107] MRC: MSS 200/C/3/EMP/5/21, Government Green Paper on Sick Pay—Effect on the Retail Sector of the Brewing Industry, undated but almost certainly September or August 1980.

[108] Ibid.

While pubs concentrated on ghostbusting, criticism also came from groups representing claimants and workers. The TUC, CPAG, and The Disability Alliance (DA) all attacked SSP in poverty-lobby terms.[109] The parts of this critique that related most strongly to sick notes concerned confidentiality. Self-certification was to become the norm for week-long absence, but sick notes would still need to be written for longer spells. For the TUC:

The transfer of the decision making entirely to employers would also involve the necessity for workpeople to disclose medical evidence to their employer in all cases of sickness absence....But there is a flexibility in the present positions which will be lost under the Green Paper so that, for example, evidence of absence due to sickness could be the DHSS notification that sickness benefit has been awarded rather than the doctor's statement itself. The virtually automatic disclosure to a person's employer...of the nature of his condition, while often unexceptional, will mean in some cases that employers will get to know of conditions which may have no relevance even to the person's capacity to do his job but knowledge of which is embarrassing or distressing to the person concerned eg, certain mental illnesses, or which may lead the employer to argue that it is not something which he should pay for eg absence due to operations for and recovery from an abortion or a vasectomy.[110]

CPAG's response echoed these sentiments.[111] DA added that disabled people, who were already discriminated against in the worlds of employment and social security, could be even more vulnerable under the Green Paper's proposals.[112] If the risks of population-level sickness were passed to the employer, then companies would in turn pass these to the worker.

Small employers especially are bound to attach more importance to a person's state of health when they know that the responsibility of paying sick pay will be

---

[109] On 'poverty lobby' groups such as this and the campaigning tactics of groups like CPAG and DA, see: Paul Whiteley and Steve Winyard, *Pressure for the Poor: The Poverty Lobby and Policy Making* (London: Methuen, 1987); Pat Thane, 'Voluntary action in Britain since Beveridge', in *Beveridge and Voluntary Action in Britain and the Wider British World*, edited by Melanie Oppenheimer and Nicholas Deakin (Manchester: Manchester University Press, 2011), pp. 121–34; Matthew Hilton et al., *A Historical Guide to NGOs in Britain: Charities, Civil Society and the Voluntary Sector since 1945* (Basingstoke: Palgrave Macmillan, 2012); Jameel Hampton, *Disability and the Welfare State in Britain: Changes in Perception and Policy 1948–1979* (Bristol: Policy Press, 2016); Gareth Millward, 'Social security policy and the early disability movement – expertise, disability and the government, 1965–1977', *Twentieth Century British History* 26, no. 2 (2015): pp. 274–97.

[110] MRC: MSS 200/C/3/EMP/5/21, Trades Union Congress, 'Government Green Paper: "Income During Initial Sickness"', 30 September 1980, pp. 11–12.

[111] MRC: MSS 200/C/3/EMP/5/21, Child Poverty Action Group, 'No Way To Treat The Sick: A response to the Green Paper "Income during Initial Sickness: A New Strategy"', August 1980.

[112] CPAG and DA had close links, most evident through the work of the sociologist Peter Townsend who had been chair and co-founder of both. See the Peter Townsend Collection, University of Essex.

theirs....Existing prejudice will be reinforced and people with disabilities are at best likely to face intrusive inquiries when applying for a job.[113]

Any sick note that gave the impression that an illness might recur regularly could weaken the position of the claimant.[114] Even Remploy, the nationalized sheltered employment company that reported to the Manpower Services Commission, warned the government that the new regulations would increase its wage bill by around £1 million, a cost that could only be recovered by increased central funding or by reducing the number of 'severely disabled' employees who were at greater risk of requiring sick pay.[115] This threat appeared to be backed up by the Chairman of the Sevenoaks Branch of the National Federation of Self Employed and Small Businesses:

> Employers will naturally take steps to avoid high risk employees and will tend not to employ those who have a high risk of claim e.g. certain age groups, those with certain disabilities or conditions, those with pre-dispositions and habitual lead swingers. This will throw the burden of providing sick pay back on the State thus negating any saving to the Social Services.[116]

The TUC concluded that, aside from the moral case against breaches of confidentiality, the other benefits that sick notes provided to the welfare state would be further undermined. The changes might further 'persuade doctors to not disclose the true nature of their diagnoses on statements'. Any organization hoping to use sick notes to trace morbidity trends would be working with even less reliable data; moreover, the vaguer the diagnosis provided the more likely it would be that the employer would challenge the evidence and hold back on paying sickness benefits.[117] Such questions would become even more charged as rehabilitation and 'reasonable adjustments' for disabled and sick employees became a key battleground of employment rights discourse in the 1990s and 2000s.[118]

---

[113] MRC: MSS 200/C/3/EMP/5/21, Disability Alliance, 'The wrong strategy: The Disability Alliance's response to the Government's Green Paper on income during initial sickness', September 1980, p. 9.

[114] Similar objections were raised in the 1960s when it had been proposed sick notes could be automatically forwarded to employers. J. Herbert-Burns, 'Certification', British Medical Journal 1, no. 5484 (1966): p. 424.

[115] TNA: T 430/11, T. A. True, Company Personnel Manager, Remploy to A. Kidd, Manpower Services Commission, 5 August 1980. On the history of Remploy see Andrew Holroyde, 'Sheltered employment and disability in the classic welfare state: Remploy c. 1944–1979' (PhD thesis, University of Huddersfield, 2019); Andy Holroyde, 'Sheltered employment and mental health in Britain: Remploy c. 1945–1981', in Healthy Minds in the Twentieth Century: In and Beyond the Asylum, edited by Steven J. Taylor and Alice Brumby (Cham: Springer, 2020), pp. 113–35.

[116] MRC: MSS 200/C/3/EMP/5/21, Richard Morel to T. J. Wells, 4 July 1980.

[117] MRC: MSS 200/C/3/EMP/5/21, Trades Union Congress, 'Government Green Paper: "Income During Initial Sickness"', 30 September 1980, p. 12.

[118] See Chapters 6 and 7.

Conclusion

The incremental changes in the way sick notes were used in the welfare state from the 1960s to the 1980s show that policy does not change simply because the existing procedure is flawed. Sick notes were always a problem, especially for the BMA. Reform only happened when opportunities were created around wider problems in health and social security policy: such as the negotiations over the GPs' contract or the massive structural reforms to the NHS. The lack of compelling alternatives to sick notes meant that even though change was possible, their outright removal was not. Besides, certification was adaptable. In 1982, self-certification was a radical departure from the DHSS's and business interests' prior insistence that short-term sick notes were necessary; but beyond seven days' illness they remained.

This story exemplifies many changes in the welfare state over this period that went well beyond sick notes. As historians have noted, Conservative governments after 1979 began to favour means-tested benefits that departed from the insurance principle. The privatization of sickness benefit reflected wider commitments to a retrenchment of the welfare state and passing of responsibility for state functions from the public to the private sector. At the same time, the debates around sick notes show that the role of 'private' interests in providing welfare did not begin in the 1970s. Employers had been providing greater access to occupational sick pay since at least the 1940s. This created the conditions that allowed the DHSS to co-opt existing private payroll administrations for paying sickness benefit. Similarly, GPs—as independent contractors within the NHS system—regularly charged for private sick notes in response to demand from employers. As the perceived need for the 1940s Beveridgean welfare system declined it became possible for the opponents of Keynesean style social democracy to present and enact alternatives. Still, we see that businesses were not always enthusiastic about privatization. There were still welfare state functions built around the collectivization of risk that directly benefited employers as much as employees. The NHS, even if some of its services required a nominal payment, was a useful well of expertise for combatting absenteeism. There was always a mix of public and private provision of welfare; but gradually, over many decades, the relative burden on the various institutions with responsibilities in this area shifted. This is significance for the history of sick notes in two ways. First, as we have seen, they were adaptable to these new forms of welfare and the changing balance of public and private. Second, we can see through these changes and the everyday operation of medical certification that various welfare logics could operate at the same time depending on the relationships between the actors using these sick notes.

To emphasize the plurality of relationships and logics during the welfare state's evolution, even within the 'public' side of this equation we see that there was no singular 'government' response to these changing circumstances. The health and social security sides of the DHSS and its predecessors had differing priorities. Industrial relations with doctors were as important as maintaining the surveillance and disciplinary structures within the National Insurance system—and this is before one considers the role of multiple departments as employers of thousands. Chapters 3 and 4 similarly showed these conflicts, but 'privatization' did not remove them. Rather, it shifted the balance and helped to explain why certain departments were (or were not) willing to fight the BMA's demands for self-certification at different times.

These created two significant consequences that inform the final two chapters of this book. On the one hand, the increased responsibility for employers to monitor absenteeism meant that business groups were more vocal about sick notes and productivity than they had been in other decades. There was now a direct financial and administrative incentive to investigate the causes and effects of absenteeism, publish findings and enact recommendations on the shop floor. Combined with the changing nature of work in the post-industrial 1980s and 1990s, we see that discourse around sick notes and workers, especially in the tabloid press, took on a new character. This rhetoric was to evolve into the explicit accusations that the nation was becoming 'Sick Note Britain'.

On the other hand, the government's interest in short-term sickness waned along with its responsibility for paying benefits. Instead, the DHSS and its successor departments considered the financial burden of chronic sickness, disability, and unemployment. In its attempts to reduce the costs of social security, new ways of measuring and policing the border between capacity and incapacity led to significant reforms to disability benefits and increased political condemnation of 'scroungers'. Although new functioning tests would replace the traditional 'sick note' for such purposes, the rhetorical invocation of 'sick note' to describe these processes showed just how ingrained medical certification was in public understanding of the welfare state.

6

Chronicity and Capacity towards the New Millennium

The introduction of Statutory Sick Pay (SSP) in 1983 was just the beginning of Conservative reforms to sickness benefits. The 1980s and 1990s saw the Department of Health and Social Security (DHSS)—and its successor, the Department of Social Security (DSS)—push progressively more responsibility for the administration and payment of sick pay onto employers.[1] This reflected the rise in the percentage of firms that offered occupational sick pay schemes and the government's commitment to divest the state of functions that could be performed by the private sector. At the same time, the rise of civil rights campaigning by disabled people, coupled with increasing state expenditure on out-of-work benefits, led the DSS to fundamentally restructure the gatekeeping procedures for the new Incapacity Benefit which launched in 1995.

This chapter is about how discourses around disability and chronicity manifested in the British media and policy debates. It shows how new capacity testing regimes were introduced in the mid-1990s to replace the sick note for determining access to long-term sickness support. This was considered politically necessary because of reforms to the welfare state and British economy encouraged by Margaret Thatcher and John Major's governments. On the one hand, SSP was effectively fully privatized in 1994, meaning the social security authorities could shift their gaze solely to the matter of long-term sickness. As visibly the largest working-age benefit, demands from right-wing commentators and politicians to reduce the burden of Invalidity Benefit were loud and sustained. On the other hand, the increase in disability benefit claims had resulted from deliberate economic and social security policy. De-industrialization had caused unemployment in many parts of the United Kingdom, meaning thousands of sick and disabled people now qualified for Invalidity Benefit. Once the political benefits of 'hiding' unemployment figures in this way wore off, it became necessary for the Conservative government to attack 'scroungers' in order to reduce the social security budget.

Alongside this focus on chronicity, however, was a reappraisal of short-term sickness. It is during this same period of market liberal welfare policy that we see

---

[1] The DSS was formed after the DHSS was split into the DSS and Department of Health in 1988.

the emergence of 'sick note' as a nickname or rhetorical pejorative in the print media. The phrase echoed numerous concerns about the long-term future of the welfare state and economic health of the country. Tied into ableist narratives of productivity and obligations to the nation, they both reflected neoliberal criticism of the working-age population as well as offering a form of ironic resistance to the economic, cultural, and political changes experience in Britain over the 1980s and 1990s.

This is not to say that there was a clear cause-and-effect relationship between the cultural representation of the sick note and DSS sickness policies. Neither directly led the other. Rather, the emergence of these two discourses at the same time tells us something about the British state's anxieties around sickness from multiple constituencies. Concerned with industrial inefficiency, poor economic performance compared to its major trading partners, and rising social security expenditure, Britain looked to restructure its sickness policies and disparage those who did not perform their duties by using ill health as an excuse. Contemporaneously, the often light-hearted and diminutive use of 'Sicknote' to describe individuals was not entirely hostile. Indeed, the humour in how the phrase was often used said something about how Britain could also be critical and mocking of the sickness gatekeeping procedures and policing regimes that were becoming stricter as the millennium ended.

To show these changes, this chapter is split into three parts. The first explores the policy context of how the government gradually withdrew support for SSP, showing how official attitudes towards sickness, occupational health, and absenteeism changed over the 1980s and 1990s. When SSP was introduced, employers could claim back some of their costs from the DHSS. After 1994, the government provided no reimbursement. By design, this coloured employers' attitudes towards sickness and sick workers. Despite opposition from business federations, the Trades Union Congress (TUC), and other voluntary organizations, the government was able to force through its changes. In the second section, the chapter considers how the media began to use the term 'sick note' in new ways. It shows that the phrase expressed how some individuals were suspected of shirking responsibility by abusing sickness mechanisms. Yes, sickness was a legitimate reason for missing a court date, pulling out of a tennis tournament, or spending a day off work—but was the holder of the sick note really so incapacitated that they could not perform their duties? What if they had more moral fibre? Although these questions were often asked of high-profile cases and celebrities, particularly from the world of sport, the jokes and inference would not have worked if the term 'sick note' did not have a fundamental relevance to readers' everyday lives. In the third and final part, these attitudes towards short-term sickness are compared with the developments in long-term sickness policy. The DSS could not so easily place the burden of long-term sickness on employers as it has short-term sickness with SSP. Contemporaneously, a growing disability movement had turned any policy that could disproportionately disadvantage disabled people into a political minefield. As the government attempted to reduce social security expenditure by limiting access to various out-of-work sickness benefits across the 1980s and 1990s, alternatives to the sick note emerged. The rise of capacity testing showed how medical statements like the 'Med 3' were no longer a viable form of gatekeeping for the state, at least for managing chronic sickness. Nevertheless, the sick note and the doctor–patient relationship could provide moral justice and a richer understanding of incapacity that the British people still admired and expected to remain.

Statutory Sick Pay and Absenteeism

As discussed in the previous chapter, SSP had been introduced to reduce the state's responsibility for paying short-term sickness benefits. Over the course of the 1980s and 1990s, this process accelerated. In 1986, the length of time employers covered SSP payments went from the eight weeks mandated in the original scheme to 28 weeks. Then in 1991, employers were only allowed to claim back 80 per cent of their SSP costs; with this being reduced to zero per cent in 1994.[2] Business groups and voluntary organizations representing workers and citizens had opposed each of these moves, echoing arguments from when SSP was introduced in 1983.[3] The Confederation of British Industry (CBI) provided evidence that the costs to businesses would be too great, while the TUC, Child Poverty Action Group, Disability Alliance, and other poverty lobby organizations were concerned that people with long-term health conditions would overlooked in recruitment or forced out of their jobs.[4] There was dissent even within government. Michael Howard, the Secretary of State for Employment in 1990, had told the Treasury and DSS that removing SSP reimbursement would penalize small businesses, backed by Lord (Patrick) Jenkin who had been one of the key architects of the original SSP.[5] The National Advisory Council on Employment for Disabled People, which reported to Howard, had similar criticisms to the

[2] TNA: BN 118/197/1, Questionnaire from the European Commission on the Right to Payment of Wages on Public Holidays During Illness, 29 January 1996; Viscount Astor, 'Statutory Sick Pay Bill', *House of Lords Official Report (Hansard)*, 11 January 1994, vol. 551, cc. 79–112, at cc. 79–80.
[3] For these discussions, see Chapter 5.
[4] These arguments were made across the period. See for example, TNA: BN 118/168, Reductions of burdens on business—Statutory Sick Pay aspects, early 1986; TNA: BN 118/183, Joint letter from Association of Independent Businesses, CBI, Forum of Private Business, National Farmers Union and Union of Independent Companies to Tony Newton, 7 December 1990; TUC to Tony Newton, 11 December 1990; TNA: BIN 118/197/2, Statutory Sick Pay—Employers Reimbursement, 15 November 1993.
[5] TNA: BN 118/183, Michael Howard to Tony Newton, 14 December 1990; ibid., Lord Jenkin to Lord Henley, 7 December 1990.

poverty lobby.[6] Likewise, the state was an employer in its own right. The Northern Ireland departments for education and agriculture reminded the DHSS in 1985 that extending SSP would increase the government's own administration and payroll costs.[7] The DHSS and DSS continued to defend its policies, arguing that National Insurance contribution rebates would benefit industry overall and that there was no statistical evidence that disabled people were being denied employment as a direct result of SSP. A 'Percentage Threshold Scheme' was introduced in 1995 to help smaller businesses claim back extraordinary costs in acknowledgement of the disproportionate risk they faced relative to their turnover.[8]

Much to the DSS's chagrin, the press reported these changes as 'privatization'.[9] The Department found this rhetoric unhelpful as it had galvanized opposition. Businesses and employees still valued the collectivized protection provided by social security and resisted its removal. In its defence, the DSS argued that citizens remained covered by sick pay and that 'the Government regards the coverage of short-term sickness very much as a partnership between the State and employers'.[10] However, this privatization process was not just about state expenditure; it was part of the wider 'Thatcherite' reform of welfare state governance.[11] By continuing to increase the direct, immediate costs of sickness for employers, industry had new incentives to reduce rates of absenteeism through better preventative measures, increased monitoring, and stricter control measures.[12]

While this process enshrined the government's commitment to divest the Treasury of its responsibilities for short-term sickness, it also maintained the Thatcher and Major governments' commitments to welfare reform that upheld the 'breadwinner model' structures described in Chapter 4. SSP affirmed a sense of 'self-reliance' since access to sickness benefit required the procurement and maintenance of steady employment (and, by extension, good relations with the employer so that sickness claims would not be contested).[13] Peter Sloman has

[6] TNA: BN 118/183, Alan Smith [Chairman, National Advisory Council on Employment for Disabled People] to Michael Howard, 29 November 1990.

[7] TNA: BN 118/168, Department of Education, Northern Ireland to DHSS, 4 October 1985; ibid., Department of Agriculture, Northern Ireland to DHSS, 4 October 1985.

[8] Ibid., and TNA: BN 118/197/1, Barbara Roche, 'Government is accused of stifling competition', *Daily Express*, 5 July 1996, p. 60.

[9] TNA: BN 118/197/2, Statutory Sick Pay—Employers Reimbursement, 15 November 1993.

[10] TNA: BN 118/183, Background note on the SSP Act 1991, December 1990; BN 118/197/2, SSP—Employers Reimbursement, 15 November 1993.

[11] See Chapter 5 and Department of Health and Social Security, *Income during Initial Sickness: A New Strategy (Cmnd 7864)* (London: HMSO, 1980).

[12] See Peter Lilley commenting the Statutory Sick Pay Bill 1993 to the House at Second Reading: *House of Commons Official Report (Hansard)* (hereafter *Hansard [Commons]*), 15 December 1993, vol. 234, cc. 109–114.

[13] On 'breadwinner' models after 1980, see: Ben Jackson, 'Free markets and feminism: The neo-liberal defence of the male breadwinner model in Britain, c. 1980–1997', *Women's History Review* 28, no. 2 (2019): pp. 297–316.

detailed how in the 1980s and 1990s processes of 'Redistributive Market Liberalism' shifted benefits away from National Insurance towards means tested benefits for the poorest and a reliance upon 'the market' for the provision of other social security.[14] Workers were theoretically free to choose better employers who provided more comprehensive sick pay, if that was what they wanted; just as they were encouraged to buy their own homes and take out private pension arrangements to provide financial security over the life cycle.[15] These commitments to workplace, private benefits on the one hand and the maintenance of incentives to home-owning, nuclear family, 'breadwinner' economic units on the other, were best expressed through the introduction of Statutory Maternity Pay (SMP) in 1987. No longer able to deny women access to core benefits because of changing expectations in the wake of second-wave feminism and increased female full-time employment,[16] SMP provided a parsimonious statutory minimum upon which 'good' employers could build or individuals could privately top up. After the European Union directive on pregnant workers was implemented in 1994, SMP provided eight weeks of full pay with a further 12 weeks at the regular SSP rate.[17] Women's organizations were critical at this level of support, arguing it fell well below the statutory minimums guaranteed in the rest of Europe.[18] Pregnancy was not seen as a 'condition' that employers could (or, indeed, *should*) police. Employers could thus claim back 105 per cent of the costs of SMP to account for the expense of administering the benefit and in recognition that most employers did not provide adequate occupational maternity cover (unlike occupational sick pay).

Employers' prejudices towards women of child-bearing age, mothers, and pregnant women did not, obviously, dissolve because of this policy.[19] But it was not the expressed intention of SMP to act as a policing mechanism in the same way as SSP was designed. As with the maternity grant dilemmas of the 1950s and 1960s seen in Chapter 4, maternity was in a hinterland between being part of the government's sick note problem and being something separate from 'normal' working life; despite the significant increase in women in employment and the visibility of women's rights discourse.[20] But it was also something that could be

[14] Peter Sloman, 'Redistribution in an age of neoliberalism: Market economics, "poverty knowledge", and the growth of working-age benefits in Britain, c. 1979–2010', *Political Studies* 67, no. 3 (2019), pp. 732–51.

[15] Avner Offer, 'The market turn: From social democracy to market liberalism', *Economic History Review* 70, no. 4 (2017): pp. 1051–71.

[16] Jackson, 'Free markets and feminism'.

[17] European Council, Council Directive 92/85/EEC, 19 October 1992.

[18] TNA: BN 118/197/1, 1995 Social Security Statement, 13 November 1995; M.-J. Saurel-Cubizolles, P. Romito and J. Garcia, 'Description of maternity rights for working women in France, Italy and in the United Kingdom', *European Journal of Public Health* 3, no. 1 (1993): pp. 48–53.

[19] Helen McCarthy, *Double Lives: A History of Working Motherhood in Modern Britain* (London: Bloomsbury, 2020).

[20] Laura King, 'How men valued women's work: Labour in and outside the home in post-war Britain', *Contemporary European History* 28, no. 4 (2019): pp. 454–68.

passed onto employers as a way of reducing the state's direct involvement with administering key social security benefits.

Phil Taylor and colleagues argue that, because of the 1994 changes, businesses became increasingly preoccupied with collecting data, conducting research, and sharing information on how to discipline employees to reduce rates of absenteeism. As discussed in the next chapter, this was a feature of how sickness was portrayed and understood during the New Labour years, and certainly accelerated in the twenty-first century.[21] Nevertheless, these processes began before reimbursement for SSP ceased in 1994, informed by (and, in turn, informing) the discourse around sick notes and absenteeism. Businesses could no longer lean on free NHS sick notes for the first week of absence or the third-party National Insurance sickness benefit control measures, meaning there was greater incentive to understand sickness as a management problem. In 1993, the Labour Force Survey began its long-term monitoring of such economic metrics, but this surveillance process was already underway.[22] In October 1987, the CBI produced the first of what would become annual reports on workhour and productivity losses due to absenteeism.[23] The same week, the Industrial Society published a report on the effect of absenteeism on business.[24] Both were covered in the national press, and the CBI document was particularly influential on the DSS's policy approach in the Statutory Sick Pay Act 1991 which reduced reimbursement to 80 per cent.[25] The Department took particular note of the headline figure of £5 billion, the supposed cost of absenteeism to British industry, and how rates of non-attendance compared unfavourably to Britain's 'major trading competitors'.[26] Such narratives about absenteeism pervaded industry and government thinking. One manager in the Central Electricity Generating Board (CEGB) recalled that he instituted stricter absenteeism controls on a midlands' establishment in the 1980s. He had anecdotal evidence that workers were hungover and taking sickness absence to cover for it, but he was also able to cite CEGB statistics that showed that this plant had twice the levels of absenteeism of similar establishments, allowing him to press his case that harsher controls were needed and contend that the union and

---

[21] Phil Taylor et al., '"Too scared to go sick"—Reformulating the research agenda on sickness absence', *Industrial Relations Journal* 41, no. 4 (2010): pp. 270–88.

[22] See Chapter 1, esp. Figure 1.2, and Office for National Statistics, 'Sickness absence in the UK labour market', *gov.uk*, 3 March 2021, accessed 13 July 2021, https://www.ons.gov.uk/employmentandlabour-market/peopleinwork/employmentandemployeetypes/datasets/sicknessabsenceinthelabourmarket.

[23] Confederation of British Industry, *Absence from Work: A Survey of Non-Attendance and Sickness Absence* (London: Confederation of British Industry, 1987).

[24] The Industrial Society, *Studies of Absence Rates and Control Policies* (London: The Industrial Society, 1987).

[25] Examples of press coverage include: John Spicer, 'The high cost of absenteeism', *The Times*, 27 October 1987, p. 3; Sarah Hogg, '£5bn a year lost due to absenteeism', *Independent*, 26 October 1987, p. 20; David Norris, 'Stay-at-home workers cost firms billions', *Daily Mail*, 26 October 1987, p. 16; Andrew Cornelius, 'Absenteeism at high level', *Guardian*, 27 October 1987, p. 26.

[26] TNA: BN 118/183, 'Absenteeism', December 1990.

the workers needed to do more to self-regulate.[27] The use of such arguments was not new. Chapter 3 demonstrated how nationalized industries such as the Post Office, Royal Ordinance Factories, and the National Coal Board monitored these statistics in the 1950s. The degree to which management was willing to discipline workers had, however, increased. A steel worker in Yorkshire recounted how he felt that discipline in the industry around absenteeism had become more lax in the 1970s from how it had been when he started in the early 1960s, but it had become far stricter since privatization in the mid-1980s.[28] There was a statistical link between the level of unionization and the level of sickness absence.[29] As union power declined in the 1980s, it became easier for bosses to impose disciplinary action on workers. And while it was still possible to use sickness as a tool for collective bargaining—British Airways staff, for example, used mass sick leave to press their demands[30]—the destruction of traditionally heavy, unionized industries had significantly weakened resistance.[31] What this shows is that neoliberal policies of market-driven welfare and disciplining of workers were not simply led by 'the government'. Yes, businesses were pushed towards these actions because of the decline of the collectivist forms of National Insurance upon which they had relied in the 'classic welfare state' era—but these changes were reflective of, and caused by, wider cultural, political, and economic shifts that had been building before the 1970s and came of age in the 1980s.[32]

The Sick Note in Media Culture

At the same time as the state was pulling away from short-term sickness provision and the private sector was increasing its surveillance of sickness in the workplace, Britain's public discourse around sickness was noticeably changing. This is most evident in the way that the phrase 'sick note' began to be used more frequently in the press from the late 1980s to describe a range of behaviours, usually with a

[27] British Library Oral History Archive: Camsey, Granville (11 of 16). An Oral History of the Electricity Supply in the UK, accessed 16 July 2020, https://sounds.bl.uk/Oral-history/Food/021M-C0821X0007XX-0010V0.

[28] British Library Oral History Archive: Wood, Paul (3 of 4) National Life Story Collection: Lives in Steel, accessed 16 July 2020, https://sounds.bl.uk/Oral-history/Food/021M-C0821X0007XX-0010V0.

[29] Laszlo Goerke, 'Sick pay reforms and health status in a unionized labour market', *Scottish Journal of Political Economy* 64, no. 2 (2017): pp. 115–42.

[30] 'BA warning to staff in "sick note" strike ploy', *Daily Mail*, 7 August 1997, p. 25.

[31] Stephen Machin, 'Union Decline in Britain', *British Journal of Industrial Relations* 38, no. 4 (2000): pp. 631–45.

[32] On these processes and on the role of business in welfare provision, see: J. Vernon, 'Heathrow and the making of neoliberal Britain', *Past & Present* (2021). Jeppe Nevers and Thomas Paster, 'Business and the Nordic Welfare States, 1890–1970', *Scandinavian Journal of History* 44, no. 5 (2019): pp. 535–51.

light-hearted, but negative, tone.[33] 'Sicknote' became a nickname. *The Times* ran a series of pocket cartoons by Mel Calman under the title 'Sick Note' in 1987. They depicted a man complaining about his health anxieties, usually to his long-suffering wife.[34] Calman's work here and elsewhere was intended as a commentary on everyday life. According to his *Times* obituary, 'his worried Everyman was the man on the Clapham omnibus',[35] and that 'future historians will develop a truer picture of the past generation from Calman's little commentaries than from bigger memoirs and official statistics'.[36] The character Bert Quigley in ITV serial drama *London's Burning* was given the name in the pilot episode in 1986 due to his hypochondria.[37] The reference would not have worked if it did not tap into something present in workplace culture in the 1980s.

It was nevertheless on the back pages that the term appeared most frequently. The highest profile 'Sicknote' was Darren Anderton, the England international footballer who played for Portsmouth and Tottenham Hotspur in the 1990s. 'He's prone to more than his fair share of illness', explained journalist Trevor Haylett in 1992.[38] Anderton suspected the reason the name became public was because a local Portsmouth journalist had moved to a national title and repeated it enough for it to stick.[39] Aston Villa forward Dalian Atkinson had also been 'dubbed "Sicknote" by the Villa fanzine because of his past tendency to absenteeism'.[40] In these cases, the nicknames were ribbing by teammates and fans of the players' own clubs. The joke worked because it referenced behaviour seen in everyday life. But it could soon wear off when hurled by frustrated supporters, especially as the perception of being 'injury prone' could affect a player's value in the eyes of potential employers.[41] To be injured was to fail to live up to the masculine ideal of sport. Bodies were supposed to be robust and players were expected to play through pain. In an era where English football was in transition from an idealized masculine space of hard-but-fair play, terraces, and muddy pitches to the Premier League's global, family-oriented television product, it is perhaps unsurprising that

---

[33] A search of the digital archives of *Daily Mail*, *Independent*, *The Times*, *Sunday Times*, *Guardian* and *Observer* for the period after 1985 produces these results.

[34] The strip first appears at: Calman, 'Sick note', *The Times*, 26 March 1987, p. 14.

[35] While adding, 'except that Calman would not have known how to catch a bus or where Clapham was'.

[36] 'Obituaries – Mel Calman', *The Times*, 12 February 1994, p. 19.

[37] 'Bert "Sicknote" Quigley', Fandom—London's Burning Wiki, accessed 31 January 2019, https://londons-burning.fandom.com/wiki/Bert_per cent27Sicknoteper cent27_Quigley.

[38] Trevor Haylett, 'Shy assassin has Wembley in his sights', *Daily Mail*, 3 April 1992, p. 62.

[39] See the Introduction to this book and Andrew Murray, 'A warning for Mourinho? Anderton bemoans having to pay through injury', *FourFourTwo*, 9 November 2016, accessed 31 January 2019, www.fourfourtwo.com/features/be-careful-forcing-players-play-through-injury-mou-darren-anderton-told-us.

[40] Phil Shaw, 'Saunders lands the inevitable sucker punch', *Independent*, 21 September 1992, p. 26.

[41] Anderton himself has been critical at the mockery in the press and from fans. Murray, 'A warning for Mourinho?'

such nicknames developed around this time.[42] The irony is that Sicknote's desire to play through pain and disprove the moniker undoubtedly contributed to the very injuries for which players were mocked.[43] As Jasbir Puar has argued, globalized capitalism contains within it forces that can injure people while at the same time demanding productivity from those same people its health services keep alive. These processes of 'debility' have implications for disability rights movements and discourses, as discussed later in this chapter and the next.[44] But here, the mocking of 'Sicknote' was part of the very same economic pressures on Anderton's body that caused him to fail to meet the expectations of his 'employers'. The problems of the 'acute' could thus never be separated from the 'chronic' stresses that employment caused for workers.

Although the term was overwhelmingly used for male athletes, 'Sicknotes' were not just about masculine bodies. In tennis, where there was higher-profile female representation than in major team sports, both men and women came under scrutiny. Yugoslavia's Monica Seles—the women's world number one—was banned from the Barcelona Olympics for pulling out of the Federation Cup in 1991 after her reason for withdrawal was considered unsatisfactory. British number one Jo Durie also withdrew but, noted the *Independent*, she had 'a legitimate sick note'.[45] Similarly, Boris Becker, the German three-time men's Wimbledon champion, had to travel to Rome to prove that he 'really' did have an injury that had forced him out of the 1992 Italian Open. The Association of Tennis Professionals compelled players to attend in person to verify injuries after a spate of withdrawals had caused embarrassment for sponsors and television partners. If players wanted to take part in the high-prestige Grand Slams they had certain obligations to the rest of the tour.[46] The idea of sick notes being a release from obligations pervaded this discourse, but there was a clear undertone that the mere possession of a sick note—even if 'legitimate'—was not enough. If players had a duty to sponsors and television partners, they also had a duty to the fans. Individuals could not pick and choose which work they performed in this globalized sporting environment.

Seles and Durie also highlighted that the British press was particularly scathing of athletes who shirked their responsibilities to national representative teams and,

---

[42] Hans Westerbeek and Aaron Smith, *Sport Business in the Global Marketplace* (London: Palgrave Macmillan, 2003); Tony Collins, *Sport in Capitalist Society: A Short History* (New York: Routledge, 2013).

[43] Murray, 'A warning for Mourinho?'. See also the treatment of Michael Owen, a generation after Anderton: Richard Arrowsmith, 'Fergie's right! Michael Owen blames Liverpool for his injury strewn career', *Mirror*, 7 December 2012, accessed 21 February 2021, https://www.mirror.co.uk/sport/football/news/michael-owen-agrees-with-alex-ferguson-1478102.

[44] Jasbir K. Puar, *The Right to Maim: Debility, Capacity, Disability* (Durham: Duke University Press, 2017). On disability as a creation of modernity and industrialization, see: Michael Oliver and Colin Barnes, *The New Politics of Disablement* (Basingstoke: Palgrave Macmillan, 2012).

[45] 'Olympic ban for Seles', *Independent*, 17 August 1991, p. 40.

[46] Mike Dickson, 'Becker trek to prove sick-note is genuine', *Daily Mail*, 14 May 1992, p. 51.

by association, the country at large. Players were regularly chastised for 'sick notes' sent to the England men's team's international soccer fixtures, with the implication that players prioritized more-lucrative club games. (Although Ryan Giggs of the Welsh football team and several members of the English cricket side were not immune to this accusation.)[47] Still, it seemed some were better at the grift than others. 'Are women athletes less susceptible to injury than men or are men just better at making excuses?' asked David Powell in *The Times*.[48] Thirteen track and field athletes had withdrawn from the 1995 national trials in Birmingham, many at short notice, meaning that there was little time to give a full medical exam and verify the injuries. Of those, nine were men. The advantage for the skivers was that athletes' performances across recent events would be considered for selection rather than their result in the trials—which, if they lost, could mean they were not selected for the upcoming World Championships. Powell added, 'it may be time to clamp down on athletes who, by taking the route that permits their absence...circumvent the British Athletic Federation's insistence that they must compete in the trials if they want to be selected'.[49] The incident infuriated selectors and National Championships organizers, especially as they had made concessions to world champion 100 metre sprinter Linford Christie to satiate the television audience, even though he had lost in the first round.[50]

Sick notes represented technical evasion, with ever-rising stakes as the money around sport—and the expectations from fans—increased in the global television era. Nothing exemplified this more than the Tonya Harding saga, which had transcended American sport to become an international celebrity gossip story. 'Harding now claims to have been attacked while walking alone across a park at midnight', noted Alan Hubbard in the *Observer*. She was due to give evidence to the US Figure Skating Association's ethics committee after her rival Nancy Kerrigan was attacked with a baton before the 1994 Winter Olympics. Most suspected Harding and her ex-husband had arranged it.[51] 'No doubt she will be sending them a sick note', Hubbard joked.[52] Somewhat ironically, Kerrigan was

[47] Martin Johnson, 'Gower gripped by a grey depression', *The Times*, 31 July 1989, p. 29; Alan Lee, 'England turn to young bowlers', *The Times*, 7 September 1990, p. 38; Jeff Powell, 'European League will hold the aces in battle between club and country', *Daily Mail*, 27 April 1992, p. 36; Rob Hughes, 'Club versus country controversy rages on', *The Times*, 10 September 1994, p. 40; Rob Hughes, 'Sick notes claim fantasy first eleven', *The Times*, 24 March 1997, p. 25.

[48] David Powell, 'Women impress Cropper by a distance', *The Times*, 18 July 1995, p. 40.

[49] Ibid.

[50] David Miller, 'Christie and Jackson run foul of Radford', *The Times*, 18 July 1995, p. 40; John Rodda, 'Christie runs into another controversy', *Observer*, 16 July 1995, p. B2.

[51] Stephanie Foote, 'Making sport of Tonya: Class performance and social punishment', *Journal of Sport and Social Issues* 27, no. 1 (2003): pp. 3–17; Craig Gilespie (dir.), *I, Tonya* (Neon, 2017).

[52] Alan Hubbard, 'New twist in the tale of the tape', *Observer*, 6 March 1994, p. 57.

given one of the two USA berths at the Olympics despite missing the national trials with the injury. Her sick note—and her moral desert—were accepted.

Importantly, 'sick note' was not confined to the demesne of sport. The metaphor articulated several criticisms. It implied an evasion of duty, an 'excuse' that, while technically correct, was ethically dubious, a moral failing in note's bearer. One of the more notorious examples was that of actor Stephen Fry. In 1995, Fry disappeared after a West End performance of Cell Mates, causing the show's run to be cancelled. Initially, there was speculation that Fry was merely a 'luvvie' who had run away after some negative reviews.[53] Missing for several days, he was eventually spotted in Belgium. Fry was required to give doctor's evidence—a 'sick note' as the press called it—to prove that he had in fact suffered a mental breakdown, allowing the theatre to claim on its insurance for the cancelled show.[54] This was not enough to stop legal proceedings against him for £500,000 in damages.[55] Over twenty years later, Fry would finally publicly acknowledge the severity of his illness, his subsequent diagnosis of bi-polar disorder, and that he had come very close to taking his own life.[56] Playwright Simon Gray and co-star Rik Mayall were not fully aware of this during their lifetimes and attacked Fry for his lack of fortitude. 'You don't leave the trenches', remarked Mayall in an interview in 2007. 'Selfishness is one thing, being a cunt is another.'[57] Although, as a letter to the Guardian argued with regard to Gray's attacks on Fry:

Calling Mr Fry a "skulking defector"…says more about Mr Gray than Mr Fry. The suggestion is that Mr Fry lacks "moral fibre". His upper lip isn't stiff enough. Stephen Fry is an actor; he's not leading his "chaps" out of the trenches to certain death. When are the English going to treat depression as an illness?[58]

It is not clear from the articles discussed here whether the criticisms of Fry's 'luvvie' excuses were also tied to homophobic tropes about masculinity, but there were certainly gendered critiques of 'celebrity culture' elsewhere in turn-of-the-millennium media. Six years after Cell Mates, Martine McCutcheon garnered the nickname 'sicknote' for leaving the play My Fair Lady some five months before it closed. She had contracted a throat infection that had required hospital care, but

---

[53] Richard Brooks and Marin Wroe, 'Fry's fright and flight is in rich luvvie tradition', Observer, 26 February 1995, p. 7.

[54] John Ezard, 'Fry stages return to get sick note', Guardian, 3 March 1995, p. 24.

[55] Owen Bowcott, 'Stephen Fry cast as villain as row over play's closure goes to court', Guardian, 30 March 1995, p. 7.

[56] See for example his interview in A Life on Screen—Stephen Fry, broadcast BBC Four, 14 July 2018.

[57] Mark Shenton, 'Interview with Rik Mayall', Theatre.com, 11 January 2007, accessed 24 November 2020, archived 24 November 2020, https://web.archive.org/web/20070513082433/http://www.theatre.com/story/id/3005429/.

[58] Rosie Norton and Peter Roberts letter to Guardian, 6 March 1995, p. 21.

shortly thereafter was seen in West End restaurants enjoying a night out with friends. The tabloid press took this as a sign that she was a malingerer—either she was sick and should remain out of the public gaze, or was well and should do the job she was paid to do.[59] Nick Curtis, an *Evening Standard* columnist writing for the *This Is London* website, linked her with other 'MAW (the model-actress-whatever), those who are famous for being famous', who had missed various public dates in recent months. The hard-working Carol Vorderman and Davina McCall were apparently not part of the celebrity hedonism and were better role models. Dropping casual references to two men (Michael Barrymore and Robbie Williams) among the many 'MAW' under scrutiny in the piece to show this was not exclusively an attack on women, Curtis opined that those like McCutcheon, Kate Moss, or Celeste were not really 'exhausted'. ' "Exhaustion" and its cousin "stress" are often euphemisms for something else, something chemically addictive', he claimed.[60] Meanwhile, the *Agenda* column in the *Sunday Times* gave a glowing review to McCutcheon's successor, Joanna Riding, comparing her professionalism with 'Sicknote' and noting that Riding won the Olivier Award for playing Eliza Doolittle in *My Fair Lady* in 2003.[61] This would have been quite an indictment of McCutcheon—if she had not won the same award for the same role in 2002.

Like the 1990s' sport stars and more recent cases such as that of Naomi Osaka pulling out of the 2021 French Open citing mental health issues, Fry and McCutcheon had obligations to their audience and the chain of business interests surrounding their performances. But they were not the only people whose 'excuses' for sidestepping legal duties were doubted. 'A sick note from a man accused of drug dealing listed so many ailments that the writer appeared to have run out of paper', reported the *Guardian* in June 1996;[62] while earlier that same year a pet cemetery owner had her sentence extended by three months after she used a sick note to try and flee the country while on trial for pretending to bury animals in elaborate caskets.[63]

Not all sick notes were suspected forgeries like in the cases above, but the convenience of their arrival was questioned. The metaphor extended to politicians who missed debates or votes in the Houses of Parliament. Andrew Rawnsley in his *Guardian* Sketch drew attention to Chancellor Norman Lamont's 'sick note' ('a prior engagement with the Treasury Select Committee') and Home Secretary

---

[59]   Mark Lawson, 'We assume they're faking it', *Guardian*, 14 April 2001, p. 20.

[60]   Nick Curtis, 'Exhaustion – the celebrity fad', *This Is London*, 9 March 2001, accessed 3 December 2018, archived 24 November 2001. http://web.archive.org/web/20011124215949/http://www.thisislondon. co.uk:80/dynamic/lifestyle/londonlife/review.html?in_review_id=369680&in_review_text_ id=315199.

[61]   Agenda, *Sunday Times*, 9 November 2003, p. 10.

[62]   'Drug defendant's multiple ailments leave judge unimpressed', *Guardian*, 29 June 1996, p. 5.

[63]   'Pet undertaker jailed', *The Times*, 27 February 1996, p. 2.

Robin Cook's 'pressing engagement with the Spanish Foreign Minister'.[64] But the metaphor worked because it drew on the experience of people's working lives. For instance, employers had long suspected that the increase in sick days given to workers had meant many employees saw their sick days not as emergency leave but as part of their regular holiday entitlement. An Industrial Society research paper in 1997 noted that managers were increasingly sceptical of diagnoses on sick notes, with a third of bosses attributing absenteeism to 'low morale and boredom'.[65] Yet, there was a qualitative difference between a questionable 'sick note' case and one where the medical certificate and reason for absence was genuine. One female employee at a Birmingham factory in the early 1980s recalled that when her father died she found it easy to get time off: 'but having said that, I never took time off work when I didn't need it. And I think that [management] do know the people that are genuine.... They know the ones that aren't genuine.'[66] Indeed, the knowledge that one could be seen as a malingerer could colour the relationship between the doctor and the patient looking to assuage doubt. Roy Hattersley, then Deputy Leader of the Labour Party, wrote in a *Guardian* column about going to hospital with back trouble in 1986. The piece is light-hearted, but, like Calman's cartoons, has a deeper meaning for 'future historians':

> Proper doctors always ask if you want a sick note. But they are careful not to write upon it the dreaded diagnosis 'bad back'. For nobody takes bad backs seriously.... They write 'trapped nerve' or 'displaced vertebrae' and they smile comforting smiles. At least, I think that's what they do. They may really be suppressing the laughter which is the natural reaction to the opening line 'Doctor, I've got a bad back'.[67]

Another tongue-in-cheek article gave advice on 'how to skive'. While lamenting that self-certification in the 1980s had not allowed workers to swing the lead with impunity with 'friendly "bad back" doctors', one could always dodge the boss's control procedures though 'intimidation'. 'Casually mention an array of medical advisers – specialists, physiotherapists, masseurs', it recommended, and then simply say that you need the day off to attend an appointment.[68] The joke reflected the growing number of health specialists within and outside the NHS concentrating on rehabilitation and occupational health while hinting at the ways

---

[64] Andre Rawnsley, 'Sketch', *Guardian*, 20 February 1992, p. 6; Andrew Rawsnsley, 'Andrew Rawnsley's guide to the political leaders of the left', *Observer*, 14 December 1997, p. 27.

[65] Reported in Neasa MacErlean, 'Sick and fired as firms count cost of absence', *Observer* (9 March 1997), p. A11.

[66] British Library Oral History Archive: Wellings, Olive (10 of 14). 'Food: From source to salespoint', accessed 15 July 2020, https://sounds.bl.uk/Oral-history/Food/021M-C0821X0007XX-0010V0.

[67] Roy Hattersley, 'Endpiece', *Guardian*, 13 September 1986, p. 19.

[68] 'How to skive', *Observer*, 3 October 1993, p. E3.

employers attempted to press the responsibility for health maintenance and recovery onto the individual worker.[69] Having done this, bosses could not reasonably object to visiting the physio—and who were they to overrule the expertise of a specialist?

Doubt around medical certificates could, however, be dangerous. They provided more than just technical cover for employees. They were regularly cited in employment scandals, especially around workplace bullying and unsafe working environments. It is here that the 'sick note' ceased to be euphemistic, a shorthand that allowed for personal attacks in a way that could not be confronted as head-on as Mayall and Gray were in the *Guardian*. They were literal (in the sense that they referred to actual medical reports) and a critique of the debilitating effects of overwork and partial rehabilitation that led to presenteeism and ultimate breakdown.[70]

In these stories, media outlets were quick to mention that a worker had provided a 'sick note'. By drawing attention to it, employers' poor behaviour was amplified. In the case of a nurse who took her own life after overwhelming work pressure from management, an employer wrote to her that 'he found it "disappointing" that she had submitted another sick note' for depression, threatening 'the longer she remained off work, the more difficult she would find it to return'. Ignoring the certificate and piling more pressure on the nurse was evidence of the hospital's unreasonableness and responsibility for her death.[71] So too was a Catholic school damned when it dismissed a woman who was pregnant with a priest's baby and took leave with a combination of maternity and 'nervous exhaustion'. The pressure she had been put under to keep the affair quiet was a significant contributor.[72] The *Independent on Sunday* made it very clear that it was in employers' best interests to take such diagnoses seriously. 'The cost to companies of staff buckling under strain runs into billions', wrote Tom Maddocks, turning the 'price of absenteeism' rhetoric on its head, 'but few are doing anything about it. This may change as employees sue.'[73] This would be affirmed by a case against Northumberland County Council, in which a social worker 'was twice driven to a nervous breakdown by stress and overwork' and accepted £175,000 in compensation.[74] The sick note, then, was resistance against 'debility'[75]—even if it was not always successful as a prophylactic, it could hold powerful organizations in check with the legal threats attached to it.

---

[69] For more on this phenomenon, see Chapter 7.   [70] Puar, *The Right to Maim*.

[71] Judy Jones, 'Double suicide blamed on NHS upheaval', *Observer*, 4 June 1995, p. 10.

[72] Robi Dutta, 'Church "told pregnant lover of priest to quit"', *The Times*, 11 August 1994, p. 3.

[73] Tom Maddocks, 'Employers miss the stress signals', *Independent on Sunday*, 10 October 1993, p. 6. On presenteeism, see Chapters 7 and 8.

[74] Peter Foster, 'Social worker wins £175,000 after stress ends career', *The Times* (27 April 1996), p. 6.

[75] Puar, *The Right to Maim*.

The references to mental health in these cases also highlight how views on workplace sickness were shifting. De-industrialization, changing demographics, and the rise of the service economy had altered the nature of work in Britain.[76] Inevitably, it also altered the concept of 'incapacity'. State concern for industrial injuries had shifted towards Health and Safety legislation and regulation.[77] 'Stress' was becoming a more common citation. But stress was not simply the result of bullying or acute pressures at work. Its meaning and cultural understanding, as Jill Kirby has demonstrated, changed over the course of the twentieth century.[78] Stress and other mental health conditions were becoming appreciated as legitimate reasons for short-term sickness—Curtis's 'chemical' jibe notwithstanding—and not (necessarily) disabling conditions that required early retirement. One claimant expressed pleasant surprise that her GP was sympathetic to her panic attacks. After picking up her sick note, she remarked, 'I'd expected them to say: "Pull yourself together."'[79] Other conditions were more difficult. Myalgic encephalomyelitis (ME) and chronic fatigue syndrome gained notoriety at this time but were hard to diagnose, and there was scepticism among a significant section of the medical profession about whether these were physical/neurological conditions or psychosomatic mental disorders.[80] Similarly, AIDS represented a new type of threat to the health of the nation and, potentially, the workforce. NHS staff lobbied the government in the early years of the crisis to classify AIDS as an occupational disease so that health workers could claim industrial injuries benefits if they contracted it.[81] These benefits paid at a higher rate than regular sickness benefits and could include a lump sum payment. In part, the desire to be categorized in a specific benefit category reflected the fear, unfamiliarity, and stigma around the disease in the 1980s. It was seen by many as a 'death sentence', one that those who did not engage in 'risky' behaviours (such as unprotected anal sex or

---

[76] Jim Tomlinson, 'De-industrialization: Strengths and weaknesses as a key concept for understanding post-war British history', *Urban History* 47, no. 2 (2020): pp. 199–219. See also: Blessing Chiripanhura and Nikolas Wolf, 'Long-term trends in UK employment: 1861 to 2018', Office of National Statistics, 29 April 2019, accessed 24 November 2020, https://www.ons.gov.uk/economy/nationalaccounts/uksectoraccounts/compendium/economicreview/april2019/longtermtrendsinukemployment1861to2018.

[77] Christopher Sirrs, 'Accidents and apathy: The construction of the "Robens Philosophy" of occupational safety and health regulation in Britain, 1961–1974', *Social History of Medicine* 29, no. 1 (2016): pp. 66–88.

[78] Jill Kirby, *Feeling the Strain: A Cultural History of Stress in Twentieth-Century Britain* (Manchester: Manchester University Press, 2019). See also Mark Jackson (ed.), *Stress in Post-War Britain, 1945–85* (Abingdon: Routledge, 2013).

[79] John Illman, 'The terror within', *Guardian*, 26 April 1995, p. A4.

[80] G. P. Holmes et al., 'Chronic fatigue syndrome: A working case definition', *Annals of Internal Medicine* 108, no. 3 (1988): pp. 387–9; Department of Health, *A Report of the CFS/ME Working Group: Report to the Chief Medical Officer of an Independent Working Group* (London: Department of Health, 2002). See also: Louise Sargent, 'A short history of myalgic encephalomyelitis', M.E. Support, accessed 16 July 2020, archived 17 March 2016, https://web.archive.org/web/20160317130141/http://mesupport.co.uk/index.php?page=a-short-history-of-m-e.

[81] See policy documentation in TNA: PIN 20/906/1–2 from 1985 to 1988.

intravenous drug use) could only contract by forced exposure to 'carriers'.[82] But this also exposed how inadequate social security provision was for people living with fluctuating conditions that had no prospect for full 'recovery' yet could still limit one's ability to gain and maintain a job. As one HIV-affected man in 1993 described his experiences:

> I used to be a car hire manager...but I decided to leave that job because I was becoming ill....People were becoming suspicious about my continued stays in hospital. Then I got a job with the Post Office, but shortly after that I became ill again....The doctor wrote something about "Aids-related complications" on my sick-note and that set alarm bells ringing at the Post Office. I haven't worked for two years now.[83]

Aside from the discrimination against people living with HIV/AIDS in employment, the increased risk of sickness (acute and chronic) meant claimants were less likely to have access to long-term state sickness benefits or short-term SSP. Furthermore, as a disease that disproportionately affected gay men, it was more difficult for claimants and their loved ones to gain access to carer benefits and other forms of protection that were still designed for the heteronormative nuclear family.[84] For these very reasons, as George Severs' research has shown, activists often deliberately sought employment so that they could qualify for SSP and gain access to the privatized world of 1980s social security.[85] But not all were able or willing to do this. The Terrence Higgins Trust and local campaign groups pressed the DSS in the late 1980s to improve provision for individuals and families affected by HIV/AIDS, with little success.[86]

Still, the increase in the diagnosis of 'new' conditions was treated with suspicion, especially from the political right. A sketch in the *Daily Mail* in 1995 imagined a game show where celebrities had to guess 'what's my skive?' Asking 'is there anything for which you can be sacked lawfully any more', attacks were made on Gulf War syndrome and 'malingerer's excuse' (ME), along with a homophobic

---

[82] Hannah J. Elizabeth, 'Love carefully and without "over-bearing fears": The persuasive power of authenticity in late 1980s British AIDS education material for adolescents', *Social History of Medicine* (2020).

[83] 'Michael and Kevin', *Guardian*, 17 April 1993, p. A20.

[84] The reasons for this and the relationship between secure employment and benefit entitlement are outlined in Chapter 4.

[85] I am indebted to George Severs for sharing drafts of his on-going PhD research at Cambridge University.

[86] Alex Brazier, *A Double Deficiency? A Report on the Social Security Act 1986 and People with Acquired Immune Deficiency Syndrome (AIDS), AIDS Related Complex (ARC) and HIV Infection* (London: Terrence Higgins Trust, 1989). I am thankful to Hannah Elizabeth and George Severs for discussions about this topic and their research into the relationship between HIV/AIDS families of choice and the state. For DSS policy on AIDS see TNA: BN 143/296, Act Up Nottingham leaflet, attached to memorandum 31 July 1990; Martin Eede, Chief Executive, The Terrence Higgins Trust to Gillian Shepherd, Under-secretary of State, DSS, 16 July 1990.

pastiche of Julian Clary.[87] A Richard Littlejohn column a fortnight later imagines a doctor's surgery with various hypochondriacs and malingerers coming to the surgery: a territorial army cadet who has never left the country says he has 'Gulf War syndrome'; a police officer says he has 'post traumatic stress disorder' (PTSD) and wants the sick note to time conveniently with a cricket test match; another woman claims to have 'yuppie flu' (a common derogatory euphemism for ME) despite having appeared on the gameshow *Blind Date* earlier in the week. A woman has her diagnosis upgraded from 'PMT' (pre-menstrual tension) to 'PostMenstrual Trauma' (dismissing the legitimacy of both PMT and PTSD) before telling the GP she will be back next week with a migraine. The piece ends with another woman who thinks she has been raped because she was drunk, using drugs, and 'that's what the equality officer at the Students' Union told me'. The punchline is that she cannot get help because all the police are off sick with PTSD.[88] Littlejohn's ableist and sexist jokes could only work—if indeed they ever did—because of the general suspicion that sick notes and mental health 'excuses' were regularly used by lazy workers to avoid obligations. Sick notes were also explicitly tied to other supposed ills in society such as reality game shows, female drunkenness, crime rates, reduced shame in talking about sexual assault, drug taking, and the weakening of the armed forces. These reactionary sketches did, however, hint that the common sense around sickness was shifting.[89] Even if certain conservative voices believed employee protections had gone too far, clearly a large enough section of the legal profession and progressive voices in employment disagreed.

Chronic Sickness and Capacity Testing

While the discussions about sick notes explicitly focused on short-term sickness, the rhetoric cannot be separated from wider anxieties about long-term illness and disability. 'Sick note' was a source of humour because it represented a fundamental failure of the gatekeeping system to reliably determine who was and was not 'really' sick. Reforms to SSP had been brought in to try to deal with these prob-lems with short-term conditions in the workplace by transferring the economic and administrative responsibility onto employers. However, the DSS was still responsible for unemployed sick claimants, many of whom claimed disability-related benefits. Here the focus was not on absenteeism (as with SSP) but economic inactivity and continued concerns about potential abuse of sickness

---

[87] 'The skive's the limit', *Daily Mail*, 23 June 1995, p. 13.
[88] Richard Littlejohn, 'Blind Date, blind drunk? It's time for a week off', *Daily Mail*, 7 July 1995, p. 11.
[89] Gareth Millward, '"A matter of commonsense": The Coventry poliomyelitis epidemic 1957 and the British public', *Contemporary British History* 31, no. 3 (2016): pp. 384–406.

systems. One way in which Conservative governments hoped to combat these pressures was to move away from using sick notes and GPs as the gatekeepers to out of work sickness benefits. Medical certificates were no longer seen as appropriate for disabled people as they did not adequately assess individuals' needs and could lock them into a life of benefits; even if it was not in their best physical, psychological, or financial interests. The sick note might have been useful in certain circumstances for employed people in the short-term, but the DSS needed a new form of assessment to draw a distinction between its bureaucratic categories of 'the sick' (who were incapable of work) and 'the disabled' (who were not).[90]

Concerns around chronic sickness were not new. One of the reasons sick notes had been key to the Beveridge report's plans for the postwar welfare state was their link to rehabilitation. It would be just as necessary to get people *back* to work as to preventing them from leaving. Medical certification, however, was only as useful as the regulations that used them. On the one hand, regulations could create demand for certificates that was unnecessary. The BMA's Annual Representative Meeting in 1948 pointed out the absurdity of having to write four-week and eight-week certificates for conditions that were 'obviously' not going to improve, such as permanent blindness or amputation.[91] An example of this in action comes from a London claimant in 1961 who had been in receipt of sickness benefit due to 'mental disorder' since the Appointed Day. The hospital in which he had stayed in the early 1950s certified that he was 'totally incapable of work and would remain so', but he was continually asked for sick notes to renew his claim. Frustrated, in 1955 he refused to submit any more. His local office knew the case and continued to pay anyway using discretionary powers; but such demands were not useful to anyone.[92]

Borderline cases were also difficult to resolve when the existence of a medical condition was not the fact under dispute. Two examples in the late 1960s of firefighters in Plymouth who had developed mental health conditions as a result of their work demonstrated this. There was no doubt that the two men involved were ill: one with 'nervous disability' and 'complete dependence on drugs'; the other with depression and headaches. The dispute with the National Insurance and fire brigade authorities had been not over whether the men could continue as firefighters, as it was clear even to the men themselves that they could not. The issue was whether they could work in other industries and should therefore cease

---

[90] Gordon Waddell et al., *The Scientific and Conceptual Basis of Incapacity Benefits* (London: TSO, 2005).

[91] TNA: MH 153/743, BMA, Resolutions of A.R.M., 1948. See also the BMA's requests in: National Insurance Advisory Committee, *Report of the National Insurance Advisory Committee on the Question of Doctors' and Midwives' Certificates for National Insurance Purposes (Cmnd 1021)* (London: HMSO, 1960).

[92] TNA: PIN 35/226, Report on [HT], 1 March 1961.

to receive public funds.[93] Similarly, a blind man from Lincolnshire sought help from his MP when there was a dispute over whether he was 'sick' or 'unemployed' after being made redundant in 1970. There was no work in his area and little chance, given he was in his mid-fifties, of more training. The issue was resolved, but a doctor still had to write him a sick note every 13 weeks.[94] As will be seen in Chapter 7, these borderline cases, particularly around mental illness, were never easy to settle—and the medical evidence provided was among the least of the problems. The political situation in the 1990s, however, compelled authorities to reconsider how medical evidence was used.

Expenditure on Invalidity Benefit since it was introduced in 1971 had increased significantly (Figure 6.1). Created as the first of a raft of new disability benefits by Conservative and Labour governments in the 1970s, Invalidity Benefit was designed for long-term National Insurance sickness benefit claimants who were unemployed.[95] In 1972/73, it cost the DHSS £196 million. By 1994/95 it cost £7.7 billion.[96] The reasons for this growth were complex, but a significant contributor was that thousands of people, especially from deindustrialized areas, became eligible for Invalidity Benefit when they lost their jobs in the economic downturns of the 1980s and 1990s. Their medical conditions were genuine and had been accommodated in their old employment but because they did not find new jobs they remained on the benefit rolls as Incapacity Benefit claimants (rather than contributing to the government's unemployment figures). A generally ageing population and the increasing eligibility of married women with National Insurance contributions records also added to the figures.[97] Processes of 'debility' were therefore clear.[98] The economic system had created this increase in disability, in one sense by the toll industrial work had on the bodies on those it employed, and in another by its reclassification of the economic inactivity resulting from the interaction between these impairments and industrial policy. The government was no longer willing to pay for this form of 'unemployment', simultaneously creating the disability that made it more difficult for these claimants to find work and demanding that these same individuals become self-sufficient.

[93] See discussions in TNA: PIN 35/226, esp. Chief Fire Officer Ralph Havery to the manager of Plymouth DHSS, 2 December 1969; Chief Insurance Office to GP Gent, 17 March 1969.

[94] TNA: PIN 35/435/1, R. Stott (Department of Employment) to P. G. H. Ewer (DHSS), 27 June 1974.

[95] Gareth Millward, 'Social security policy and the early disability movement – expertise, disability and the government, 1965–1977', Twentieth Century British History 26, no. 2 (2015): pp. 274–97.

[96] Department for Work and Pensions, 'Benefit expenditure tables', March 2013, accessed 17 July 2020, http://statistics.dwp.gov.uk/asd/asd4/expenditure_tables_Budget_2013.xls.

[97] National Audit Office, Invalidity Benefit: Report by the Comptroller and Auditor General (HC 91 (1989–90)) (London: HMSO, 1989); Richard Berthoud, Invalidity Benefit: Where Will the Savings Come From? (London: Policy Studies Institute, 1993); Christina Beatty et al., Hidden Unemployment in the East Midlands (Sheffield: Centre for Regional Economic and Social Research, Sheffield Hallam University, 2002).

[98] Puar, The Right to Maim.

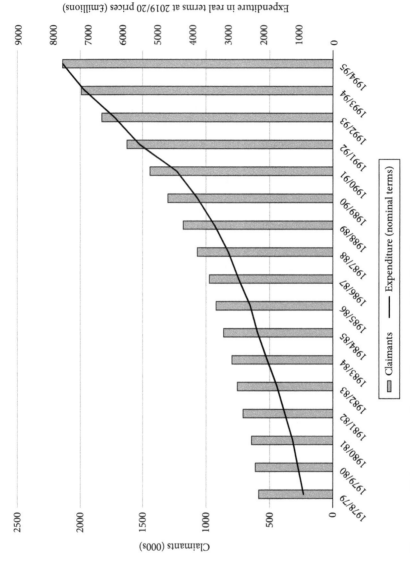

Figure 6.1 Claimants to and expenditure on invalidity benefit, UK, 1978/79 to 1994/95.

Source: Department for Work and Pensions, 'Spring budget 2020: Expenditure and caseload forecasts', gov.uk, 20 March 2020, accessed 13 July 2021, https://www.gov.uk/government/publications/benefit-expenditure-and-caseload-tables-2020.

The Secretary of State for Social Security Peter Lilley famously told the 1992 Conservative Party Conference that he, like Mikado, had 'a little list' of those who abused the welfare state, proclaiming he would be 'closing down the something-for-nothing-society'.[99] In the battle against 'scroungers' the most prominent targets were single mothers and unemployed people.[100] However, as the costliest single item after pensions, Invalidity Benefit was an area where most gains could be made in reducing social security expenditure and where prejudices against disability claimants could be exploited. The government argued that the rise in claims could not be due to the population getting less healthy.[101] As John Major told the 1993 Conservative Party Conference, 'frankly, it beggars belief that so many people have become invalid'.[102] Lilley sold the need for reform by calling Invalidity Benefit the 'bad back benefit'.[103] Consequently, he and the DSS proposed a new form of out-of-work benefit with a test that distinguished between those who needed help to find employment and those who were morally entitled to disability-related social security.

This 'All Work Test' would be different from the 'sick note' approach in two key aspects. First, it would measure the claimant against whether it would be reasonable to expect him or her to be able to perform the tasks required of a 'normal' job. It would deliberately ignore social factors such as the claimant's age, the availability of employment in the local area, and the claimant's existing training and work experience. This distinction between the 'own-occupation' condition and the 'all-work' condition was formalized in the separation of short-term Incapacity Benefit (for the first six months of sickness) and the long-term version. Second, it would apply an 'objective' functioning examination of claimants using a Benefits Agency Medical Service (BAMS) medical professional rather than relying on an assessment by the claimant's own doctor. It did not use diagnoses and a doctor's opinion on whether the patient could work. BAMS designed a test that would give scores for 'descriptors' based on how well a claimant could perform certain tasks in 'functional areas', such as standing, rising from sitting, walking, reaching, manual dexterity, speech, and seeing.[104] If the combination of scores was high enough, the claimant would qualify for the

[99] Lilley was referencing the Gilbert and Sullivan opera *The Mikado*. Robert Morgan, 'Lilley targets "scroungers"', *The Times*, 8 October 1992, p. 8.
[100] Derek Fraser, *The Evolution of the British Welfare State—A History of Social Policy since the Industrial Revolution*, 4th edn (Basingstoke: Palgrave Macmillan, 2009); Stephen McKay and Karen Rowlingson, *Social Security in Britain* (Basingstoke: Macmillan, 1999).
[101] On this 'cultural inflation' argument in the UK context see Chapter 1 and Martin Gorsky et al., 'The "cultural inflation of morbidity" during the English mortality decline: A new look', *Social Science & Medicine* 73 (2011): pp. 1775–83.
[102] Anthony Bevins, 'Tory right remains wary of Chancellor', *Independent*, 16 June 1993, p. 1.
[103] Stephen Bates, 'Reform of "bad back" benefit not an attack on the sick, says Lilley', *Guardian*, 25 January 1994, p. 6.
[104] TNA: JB 3/100, Kirby Swales and Peter Craig, Social Security Research Branch, Evaluation of the Incapacity Benefit Medical Test, December 1996.

benefit. These descriptors were based on the tasks that were considered typical for a job in the 1990s' economy and were refined in consultation with a panel of '80 experts' drawn from the medical profession, industry, and disability organizations.[105]

Historically, the government had been less worried about the threat of malingering on long-term benefits than short-term ones because the long-term sick had many more points of contact with authorities. In doubtful cases, it was easier to perform re-examinations or sick visits, while the family GP would have a better idea of the claimant's medical history and social circumstances. The rhetoric around 'scroungers'—just like that about 'abuse' around the time of the Fisher Report in the 1970s[106]—conjured images of the malingerer, and the DSS leant on example cases that showed 'common sense' failures of the system. An invalidity benefit claimant in Aylesbury, for example, was the subject of a large spread in the Daily Mail after coming 'second in the discus, third in the hammer, third in the shot put and sixth in the javelin' at a local athletics meeting.[107] Lilley himself in a speech about his benefit plans talked about claimants who were 'going on cycling holidays' and a woman who claimed she could not sit for long periods but had gone on a long haul flight to Australia.[108] Matthew Banks, MP alleged that 'the man who waved the flag at the [1993] Grand National was actually on invalidity benefit' (a claim strenuously denied).[109] These examples, even if they were reported accurately, were not necessarily malingering. Just as Martine McCutcheon's throat infection might have stopped her singing nightly in a West End musical, it was unlikely to make it impossible to eat a meal with friends. Similarly, many people had conditions that were episodic which made it difficult to hold down regular work, but where it was still possible to perform some physical tasks some of the time. Tying all incapacity to physical health was simplistic and damaging for disabled people, but not out of step with social constructions of disability at the time.[110] As for the Grand National story, the reference was to Keith Brown who had gained the nickname 'Captain Cock-Up'

[105] See TNA: JB 61/15/1, Lucy Makinson to Minister of State and Secretary of State, All-Work Test of Incapacity: Work in Progress, 26 May 1994; Waddell et al., The Scientific and Conceptual Basis of Incapacity Benefits.

[106] Henry Fisher, Report of the Committee on Abuse of Social Security Benefits (Cmnd 5228) (London: HMSO, 1972). See Chapters 4 and 5.

[107] Bill Mound and Jackie Kemp, 'Healthy display by man too ill to work', Daily Mail, 23 July 1993, p. 11.

[108] Christopher Bell, 'Tests for £750,000 to end the frauds on invalidity cash', Daily Mail, 25 January 1994, p. 2.

[109] 'Social Security (Incapacity for Work) Bill', Hansard [Commons], 24 January 1994, vol. 236, cc. 35–121, at col. 37. For the denial: Jill Sherman, '280,000 to lose benefit in new incapacity test', The Times, 25 January 1994, p. 8.

[110] Jane Campbell and Michael Oliver, Disability Politics: Understanding Our Past, Changing Our Future (London: Routledge, 1996); Miriam Corker and Tom Shakespeare, Disability/Postmodernity: Embodying Disability Theory (London: Continuum, 2002).

for being in charge of two farcical restarts of the 1993 race.[111] With no evidence to back the claim, Banks appears to have repeated an urban legend about Brown's benefit status, probably an ableist insult about Brown's mental 'capacity' to do his job. Still, the stories, combined with the anti-scrounger rhetoric, were believable to enough Conservative MPs and to enough of the population at large to allow the government room to claim that reform of out-of-work benefits was necessary.

Regardless of tabloid tittle-tattle, the All Work Test was not designed as a diagnostic tool to weed out malingerers, even if the DSS hoped this would be a welcome side effect. There was little doubt in any of the contemporary research that most existing Invalidity Benefit claimants genuinely had a health condition.[112] The test was also not designed to detect disability. Disabled people could, and did, work. The placement of disabled people in work has schemes been a key part of British social security and employment policy since the 1910s. The DSS even attempted to encourage this through a new Disability Working Allowance which augmented the wages of disabled people.[113] Instead, the All Work Test was to measure 'restriction[s] or lack of ability to perform the activities involved in working where it would be unreasonable to expect people to work'.[114] The DSS claimed that it would be more 'objective' than a doctor's note and would ensure that those who could not work would receive support, while those who could work would receive unemployment benefit and help to find a new job.[115] This process would accelerate in the 2000s, as seen in the following chapter.

The idea of applying a functioning test was not new to the 1990s, nor were Conservative government attempts to reform disability benefits. The Thatcher government had initially decided not to target disability benefits for the large cuts and reorganizations that would happen to unemployment and Supplementary Benefits, in part because disabled people were seen as 'the deserving poor' for whom a residual social security system was considered fair.[116] However, in 1984 a

[111] Edward Marriott, 'Vices & virtues', *The Times*, 1 January 1994, p. 11; June Southworth, 'The only certain non-starter in this National', *Daily Mail*, 8 April 1994, p. 9.
[112] Most notably in *HC 91 (1989–90)*. See also Berthoud, *Invalidity Benefit*; Angela Hadjipateras and Marilyn Howard, *Worried Sick: Reactions to the Government's Plans for Invalidity Benefit* (London: Disability Benefits Consortium, 1993); Beatty et al., *Hidden Unemployment in the East Midlands*.
[113] Department of Social Security, *Disability Benefits: The Delivery of Disability Living Allowance and Disability Working Allowance Reply by the Government to the Third Report from the Social Security Committee (Cm 2282)* (London: HMSO, 1993); Helen Bolderson, *Social Security, Disability and Rehabilitation* (London: Jessica Kingsley, 1991); Julie Anderson, *War, Disability and Rehabilitation in Britain: 'Soul of a Nation'* (Manchester: Manchester University Press, 2011); Andy Holroyde, 'Sheltered employment and mental health in Britain: Remploy c. 1945–1981', in *Healthy Minds in the Twentieth Century: In and Beyond the Asylum*, edited by Steven J. Taylor and Alice Brumby (Cham: Springer, 2020), pp. 113–35.
[114] TNA: PIN 35/978, IB Report—Briefing Pack, 21 September 1994.
[115] TNA: JB 61/15/1, Lucy Makinson to Minister of State and Secretary of State, All-Work Test of Incapacity: Work in Progress, 26 May 1994.
[116] Gareth Millward, 'Invalid definitions, invalid responses: Disability and the welfare state, 1965–1995' (PhD thesis, London School of Hygiene and Tropical Medicine, 2014); Conservative Party, *1979 Conservative Party General Election Manifesto* (London: Conservative Party, 1979).

combination of campaigning and regulations from the European Economic Community meant that Non-contributory Invalidity Pension (NCIP) and its peculiar variant Housewife's Non-contributory Invalidity Pension (HNCIP) were disbanded and merged into a new Severe Disablement Allowance (SDA). HNCIP had included a 'household duties test', as discussed in Chapter 4. The doctor provided a certificate similar to a sick note alongside an assessment of a married woman's ability to perform key tasks in the categories 'shopping', 'meals', 'washing and ironing', and 'cleaning'.[117] In effect, therefore, married women were tested twice. Single women and men did not have to provide anything more than the sick note (assuming they met the other administrative, non-medical criteria). This was discrimination according to the European Council directive on equal treatment for men and women in social security.[118] Rather than simply removing the duties test, SDA was created to merge NCIP and HNCIP while ensuring that eligibility was restricted and thousands of married women did not suddenly become eligible for the benefit.[119] It included a new medical criterion—all claimants would have to be incapable of work *and* assessed as '80 per cent disabled'. This judgement would be made by DHSS assessors using the medical evidence supplied by the claimant's doctor. Although not a functioning test per se, in the case of disagreements DHSS staff would take into account a range of functional limitations that had been used in the Industrial Injuries and War Pensions schemes to determine rates of benefit for victims of workplace injuries since 1948.[120]

Across the 1980s and 1990s, then, attempts to restrict access to government funds on the grounds of sickness were accelerated both in short- and long-term benefit schemes. The rise of the term 'sick note' in the press around this period reflected anxieties that were also seen in policy changes. Long-term sickness, however, was inevitably also bound up in contemporary debates about disability, making it a thornier issue for the DSS to take on. Over the 1980s, a new disabled

---

[117] TNA: PIN 15/4481, DHSS Leaflet NI 214, NCIP for Married Women, June 1977, pp. 1–2. Copy also consulted in Peter Townsend Collection, University of Essex: 78.19.

[118] European Council, Council Directive 79/7/EEC, 19 December 1978. Although never tested in court, the DHSS was given confidential legal advice that HNCIP broke the directive and that they would lose if challenged. TNA: PIN 35/96, Introduction of Severe Disablement Allowance, December 1983. See also: Department of Health and Social Security, *Review of the Household Duties Test* (London: HMSO, 1983).

[119] See Jackie Gulland, 'Extraordinary housework: Women and sickness benefit in the early-twentieth century', *Women's History Magazine* 71 (2013): pp. 23–30. The DHSS estimated that this would have cost £275 million per annum, or around 8 per cent of all social security expenditure on disability benefits. TNA: PIN 35/96, Ministers' SDA Q&A briefing, attached to memorandum 1 December 1983. Anyone claiming HNCIP when SDA was introduced would continue to receive benefit.

[120] TNA: PIN 35/96, R. H. Smith to M. E. H. Platt, 20 December 1983; TNA: PIN 35/658, K. A. Cameron, SDA—Assessment of mental illness/handicap, 16 March 1984. On the definition and measurement of incapacity see Jackie Gulland, *Gender, Work and Social Control: A Century of Disability Benefits* (London: Palgrave Macmillan, 2019).

people's movement grew.[121] While the voluntary organizations that emerged in the 1960s and 1970s had focused on social security, the generation in the 1980s and 1990s took its lead from other equalities issues such as LGBT campaigning, feminism, and anti-racism.[122] Across the 1990s there were several attempts to pass a Civil Rights (Disabled Persons) Bill through parliament using private members' bills. A ham-fisted attempt to block the 1994 version led to major embarrassment for DSS ministers and the government, leading to the passing of the 1995 Disability Discrimination Act.[123] The 'disability lobby' therefore had to be treated carefully and policies that were seen to be discriminatory against disabled people could generate unwelcome headlines. Voluntary organizations and the opposition benches in parliament argued that Incapacity Benefit was more a cost-saving exercise than one concerned about fair distribution of resources. The National Association of Citizens Advice Bureaux (NACAB) was particularly scathing, noting that simply moving disabled people onto unemployment benefit would not solve the problem of the lack of suitable work.[124] Although the right-wing press and Conservative back benchers were keen to cut social security spending for financial and moral reasons, even they were cautious once it became clear that many thousands of present and future claimants would be excluded from Incapacity Benefit despite fitting a common-sense definition of disability. Torn between a perceived moral duty to provide for the 'deserving poor' at the same time as driving out 'scroungers', the All Work Test was not a perfect solution.[125] As a *Daily Mail* editorial conceded, 'the well-meaning effort to stamp out abuses in the system is creating a political nightmare'.[126]

To avoid these criticisms, the DSS repeatedly referred to its new capacity test as 'objective'. In part, this was a defence of the accuracy of the test—but it also promoted the notion that *only* capacity for work should be a factor in benefit decisions, not other subjective social factors.[127] The Department was also correct that

[121] Mike Oliver, 'The disability movement is a New Social Movement!', *Community Development Journal* 32 (1997): pp. 244–51.

[122] Campbell and Oliver, *Disability Politics*; Tom Shakespeare, *Disability Rights and Wrongs* (Abingdon: Routledge, 2006); Millward, 'Social security policy and the early disability movement'.

[123] Alice Thomson and Jonathan Prynn, 'Minister forced to talk out Bill for disabled', *The Times*, 21 May 1994, pp. 1, 2; Nicholas Scott, 'Personal statement', *Hansard [Commons]*, 10 May 1994, vol. 243 c. 155; Nikki Fox, 'The Disability Discrimination Act: 20 years on', *BBC News*, 6 November 2015, accessed 24 November 2020, https://www.bbc.co.uk/news/av/health-34743197; Millward, 'Invalid definitions'.

[124] For example, see: Alice Thomson, 'Benefit curb may create more jobless', *The Times*, 24 January 1994, p. 2; Cllr Muriel Green, letter to *Daily Mail*, 31 January 1994, p. 32; Rosie Waterhouse, 'Disabled "under attack from Tory right wing"', *Independent*, 31 August 1994, p. 4; David Brindle, 'New benefit "will anger disabled"', *Guardian*, 13 April 1995, p. 6.

[125] Alan Duncan et al., *Who Benefits? A Plan for Social Security: Reinventing Welfare* (London: No Turning Back Group, 1993); Iain Duncan-Smith, 'Every day, every working Briton pays £13 in tax to those on State benefit. And it's going to get worse', *Daily Mail*, 13 April 1994, p. 8; Paul Eastham, 'Tory panic over curb on benefits', *Daily Mail*, 30 December 1994, p. 2.

[126] 'Paying the price of welfare madness', *Daily Mail*, 30 December 1994, p. 8.

[127] TNA: PIN 35/978, IB Report—Briefing Pack, 21 September 1994.

elements of social security that did 'trap' claimants. The logic of Invalidity Benefit and other social security benefits required claimants to present themselves as sick or as needy as possible to ensure they met the qualification criteria. This contradicted social model disability rights campaigning but was a necessary coping mechanism in a disabling society where access to resources was restricted.[128] As with Roy Hattersley's 'bad back', doctors were encouraged by their patients and the system to ensure diagnoses appeared at face value to be severe; a status that could easily be internalized. For those on the margins of employment, being labelled an 'invalid' had a psychological effect and could be especially damaging to men who believed in masculine ideals of the 'breadwinner model'.[129] One woman wrote in a diary of her family life after her husband was made redundant in the *Daily Mail*:

> Bill had an appointment at the doctor's...When he arrived home, his eyes are red. I know he has been crying...He thrusts a sick note into my hand. 'What does it mean?' I ask. Bill shakes his head. 'But you're ill', I remind him, irritably. 'Well they [potential employers] don't need to know....Not only am I redundant but I'm a write-off', Bill says, and the tears come again.[130]

The *Independent on Sunday* ran a feature on a mining village in which similar stories of men with depression are signed onto invalidity benefit—though, as with Stephen Fry, there is some doubt as to the genuineness of the claims. Regardless, it was clear that many of the men in the village were sick, unemployed, and their prospects of retraining for new work were remote, especially as many were in the later stages of their working lives.[131]

To be sure, if removing these social considerations was the aim of the exercise, sick notes would no longer be sufficient. There was plenty of anecdotal and social science evidence that GPs were sympathetic to the needs of their patients beyond strictly medical criteria.[132] Moreover, as had been argued from at least the 1940s, GPs were not necessarily experts in occupational health and therefore did not possess the expertise to judge an individual's capacity to do their (or anyone else's) job.[133]

---

[128] Campbell and Oliver, *Disability Politics*; B. Watermeyer, 'Claiming loss in disability', *Disability & Society* 24 (2009): pp. 91–102.

[129] See Chapter 4 and Jane Lewis, 'Gender and the development of welfare regimes', *Journal of European Social Policy* 2, no. 2 (1992): pp. 159–73; King, 'How men valued women's work'.

[130] Elizabeth Alty, 'Hope and despair of life after redundancy', *Daily Mail*, 8 April 1993, pp. 44–5.

[131] Esther Oxford, 'The village that is sick of living without a future', *Independent on Sunday*, 15 August 1993, p. 5. See also: Beatty et al., *Hidden Unemployment in the East Midlands*; Berthoud, *Invalidity Benefit*.

[132] See: David Hughes, 'Jobless "quite the dole queue to go on the sick list"', *Daily Mail*, 10 March 1995, p. 2. The DSS also commissioned research on the phenomenon: Jane Ritchie, Kit Ward, and Wendy Duldig, *A Qualitative Study of the Role of General Practitioners in the Award of Invalidity Benefit* (London: Social and Community Planning Research, 1993).

[133] See Chapter 2 and Waddell et al., *The Scientific and Conceptual Basis of Incapacity Benefits*.

Still, to ignore such social and cultural factors flew in the face of the social model of disability that the DSS leant on to justify pushing disabled people towards employment. Disability organizations had long campaigned for the right to work. Not only would this provide financial reward, work was shown to have a psychological and cultural benefit by giving people a sense of purpose and allowing them to fully participate in society.[134] Retesting, however, only focused on the medical barriers to employment and not the social ones: the attitudes of employers, unwillingness to make workplaces accessible or make reasonable adjustments to working practices, and the disabling effects of the built environment.[135] If disabled people could find work, it was likely to be unsuitable and poorly paid.[136] Various organizations made these concerns known during the consultation process for Incapacity Benefit, including Mind, MENCAP, the Disability Alliance, the Royal Association for Disability and Rehabilitation, and NACAB.[137] The very concept of the 'objective' test was attacked, especially given the obviously 'subjective' measures in place. There was no objective average job, level at which it was 'unreasonable' to expect a sick person to work, or measure of combinations of mental and physical health capacities.[138]

The DSS and the key architect at BAMS, Mansell Aylward, continued to defend the approach and would work on refinements into the next millennium.[139] But even GPs themselves were sceptical. Despite decades of campaigning to reduce their sick note obligations, the BMA expressed concern that the medical professionals hired by BAMS to assess claimants would not be trained well enough to cope with the demands of the job and volume of claims that would pass their desks.[140] There were also anxieties about maintaining doctor-patient confidentiality when passing medical records between different agencies.[141]

[134] Committee on Restrictions Against Disabled People, *Report by the Committee on Restrictions Against Disabled People* (London: H.M.S.O., 1982); Chris Grover and Linda Piggott, 'Disabled people, the reserve army of labour and welfare reform', *Disability & Society* 20 (2005): pp. 705–17; Richard Berthoud, *Trends in the Employment of Disabled People in Britain* (Colchester: Institute for Social & Economic Research, 2011).

[135] Vic Finkelstein, 'Phase 2: Discovering the Person in "Disability" and "Rehabilitation"', *Magic Carpet* 27 (1975): pp. 31–8; Campbell and Oliver, *Disability Politics*; Oliver and Barnes, *The New Politics of Disablement*.

[136] Jull Insley, 'Long-term sick face poverty', *The Times*, 15 January 1994, p. 26.

[137] See correspondence in TNA: PIN 35/978 and TNA: JB 61/15/1, New Medical Assessment for Incapacity Benefits—Handling and Publication of Report, 5 July 1994.

[138] Ministers were told to defend the objectivity of the test and to reject complaints, though there is little actual argument, simply rebuttals. See: TNA: PIN 35/978, IB Report—Briefing Pack, 21 September 1994.

[139] Mansel Aylward, 'Certifying incapacity for work', *British Medical Journal* 310, no. 6974 (1995): p. 261; Waddell et al., *The Scientific and Conceptual Basis of Incapacity Benefits*. See also: Chapter 7.

[140] TNA: PIN 35/978, Aylward's response to BMA criticism in *Pulse* 28 October 1994; David R. J. Penney and G. H. Heyse-Moore letters to *Guardian*, 11 October 1994, p. 21.

[141] Although there were long-standing legal and bureaucratic links between the DSS (and its predecessors) and NHS doctors, BAMS was technically a third-party and some procedures had to be reworked. See: TNA: PIN 35/978, Confidentiality, Use and Disclosure of Personal Health Information, 10 August 1994.

The most problematic aspect was for those with long-term health conditions of an episodic nature. The worry was that a one-off test would catch a claimant on 'a good day' whereas the family doctor would know about recurrent episodes that made it difficult for their patient to sustain employment.[142] Disability groups also noted that while a certain task might be possible there was little reference to how long or how much effort it might take to complete that task.[143] The 'subjective' link between the doctor and the patient, therefore, still had its uses.

Conclusion

The 1980s and 1990s saw two key changes that resonate in the British sickness systems today. First, 'sick note' was popularized as a humorous way of describing absenteeism within the workplace and outside it. Second, capacity testing became an integral part of the long-term sickness system that would eventually inform the 'fit note' when it was introduced in 2010. This 'biopsychosocial model' of disability, which adopted some arguments from disability campaigners while somewhat paradoxically placing greater emphasis on individuals' responsibility for their own health and employment prospects, would become a feature of the New Labour years discussed in the following chapter.[144] These changes might have occurred under a Conservative government, but even in opposition Labour promoted a 'tough love' approach to social security.[145] How it dealt with the contradiction of committing to greater rights for disabled people while supporting sickness regimes that disproportionately affected them can only be understood with reference to the changes seen here in the 1990s.

These events reflected a wider anxiety in the political establishment and the wider country about absenteeism, relative economic weakness compared to similar nations and a decline in moral fibre. At the same time, the humour around sick notes suggested that, despite the decline in union activity and rise in unemployment, workers and the working classes could still resist bad practices by employers and poke fun at the absurdities in the gatekeeping system. The Bert Quigleys of the world may have been teased—or, in some cases, bullied—by their workmates for taking days off as staff attempted to assert discipline among each other. But there was also an inherent criticism of the sick note regime in place. It had, despite undergoing some evolution over the years, retained much the same

---

[142] TNA: PIN 35/978, Incapacity Benefit—Comments Received on Proposals for the New All Work Test, 21 November 1994.
[143] Peter Townsend Collection, University of Essex: 76.07, Fred Reid to Ian McMaster, 6 January 1988.
[144] Waddell et al., *The Scientific and Conceptual Basis of Incapacity Benefits*.
[145] Andrew Grice, 'Blair's "tough love" plan to outflank timid Tories on welfare', *Sunday Times*, 13 November 1994, p. 34.

character as the one instituted in the 1940s. It had not removed the 'ipse dixit' problem, nor had it provided an adequate curb on absenteeism, hence the need to reform SSP. The petty bureaucracy of needing a sick note to prove illness was, at face value, a box ticking exercise worthy of mockery: both because it was so easily exploitable and because, even when genuine, all the constituencies involved in the process doubted its validity. And yet it remained as the lest terrible option for most actors most of the time.

In the next chapter, these themes will be explored further. In the post-Disability Discrimination Act, New Labour era, the internet provided new communication tools to educate workers and claimants about their rights. The government and employers, however, were now adapting to sickness regimes that required greater private-sector surveillance of absenteeism alongside an increased government commitment to reducing economic inactivity by 'rehabilitating' chronically sick people into paid employment. As more money was spent on developing expertise on the management of sickness, the government would draw on the lessons of the 1980s and 1990s to steer its future activity.

7

The 'Death' of the Sick Note?

The use of 'sick note' as a rhetorical device did not end in the mid-1990s. In fact, as Britain entered the new millennium with a New Labour government, use of the term accelerated. The *Daily Mail* ran headlines about 'Sick-note Britain' in 1998, though the phrase became more common in the late 2000s, especially after the 2007 economic downturn. It was not just the individual benefit claimants and absentees who were 'sick notes'—something was rotten with the whole nation.

This chapter covers the developments in the rhetoric around sick notes in the New Labour years. The logic that had driven the All Work Test and Incapacity Benefit in the mid-1990s was built upon and extended to medium-term sickness. Whereas the Major government had focused on driving down claims, New Labour's active labour market policies sought to encourage unemployed disabled people into work. For employed people, both the government and employers expended great energy on getting people with medium-to-long-term sickness back to their jobs as soon as possible, with stricter discipline and a rhetorical emphasis on preventing sickness in the first place. The lines between capacity and incapacity became blurred, undermining the worth of the sick note as a method of determining sickness. And yet, despite these changes, medical certification and the logic that underpinned it were able to adapt. Replacing the 'Med 3' with the 'fit note' in 2010 could be seen as the 'death' of the sick note—but the everyday experience of seeking support for short-term sickness was, in effect, the same in the 2010s as it had been for decades.

During the early years of the twenty-first century two key policy changes affected Britain's relationship with the 'Med 3' that has been central to the previous chapters. First, the introduction of Employment and Support Allowance (ESA) in 2008 created a new form of out-of-work sickness benefit to replace Incapacity Benefit. Built on the same testing principles as those seen in the previous chapter, it was repurposed to better fit the active labour market policies of the New Labour government. Second, in 2010 the Brown administration replaced the sick note with a new electronic 'fit note'. Implementing recommendations from the 2008 Black Report, this new note gave space for professionals to assess what the patient *could* do in a workplace, intending to help workers and employers negotiate a return to work that could fit around the employee's symptoms.[1] With both these policies, the government sought to bring those on the margins of

---

[1] Carol Black, *Working for a Healthier Tomorrow* (London: TSO, 2008).

incapacity into paid employment and cease reliance upon benefits and occupational sick pay. However, the quality of the work available, the flexibility of employers and the arbitrary nature of 'incapacity' decisions meant the implementation of these ideas was far from smooth.

Nevertheless, none of this can be understood without reference to British attitudes towards sickness and wider economic changes over the 1997 to 2010 period. Through global economic processes and active choices by government and business leaders, work in Britain was increasingly digital, service-based, and precarious. Now that employers were almost entirely responsible for sick pay, sickness absence became less and less acceptable.[2] Thus, think tanks, business confederations, and insurance companies dedicated resources to identifying the scale and nature of the problem while providing advice on how to combat it. Their subsequent reports were promoted in the national and trade press, who were also convinced that too much absenteeism and disability-benefit claiming was stifling the economy and indicative of failures in the country at large. The phrase 'Sick-note Britain' was born, amplified, and reinforced by the cycle of news coverage and responses from various constituencies.[3]

This period was one of paradoxes. The government increased sanctions on benefit claimants, while also making tangible commitments to anti-discrimination legislation for disabled people. Employers regularly demanded private sick notes and 'proof' of sickness but pronouncements in the media suggested they did not think the GP's signature was worth the paper it was scrawled upon. Employees found themselves in ever-increasing precarity, with weaker and smaller trades unions unable to resist 'flexible' working practices imposed from above; yet the internet offered new ways for workers to express solidarity, find advice, and use British and European Union employment law to assert their rights. It was a continuation and evolution of the years of Conservative rule—and something quite different.

This chapter tackles these issues in four main sections. First, the politics of New Labour and social security policy explain how, why, and when the Blair government decided to reform sickness and disability policy. Built on 'Third Way' principles of an active labour market and a market liberal social security system, the Department of Social Security (DSS)—from 2001 the Department for Work and Pensions (DWP)—strove to 'make work pay' by increasing punitive sanctions on certain groups of benefit claimants while providing training and placement services to open 'Pathways to Work'.[4] The second section of this chapter details the

---

[2] See Chapter 6 and Phil Taylor et al., '"Too scared to go sick" – Reformulating the research agenda on sickness absence', *Industrial Relations Journal* 41, no. 4 (2010): pp. 270–88.

[3] David Jones, 'Sign up here for Sick-note Britain', *Daily Mail*, 14 April 1998, pp. 22–3.

[4] Peter Hill, 'Working hard or hardly working? Evaluating New Labour's active labour market policy' (PhD thesis, University of Warwick, 2016); Peter Sloman, 'Redistribution in an age of neoliberalism: Market economics, "poverty knowledge", and the growth of working-age benefits in Britain, c. 1979–2010', *Political Studies* 67, no. 3 (2019): pp. 732–51.

changes to out-of-work disability benefits, notably the creation of ESA and a new functioning test: the Work Capability Assessment. The government's attempts to reduce expenditure and 'benefit dependency' by rehabilitating those on the borderline of incapacity shows how New Labour's attitudes towards social security clashed with the sick-note approach to determining eligibility for support. This process was informed by contemporary debates about 'scroungers' and other types of welfare recipient while jarring with traditional social security approaches: the social democratic principle of providing equality of opportunity to disadvantaged groups such as disabled people; and the conservative and liberal concepts of helping 'the deserving poor'. Treading this line between contradictory public opinion (i.e., that disabled people should be supported by the state *and* that the state should be tougher on disability claimants) was evident in the compromises made in ESA policy.

The third section shows how these discussions around employment and state benefits could not be separated from the wider 'sick note Britain' discourse vis à vis employment and absenteeism. Many doubted sick notes, the ability of GPs to write objective certificates of 'real' incapacity, and the reasons given by employees for missing work. The sick note system encouraged doctors, employers, and workers to see a binary line between 'capacity' and 'incapacity', obscuring the possibility of adjusting working patterns to reduce long-term absence. At the same time, the unfairness of policing regimes around absenteeism drew heavy criticism, especially from workers subjected to them. These debates lead to the fourth and final section on the creation of the 'fit note'. Designed to replace the Med 3 with a new electronic statement of what work a patient could engage in, the policy sought to keep people at work for longer, get them back quicker, and, by extension, reduce the number of sick people leaving their jobs and becoming state benefit claimants themselves. Sold as a way to improve industrial efficiency, public health, and industry-wide occupational health statistics, this cannot be understood without the wider context of Britain's attitudes towards absenteeism and DWP's active labour market policies. But while the sick note 'born' in 1948 might technically have 'died', in practice it lumbered on. It remained the least terrible option on offer for Britain's private and public sickness welfare systems.

New Labour and Active Labour Management

We should not forget why reform is right, and why, whatever the concerns over individual benefits, most people **know** it is right. Above all, the system must change because the world has changed, beyond the recognition of Beveridge's generation. The world of work has altered—people no longer expect a job for life; traditional industries have declined; new technologies have taken their place. There is a premium on skills and re-skilling throughout life. The role of women has been transformed. Family structures are different. We live longer, but work for fewer years. And the expectations of disabled people have changed out of all recognition, from half a century ago. We need a system designed not for yesterday, but for today.[5]

Tony Blair's introduction to *A New Contract for Welfare* set out a Green Paper for radical reforms to social security policy. The New Labour government sold itself as committed to fighting 'social exclusion'. At the same time, it signalled that it could be trusted with public funds by clamping down on 'scroungers'. Reforms to the sick note in the 2000s—for short-term and long-term illness—can only be understood within New Labour's preoccupation with work and worklessness.

One way of understanding New Labour's welfare policy is through its approaches to inequality. Ruth Levitas identifies 'three discourses of social exclusion' that typify British social policy. First, a 'redistributive' approach which focuses on poverty. Second, a 'social integration' approach that focuses on access to work and services. And third, an 'underclass' approach which focuses on the behaviour and customs of disadvantaged groups.[6] While Levitas cautions that these are Weberian ideal types rather than concrete proposals for action, they do serve as useful analytical frames for the various parts of Labour's social policy in both the twentieth and twenty-first centuries. Taking a redistributive approach would suggest the solution to combatting exclusion would be to provide unemployed people with more money; but this could create welfare dependency in the 'underclass' by encouraging people to claim and stay on benefit. This had, in effect, been the crude dividing line between New Right benefit policy (designed to make benefit harder to claim and less attractive to live on to force people to find paid employment) and a supposedly over-generous welfare system that had been part of the failed Keynesian economics of the previous age.[7] Whether true or not, this analysis resonated. For Conservatives, it was a necessary foundational myth for Thatcherite economics; for New Labour, rejecting the imagined 1970s was important for re-establishing economic credibility in post-Thatcher British politics.[8] For a party still concerned with 'exclusion' which had eschewed redistribution as a primary solution, integration offered a potential answer. By

[5] Emphasis original. Department of Social Security, *A New Contract for Welfare (Cm 3805)* (London: TSO, March 1998), p. iv.
[6] Levitas refers to these models as RED, SID, and MUD. See: Ruth Levitas, *The Inclusive Society?* (London: Palgrave Macmillan UK, 2005), esp. pp. 7–28.
[7] See the justification for SSP in Chapter 5, Incapacity Benefit in Chapter 6 and Stuart Hall, 'The great moving right show', in *The Politics of Thatcherism*, edited by Stuart Hall and Martin Jacques (London: Lawrence &Wishart, 1983), pp. 19–39.
[8] Glen O'Hara and Helen Parr, 'Conclusions: Harold Wilson's 1964–70 governments and the heritage of "New" Labour', *Contemporary British History* 20 (2006): pp. 477–89. See also the way the 'Winter of Discontent' was constructed and reconstructed across time: Colin Hay, 'Chronicles of a death foretold: the Winter of Discontent and construction of crisis of British Keynesianism', *Parliamentary Affairs* 63 (2010): pp. 446–70.

promising 'work for those who can; security for those who cannot,'[9] Tony Blair and New Labour could pledge redistribution to the 'deserving poor' while tackling the 'welfare dependency' underclass via back to work schemes, tax credits, the minimum wage and better child care.[10] This 'Third Way' thinking, inspired by sociologist Anthony Giddens and the Clinton administration's 'workfare' schemes in the United States was central to New Labour's employment policy, and, by extension, its treatment of sickness.[11]

Biopsychosocial models of disability were also central to New Labour policy. These models stressed the importance of paid employment to the well-being of sick and disabled people. As Waddell and Burton argued in their DWP review of the evidence on work and disability in 2005, 'the beneficial effects of work outweigh the risks of work, and are greater than the harmful effects of long-term unemployment or prolonged sickness absence. Work is generally good for health and well-being.'[12] This approach had justified increasingly punitive measures and stricter eligibility criteria around the Major government's Incapacity Benefit and Jobseekers Allowance.[13] Labour continued with these assumptions. It committed to the outgoing Conservative government's budget plans for social security, refusing to roll back cuts to out-of-work benefits.[14] Indeed, Iain Duncan Smith dubbed the 1997 Social Security Bill 'the Peter Lilley Memorial Bill' given that many of the measures proposed by the ex-Secretary of State, such as cuts to benefits for single parents, were now being enshrined in law by the new government.[15]

Given its intellectual roots and party base, however, the new government was unable to ignore the structural discrimination that disproportionately punished people with certain characteristics from having equal opportunities to leave benefit and find meaningful work.[16] The Disability Discrimination Act was strengthened with the creation of a Disability Rights Commission that performed

---

[9] Cm 3805, p. iii.

[10] Martin Hewitt, 'New Labour and social security', in New Labour, New Welfare State? The 'Third Way' in British Social Policy, edited by Martin A. Powell (Bristol: Policy Press, 1999), pp. 149–70; Hill, 'Working hard or hardly working?'

[11] Anthony Giddens, Beyond Left and Right: The Future of Radical Politics (Cambridge: Polity Press, 1994); C. Grover and L. Piggott, 'Social security, employment and Incapacity Benefit: Critical reflections on A New Deal for Welfare', Disability & Society 22, no. 7 (2007): pp. 733–46; Martin A. Powell, 'Introduction', in New Labour, New Welfare State? The 'Third Way' in British Social Policy, edited by Martin A. Powell (Bristol: Policy Press, 1999), pp. 1–28.

[12] Gordon Waddell and A. Kim Burton, Is Work Good for Your Health and Well-Being? (London: TSO, 2006).

[13] See Chapter 6 and Waddell and Burton, Is Work Good for Your Health and Well-Being?; Tom Shakespeare, Nicholas Watson, and Ola Abu Alghaib, 'Blaming the victim, all over again: Waddell and Aylward's biopsychosocial (BPS) model of disability', Critical Social Policy 37, no. 1 (2017): pp. 22–41.

[14] Hewitt, 'New Labour and Social Security'.

[15] 'Social Security Bill', House of Commons Official Report (Hansard), 22 July 1997, vol. 298, cc. 783–857, at col. 793; Powell, 'Introduction'.

[16] Powell, 'Introduction'.

similar functions for disability discrimination as the Equal Opportunities Commission and the Commission for Racial Equality had for gender and racial discrimination.[17] Further, Blair appointed long-time anti-poverty campaigner Frank Field as Minister for Welfare Reform.[18] However, the exercise ended with Field's resignation. He had pushed for universal benefits provided on the condition that people sought work and an end to means testing. Too punitive for many in the party and too expensive for others, Blair later commented that 'the problem was not so much that his thoughts were unthinkable as unfathomable.'[19] Yet, Labour did not completely ignore the caveats in Waddell and Burton's evidence review. *Good* work might be good for you—but bad work, poorly suited to the employee, could cause physical and mental health problems that could themselves lead to worklessness.[20] Acknowledging these issues had two consequences. First, as already outlined, the government introduced a series of policies designed to 'make work pay', increasing the gap between benefit rates and wages by raising the effective take-home pay of workers through tax credits, the minimum wage and access to services such as childcare, rehabilitation, and work training. This approach, which Peter Sloman describes as 'redistributive market liberalism', entrenched many of the aspects of neoliberal social security reforms of the 1980s and early 1990s; but at the same time, there was a greater commitment than during the Conservative years to using 'the market' and state apparatus to measure and attack acute poverty.[21] Second, this mix of a market liberal approach and the social democratic roots of the Labour party meant that the government acknowledged that there were still groups of the 'deserving poor' who were targeted less stringently and more slowly than other groups of benefit claimants. Consciously, New Labour only began to consider radical reforms to disability benefits in the early 2000s and did not draft concrete plans until the run up to the 2005 General Election.[22]

While the headline targets of benefit reform were the unemployed, 'undeserving' benefit claimants, and those on the margins of employment who could be reskilled and rehabilitated, there were knock-on consequences for in-work sickness. The focus on getting claimants into work—any work—meant that people were often fitted to jobs that did not suit their experience, qualifications, or personal preferences. The 'world of work' had indeed 'altered', as Tony Blair

---

[17] Disability Rights Commission, *Annual Report and Accounts April to September 2007* (London: TSO, 2009).

[18] Field had been chair of the Child Poverty Action Group, whose responses to SSP are covered in Chapters 5 and 6.

[19] In reference to Field's remit which had been 'to think the unthinkable'. Tony Blair, *Tony Blair: A Journey* (London: Stanley Paul, 2010), p. 217.

[20] Waddell and Burton, *Is Work Good for Your Health and Well-Being?*

[21] Sloman, 'Redistribution in an age of neoliberalism'.

[22] See below and Hill, 'Working hard or hardly working?'

declared, and would continue to do so as a result of government policy. A greater proportion of people worked in service industries, with more women and more part-time work in the economy (Figure 7.1).[23] But if 'people no longer expect[ed] a job for life', then it was because they had little choice but to accept jobs that would only ever be temporarily satisfactory for them and their employer. The global move towards 'flexible' employment—where companies employed people on short-term, insecure contracts so that they could hire and dismiss workers according to acute needs rather than having to make long-term investments— produced a glut of low-paying work requiring few qualifications, but made it harder to secure jobs with long-term prospects.[24] Further, while the minimum wage and tax credits increased the potential take-home pay of a worker versus an out-of-work benefit claimant in the same situation, it also encouraged a 'Speenhamland' system of wage supplementation by the state that allowed businesses to hire people on a statutory minimum with little prospect of career advancement.[25] Underemployment and precarity became increasingly common in the new millennium, and this was reflected in the way workers responded to absenteeism policing and the sick note.

If sickness welfare were to change, so too would the sick note. Rather than being a certificate that an individual had met the eligibility criteria for benefit—a binary distinction between capacity and incapacity—the state required something new. Public and private institutions needed to assess those in the hinterland of employability, people with health conditions yet capable of some kind of work. As a result, the methods of assessing and categorizing benefit claimants underwent significant reform in the 2000s.

[23] Jim Tomlinson, Jim Phillips, and Valerie Wright, 'De-industrialization: A case study of Dundee, 1951–2001, and its broad implications', *Business History* (2019): pp. 1–27. For other long-term employment trends, see Blessing Chiripanhura and Nikolas Wolf, 'Long-term trends in UK employment: 1861 to 2018', Office of National Statistics, 29 April 2019, accessed 24 November 2020, https://www.ons.gov.uk/economy/nationalaccounts/uksectoraccounts/compendium/economicreview/april2019/longtermtrendsinukemployment1861to2018.

[24] See Chapter 8 and Il-Ho Kim et al., 'Welfare states, flexible employment, and health: A critical review', *Health Policy* 104, no. 2 (2012): pp. 99–127; Jill Rubery, Arjan Keizer, and Damian Grimshaw, 'Flexibility bites back: The multiple and hidden costs of flexible employment policies', *Human Resource Management Journal* 26, no. 3 (2016): pp. 235–51.

[25] 'Speenhamland' was a system of poverty relief in the early nineteenth century which topped up poor people's wages. It was criticized for allowing employers to simply pay less, effectively making local rate payers subsidize businesses' labour costs. Poor Law Commissioners, *Report from His Majesty's Commissioners for Inquiring into the Administration and Practical Operation of the Poor Laws* (London: B. Fellowes, 1834), esp. pp. 128–34. For more on these criticisms of tax credits and wage supplementation, including the Family Income Supplement policies of the Heath government in the 1970s, see: Hill, 'Working hard or hardly working?'; Grover and Piggott, 'Social security, employment and Incapacity Benefit'; Hewitt, 'New Labour and social security'; Sloman, 'Redistribution in an age of neoliberalism'.

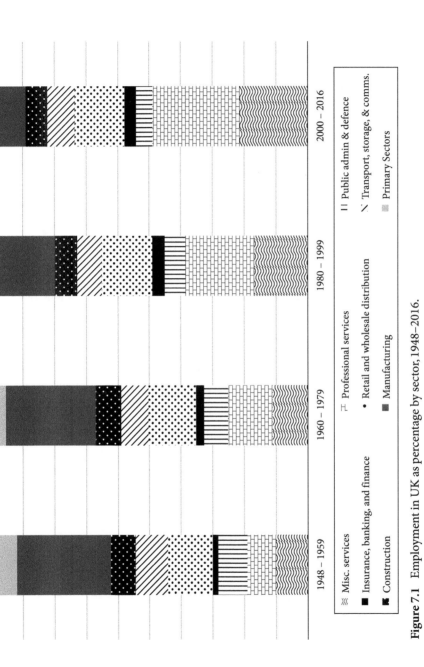

Figure 7.1 Employment in UK as percentage by sector, 1948–2016.

'Misc. services' includes hotels and careering. 'Professional services' includes scientific and technical services (including education and health).

Source: Blessing Chiripanhura and Nikolas Wolf, 'Long-term trends in UK employment: 1861 to 2018', Office of National Statistics, 29 April 2019, accessed 24 November 2020, https://www.ons.gov.uk/economy/nationalaccounts/uksectoraccounts/compendium/economicreview/april2019/longtermtrendsinukemployment1861to2018.

Employment and Support Allowance

'Merthyr has become the "sick-note capital of Britain" – with 24 pc of working-age adults claiming disability benefits' reported the *Daily Mail*'s David Jones in April 1998 under a double-page spread titled 'Sign up here for Sick-note Britain'.[26] Rather than an attack on in-work absenteeism the phrase was directed at disability benefit claimants. The *Mail* asked 'what the Government can do about a problem that is diverting funds from the genuinely ill', and provided a vignette of the Welsh Valleys' town that depicted the residents as 'habitual malingerers and spineless quitters', drug addicted 'scroungers' with 'large colour television[s], expensive stereo[s], fashionable cream-coloured blinds [and] decent carpets' who spent too much time on a weekday 'milling around, chatting about nothing very much'.[27] By 2007, the press had picked up on a story that 2,000 Incapacity Benefit claimants were signed off because they were too fat to work. A further 50 had acne and ten were incapacitated by leprosy.[28] 'Little riles the taxpayer more than the thought of their hard-earned, much-needed cash being siphoned straight into the cake-stuffed pocked of a lazy benefit cheat', noted Clare Allan in the *Guardian*.[29] In many ways, this continued rhetoric seen in the late 1980s and early 1990s driven by similar economic shifts. Even the *Mail* piece acknowledged the lack of employment in Merthyr, especially after the rapid closure of the coalmines. It had been well-established in the debates over disability benefits that regions with high unemployment also experienced high levels of disability.[30] It was also not new to imply that certain demographics cheated the benefits system, or that conditions such as 'stress', 'bad backs', or morbid obesity, did not 'deserve' disability payments.[31] Still, in the late 1990s and into the new millennium there was an increase in the volume and hostility in the use of 'sick note' as a rhetorical device to attack out-of-work disability claimants; a rhetoric that government ministers were willing to endorse.

'Sick note Britain' was a curious term to employ for disability since Incapacity Benefit was no longer determined by a 'sick note' in the form of the Med 3 used for in-work sickness. The functioning assessment part of the All Work Test (by the 2000s named the Personal Capability Assessment) determined a claimant's eligibility for benefit based on the ability to perform certain work-related tasks as assessed by a Benefits Agency Medical Service-contracted professional.[32]

---

[26] Jones, 'Sign up here for Sick-note Britain'.   [27] Ibid.

[28] Richard Ford and Sam Coates, 'Too fat to work', *The Times*, 19 November 2007, p. 1.

[29] Clare Allan, 'It's my life: Those who can't work still have something to give', *Guardian*, 9 April 2008, p. 6.

[30] See Chapter 6 and C. Beatty et al., *Hidden Unemployment in the East Midlands* (Sheffield: Centre for Regional Economic and Social Research, Sheffield Hallam University, 2002).

[31] See Chapter 4 on migration and Chapter 6 on 'stress' and 'bad backs'. Also: Henry Fisher, *Report of the Committee on Abuse of Social Security Benefits (Cmnd 5228)* (London: HMSO, 1972).

[32] See Chapter 6.

Nevertheless, the idea that a flawed testing procedure was a convenient excuse for 'undeserving' people access to benefit pervaded beyond the right-wing press. As Mirko Grdešić has demonstrated, one of the attractive elements of neoliberal benefit policies was that they were about 'making "tough" but "necessary" choices', appealing to individuals and organizations from a range of ideological traditions.[33] Grotesque caricatures like Andy from the popular sketch show *Little Britain* could be read as a joke at the expense of well-meaning, naïve people trying to do the right thing (represented by his carer, Lou), exploited by canny malingerers who knew how to elicit sympathy.[34]

New Labour was also concerned with benefit 'scroungers', though initially it concentrated primarily on the general classes of 'the unemployed'. Partially, Peter Hill argues, this was because disabled people were still considered part of the 'deserving poor'.[35] Those who were 'really' and 'severely' disabled (however those states could be adequately determined) had to be supported by the state for moral and electoral reasons.[36] Such concerns had also been faced by the first two terms of the Thatcher government.[37] As Incapacity Benefit continued to consume a large part of DWP's budget and economic inactivity did not fall as much as was hoped, these issues became more politically sensitive. Like invalidity benefit in the 1990s, the number of new claimants entering the benefit remained higher than the number who left. DWP therefore followed two paths. On the one side, it launched a 'Pathways to Work' programme for disabled people, providing training and job placement for those who were capable of some form of paid work. Pilots began in the mid-2000s based around 'Work Focused Interviews' with claimants.[38] On the other, it sought to reduce entitlement to disability related benefits by redesigning the All Work Test and forcing some disabled claimants to take part in programmes that would prepare them for the world of work, moving them eventually either into employment or jobseekers allowance.[39] The result was

[33] M. Grdešić, 'Neoliberalism and welfare chauvinism in Germany: An examination of survey evidence', *German Politics & Society* 37, no. 2 (2019): pp. 1–22.

[34] The character first appears in *Little Britain—Bath of Beans*, broadcast BBC Three, 16 September 2003. The dynamic between Andy and Lou is more complex than this, but clearly exploited 'the common sense idea of a binary between true and faked disability'. Margaret Anne Montgomerie, 'Visibility, empathy and derision: Popular television representations of disability', *Alter* 4, no. 2 (2010): pp. 94–102, at 98.

[35] Hill, 'Working hard or hardly working?', p. 200. See also Grover and Piggott, 'Social security, employment and Incapacity Benefit'.

[36] Similar ideas are expressed in wider disability policy. See, e.g.: Prime Minister's Strategy Unit, *Improving the Life Chances of Disabled People* (London: Prime Minister's Strategy Unit, 2005).

[37] Gareth Millward, 'Invalid definitions, invalid responses: Disability and the welfare state, 1965–1995' (PhD thesis, London School of Hygiene and Tropical Medicine, 2014); Paul Pierson, *Dismantling the Welfare State?: Reagan, Thatcher, and the Politics of Retrenchment* (Cambridge: Cambridge University Press, 1994), p. 6.

[38] Helen Gray, Richard Dorsett, and Getinet Haile, *The Impact of Pathways to Work* (Leeds: Corporate Document Services, 2007).

[39] Department of Work and Pensions, *A New Deal for Welfare: Empowering People to Work (Cm 6730)* (London: TSO, 2006).

Employment and Support Allowance (ESA). To triage claimants, a Work-Related Activity Group (WRAG) time-limited the benefit for those considered able to become capable of work through training and rehabilitation. A Support Group remained for the rest. These categories were determined by a new Work Capability Assessment built on the same 'functioning' principles as the Personal Capability Assessment.[40]

The Work Capability Assessment has become notorious in the years after its introduction. The Ken Loach film *I, Daniel Blake* dramatized the often arbitrary way in which people with genuine medical conditions and long-standing National Insurance contributions could be denied benefit.[41] For years, disability organizations had made the same criticisms of the Conservative–Liberal Democrat coalition government, and even an independent DWP-commissioned review body noted significant failings with the way the tests were being applied and interpreted.[42] The large contracts offered to private companies to perform the testing procedures also attracted criticism, with questions about how democratically accountable such firms could be and whether the profit motives and target setting cultures of these businesses and DWP led to perverse incentives to find claimants fit for work.[43] Some of these concerns are considered in greater detail in the Conclusion to this volume. Still, it must be stressed: despite being associated heavily with the punitive policies pursued by the Treasury and the Iain Duncan Smith-led DWP during the coalition, ESA was created by New Labour for specific purposes related to its wider goals of reducing economic inactivity.[44] Therefore the creation of punitive as well as supportive mechanisms in ESA has to be seen in the context of New Labour, as does the use of outsourcing and target setting.[45] Moreover, the effects of the global recession after late 2007 coloured the Brown and Cameron ministries' approaches to ESA, even though the planning for the benefit preceded the crash. This section, therefore, considers ESA as an evolution of New Labour policy and its relationship to the sick notes seen in the

[40] Malcolm Harrington, *An Independent Review of the Work Capability Assessment* (London: TSO, 2010).

[41] Ken Loach (dir.), *I, Daniel Blake* (BFI, 2016).

[42] Gareth Millward and Peter Border, *Assessing Capacity for Work (PN 413)* (London: Parliamentary Office of Science and Technology, 2012); Jackie Gulland, *Gender, Work and Social Control: A Century of Disability Benefits* (London: Palgrave Macmillan, 2019); Paul Litchfield, *An Independent Review of the Work Capability Assessment—Year Five* (London: TSO, 2014).

[43] Debbie Jolly, 'A tale of two models: Disabled people vs Unum, Atos, government and disability charities', Disabled People Against Cuts, 8 April 2012, accessed 24 November 2020, http://dpac.uk.net/2012/04/a-tale-of-two-models-disabled-people-vs-unum-atos-government-and-disability-charities-debbie-jolly/; Jon Warren, Kayleigh Garthwaite, and Clare Bambra, 'After Atos Healthcare: Is the Employment and Support Allowance fit for purpose and does the Work Capability Assessment have a future?', *Disability & Society* 29, no. 8 (2014): pp. 1319–23.

[44] Chris Grover, 'The end of an era? The resignation of Iain Duncan Smith, Conservatism and social security benefits for disabled people', *Disability & Society* 31, no. 8 (2016): pp. 1127–31.

[45] On this form of governance see: Michael Burton, *The Politics of Public Sector Reform: From Thatcher to the Coalition* (Basingstoke: Palgrave Macmillan, 2013), pp. 163–5, 189–94, 219–24.

rest of this book rather than offering a disability studies critique informed by its operation in the 2010s.

ESA was designed as both a 'carrot' and a 'stick' to reduce dependency on disability benefits, though it was difficult to determine from the initial proposals the true size of either. Secretary of State Alan Johnson published plans to reform Incapacity Benefit in early 2005.[46] Speculation from the left-leaning press, such as in one editorial by Polly Toynbee, suggested that the stick was more a 'tiny twig', a presentational attempt to outmanoeuvre Michael Howard's Conservative Party and show that Labour could be tough on benefit abuse even though the substance of the proposals was relatively benign.[47] Business commentators also appeared quite supportive of the principles behind the plans. *Public Finance* described Johnson's plans as 'firm but fair', a necessary political move to avoid the accusation of 'being called a soft touch for feckless, workshy scroungers'.[48] But the proposals were more than presentational, being pursued by both Blair and Brown in New Labour's final term in office. Although Johnson moved to the Department of Trade and Industry after the election—very nearly earning himself the job title 'Secretary of State for PENIS'—the plans survived him in DWP.[49] His successor David Blunkett was also keen to reduce expenditure on disability benefits.[50] A 2006 green paper was published under John Hutton before implementation was taken on by Peter Hain and then James Purnell.[51] Hain, in a piece for *New Statesman* shortly before his resignation over financial irregularities in his deputy leadership campaign, argued that government needed to provide opportunity for 'British benefit claimants becoming British workers in British jobs' by 'calling time on our "sick note" culture'.[52] Unlike the Conservatives who would, Hain claimed, simply cut eligibility to benefit to allow for tax cuts, Labour would use public funds to invest in training, partnerships with employers, and other back-to-work schemes to get people off Incapacity Benefit and into paid employment. In defending these proposals, he highlighted a 'Workfare' scheme in Wisconsin

---

[46] Department of Work and Pensions, *Five Year Strategy: Opportunity and Security Throughout Life (Cm 6447)* (London: TSO, February 2005).

[47] Polly Toynbee, 'Huge carrot, tiny twig', *Guardian*, 4 February 2005, p. 23. See also: David Cracknell, 'Labour's plan is not just good economics', *Personnel Today*, 25 January 2005, p. 9.

[48] Judith Hirst, 'Birth of a salesman', *Public Finance*, 18–24 February 2005, pp. 30–2.

[49] Tony Blair had promised Johnson the ministerial post at a new trade department called 'the Department of Productivity, Energy, Industry and Science'—with some rascals in Whitehall adding the 'n' from 'energy' to the acronym. Johnson retold the story in 2016, possibly with some embellishment: Mikey Smith, 'Alan Johnson reveals he was very nearly Secretary of State for PENIS', *Mirror*, 11 September 2016, accessed 17 August 2020, https://www.mirror.co.uk/news/uk-news/alan-johnson-reveals-very-nearly-8812242. It was also reported at the time: 'Profile: Alan Johnson', *Daily Telegraph*, 18 June 2005.

[50] 'He told the Guardian that many parts of Britain had "lost the work ethic that existed in working-class estates in which I grew up in northern Sheffield"'. Patrick Wintour, 'Specialist plan to advise GPs on sick notes', *Guardian*, 11 August 2005, p. 7.

[51] *Cm 6730*; Stephen Kennedy and Wendy Wilson, *The Welfare Reform Bill (RP 06/39)* (London: House of Commons Library, 2006).

[52] Peter Hain, 'Labour and the sick note', *New Statesman* 136, no. 4873 (2007): pp. 13–14.

championed by the Conservatives which succeeded in reducing the disability benefit rolls, but did not result in claimants finding new work, leaving many reliant upon family or charity.[53] For Purnell, this was 'a cultural shift'. 'Gone are the days when writing a sick note is writing people off for life...ESA will give more financial support to the poorest, most disabled in society while extending the opportunity of employment to all those who can work'.[54]

Despite the high turnover of ministers at DWP, disputes had never been about the 'carrot', but about the relative size of the 'stick'. Reports emerged that Johnson's predecessor, Andrew Smith, had resigned because of his opposition to time limiting claims to Incapacity Benefit, though he had championed policies to 'reskill' disabled people.[55] Johnson and Blunkett were also pressured to move faster to reduce claimant numbers than either had initially wanted.[56] Disability groups were concerned that, like the All Work Test, the main goal was to cut costs rather than genuinely target resources where they could be the most effective. This target-driven 'evidence based policy' approach which had been present in the Conservative governments accelerated under New Labour and was known to throw up perverse incentives.[57] There was also apprehension at the speed at which the plans were put into motion. The Green Paper was published in January,[58] the consultation document—which gave little space for the feedback from disability organizations—was published in June,[59] while the Bill to create ESA was published in July.[60] As for the Work Capability Assessment, although it borrowed from the principles of the Personal Capability Assessment, it was deployed in a different way. All claimants would now have to undergo the Assessment, removing the 'own occupation test' for short-term Incapacity Benefit.[61] This was explicitly designed to move people into work; but, as Chris Grover and Linda Piggott noted in their contemporary analysis of the plans, 'the focus...is the quantity rather than the quality of paid employment', somewhat undermining Waddell and Burton's caveats about the need for appropriate work.[62] Moreover, it had not

---

[53] Hain, 'Labour and the sick note'; Andrew Grice, 'Crackdown to prevent the young falling into life on state benefits', *Independent*, 29 December 2007, p. 11.

[54] Sam Coates, 'Benefit claimants lose incentive to stay sick', *Times*, 28 March 2008, p. 36.

[55] David Cracknell, 'Labour's plan is not just good economics', *Personnel Today*, 25 January 2005, p. 9; James Blitz, 'Blair and Brown at odds over reshuffle', *The Times*, 7 September 2004, p. 1; Marie Woolf, 'Unflashy workhorse who won respect', *Independent*, 7 September 2004, p. 18.

[56] Polly Toynbee, 'A chance to rescue others from life's dead-end sidings', *Guardian*, 1 November 2005, p. 33.

[57] Justin Parkhurst, *The Politics of Evidence: From Evidence-Based Policy to Good Governance of Evidence* (Abingdon: Routledge, 2017). Sloman describes this process with regard to child poverty in Sloman, 'Redistribution in an Age of Neoliberalism', esp. at p. 736.

[58] Cm 6730.

[59] Department of Work and Pensions, *A New Deal for Welfare: Empowering People to Work. Consultation Report (Cm 6859)* (London: TSO, June 2006).

[60] On this timeline and the criticism from disability organizations, see: Grover and Piggott, 'Social security, employment and Incapacity Benefit'.

[61] Kennedy and Wilson, *The Welfare Reform Bill*.

[62] Grover and Piggott, 'Social security, employment and Incapacity Benefit'.

dispensed with the 'sick note' principle of signing people off work entirely. As with Invalidity and Incapacity Benefits, the process still depended on an arbitrary line dividing 'the incapable' from other types of claimant. The novelty came in explicitly acknowledging a hinterland group through the WRAG of people who were discriminated against due to impairment or temporarily incapable but who could become moulded to the needs of the economy. Those who refused to be disciplined could be denied incapacity-related support. Still, as Jackie Gulland argues (and many of the examples in this volume attest), such conditionality was not invented in 2008. There have always been expectations imposed upon claimants, with those who did not conform to ideal types regularly accused of malingering.[63]

These attitudes to chronic sickness and unemployment cannot be separated from contemporary anxieties around short-term sickness in employees. Indeed, the sick note rhetoric employed against benefit 'scroungers' had many parallels with those who 'abused' the various sick pay and employment protections that businesses were now obliged to provide. As with disability, there were concerted efforts to get people 'back to work' as quickly as possible by assessing what workers could do while living with medical conditions as well as what 'reasonable adjustments' employers could make. Similarly, there was concern that the economy needed to police the borders of 'genuine' sickness as the rise in certain conditions and employee behaviours could not be explained by authentic morbidity.

'Sick Note Britain'

While the *Daily Mail*'s 1998 article focused on the 'sick-note Britain' of Incapacity Benefit, short-term sick notes continued to be a source of tension in Britain's welfare state. The shortcomings of medical certification which this volume has detailed remained. Fifty years of daily use had further cemented behaviours, administrative apparatus, and cultural meanings that were hard to shift. The economic and political changes that had driven New Labour's reforms of long-term sickness-related benefits were reflected in the way people talked about and understood sick notes and absence from work. The government would eventually respond to criticisms from various constituencies by creating the 'fit note'. Before examining that process, the media around absenteeism and 'skivers' is instructive. Framed by business groups' preoccupations with absenteeism, there was also resistance from doctors and claimants to the demands placed upon them.

In the 1940s and 1950s, sick notes and absenteeism were linked to anxieties about national productivity and the need to rebuild the postwar economy.[64] In

---

[63] Gulland, *Gender, Work and Social Control*, pp. 80–1.
[64] See Chapter 3.

the 2000s, negative stories about absence were driven by reports commissioned by business confederations and insurance companies. According to the Confederation of British Industry (CBI), absenteeism cost £10 billion in 1998, which was up to £11.6 billion in 2003 and £17 billion by the end of the decade.[65] Norwich Union claimed this was fuelled by 9 million sick notes which were 'questionable or invalid' in 2004 (or 40 per cent of all notes).[66] This research formed part of a wider knowledge sharing ecosystem built on the identification and marketing of 'absenteeism' as a key risk for employers to manage. This had been driven by the fact that employers were now solely responsible for Statutory Sick Pay. The surveys continued to prove that absenteeism existed and that the extent of it was increasing[67]—even though other measures, such as the Labour Force Survey data outlined in Figure 1.2—contradicted these 'specialist' findings.[68] Companies facing these risks—including effects such as lost wages and productivity—could, of course, purchase insurance products from the companies that happened to sponsor the reports.[69] Human resources (HR) and absentee management could be outsourced to specialist agencies.[70] Alongside this, an economy had grown around producing and disseminating information on the best means of preventing absence. HR and business administration trade journals such as *Personnel Today* and *Employee Benefits* regularly ran pieces on the effects of absenteeism, typical cases of disputes between employers and workers, and procedures that organizations could adopt to stop people becoming sick (or helping them back to work faster if they did).[71] As Phil Taylor and colleagues have argued, employers ended up reifying a particular form of absenteeism through these attempts to define, measure, and control it. Statistics were often unreliable from one study to another but were taken as proof that the problem was both large and growing. Computerization of sickness absences, deemed necessary in

[65] Darren Behar and Gordon Rayner, 'Bogus sick days costing business £1.75bn a year', *Daily Mail*, 24 May 2004, p. 2.

[66] 'Nearly half of all sick notes are "suspicious"', *The Times*, 24 April 2004, p. 5; Matt Keating, 'Office Hours: Do everyone a favour and don't bring your cold to work', *Guardian*, 26 November 2007, p. 3.

[67] Taylor et al., 'Too scared to go sick'.

[68] See: Office for National Statistics, 'Sickness absence in the UK labour market', *gov.uk*, 3 March 2021, accessed 13 July 2021, https://www.ons.gov.uk/employmentandlabourmarket/peopleinwork/employmentandemployeetypes/datasets/sicknessabsenceinthelabourmarket.

[69] Barry Hoffman, 'The protection gap must be bridged', *Employee Benefits*, February 2009, p. S35; Helen Sandler, 'Group income protection', *Employee Benefits*, April 2010, pp. 53–6. For example, the CBI's 2003 report was sponsored by AXA, the 2010 one by Pfizer. An Engineering Employers' Federation study in 2009 was sponsored by Unum. CBI, *On the Path to Recovery: Absence and Workplace Health Survey 2010* (London: CBI, 2010); Jonathan Moules, 'Slowing economy blamed for increase in long-term sickness, says survey', *Financial Times*, 18 May 2009, p. 6.

[70] Mark Vernon, 'A new chapter in outsourcing', *Financial Times*, 21 May 2003, online.

[71] Some examples from various journals include: 'Rise in stress boosts EAPS', *Employee Benefits*, June 2003, p. 7; Ross Wigham, 'Target the bullies to beat stress epidemic', *Personnel Today*, 10 February 2004, p. 10; Sam Barrett, 'Bad back to the future', *Corporate Adviser*, December 2006, p. 26; Jacky Hyams, 'A promising prognosis', *Human Resources*, October 2008, pp. 36–8; 'Coming months will create an absence headache for HR', *Personnel Today*, 21 July 2009, p. 3.

the wake of Statutory Sick Pay reform, allowed for cross-industry data sharing, but absenteeism was rarely like-for-like from one employer, let alone one sector, to the next. Perhaps even more crucially, the relative risk of absenteeism to an individual employer increased as companies became deliberately 'leaner', employing fewer people, demanding more of them, and allowing less slack in the system to account for missed hours or underperformance.[72] It is unsurprising in these circumstances that the gateway to legitimized 'involuntary absence'—the sick note—came under attack.[73]

Individual stories helped to make sense of these statistics. Just as sensational stories of scroungers helped justify Peter Lilley's attacks on disability benefits in the 1990s, common-sense-defying stories of malingerers made the absenteeism problem more believable. There was: the Premier League assistant referee signed off from his day job as a police sergeant with 'stress'; the British Transport Police officer with a 'bad back' who was moonlighting as a double-glazing salesman; and a surgeon on sick leave from his NHS work who used the time to make money performing operations on private patients and attending the Monaco Grand Prix.[74] 'Dock the pay of the sicknote skivers', blasted the *Daily Mail* on its front page in July 2004.[75] It appeared commonly accepted that workers were prone to taking the odd 'sickie', many of which just so happened to occur on a Monday.[76] There had to be a solution, surely? Besides, getting back to work was a question of will power. If Tony Blair could return to his job soon after a heart operation, then the whole nation could play their part to end the 'sick note culture'.[77]

Within this media climate that employers' groups had helped to create, businesses sought stricter policing of absenteeism. Yet, greater awareness of complicated and fluctuating long-term medical conditions, especially those involving mental health symptoms, had made it difficult to apply hard and fast rules. Nothing exemplified this better than 'stress'.[78] On the one hand, businesses had become more aware of their workers' mental health and the negative effects that overwork and a hostile environment could engender. Stress was a 'legitimate' reason for missing work and something a business needed to manage. A 2008

[72] Taylor et al., 'Too scared to go sick'.

[73] On 'involuntary absence' and attempts to quantify, see Chapter 3.

[74] Andrew Norfolk, 'This police sergeant is off sick suffering from stress', *The Times*, 18 September 2002, p. 5; Michael Clarke, 'The sicknote squad', *Daily Mail*, 20 September 2000, p. 39; Sue Lapperman, 'Sick-note surgeon loses job plea', *The Times*, 14 January 1999, p. 3.

[75] David Hughes and Sean Poulter, 'Dock the pay of the sicknote skivers', *Daily Mail*, 5 July 2004, p. 1.

[76] Darren Behar, 'Drastic cure is prescribed for sickie epidemic', *Daily Mail*, 13 July 2004, p. 9; Carol Midgley, 'The furtive myth of Mondayitis', *The Times*, 25 January 2007, p. 14.

[77] David Charter, 'Doctors told to follow Blair and end "sicknote culture"', *The Times*, 19 October 2004, p. 12.

[78] On this history, see Chapter 6 and Jill Kirby, *Feeling the Strain: A Cultural History of Stress in Twentieth-Century Britain* (Manchester: Manchester University Press, 2019); Mark Jackson (ed.), *Stress in Post-War Britain, 1945–85* (Abingdon: Routledge, 2013).

survey (sponsored by AXA) suggested that 69 per cent of HR departments saw it as 'prevalent' in their organizations.[79] On the other hand, individuals claiming stress were treated with suspicion and, sometimes, outright hostility. GPs were regularly chastised for being far too willing to sign people off with this 'unsubstantiated diagnosis…they do not expect to be challenged'.[80] Businesses argued that GPs would write sick notes 'at the drop of a hat' and 'dish them out too freely' to patients whose tales they were too willing to take at face value.[81] The CBI further criticized doctors for being slow to give appointments and only being open during work hours, meaning employees had to wait for treatment and miss work to receive it.[82] HR commentators argued that all this made it difficult to separate malingerers from genuine cases, or, at the very least, made it tough to identify the causes of stress which would enable the employer to make reasonable adjustments.[83] Workers with mental health problems were also aware that diagnoses were 'not specific and tangible'. As author Clare Allan wrote, mental illness 'doesn't show up on scans or in blood tests or fit neatly into boxes, which must be trying for a government determined to have us all stamped and sorted and processed and put back to work'.[84] But it was not just stress. The old 'bad back' remained a bugbear, joined by the increased visibility of eating disorders, fertility treatment, and gender confirmation surgery.[85] Grief was a particularly tricky psychological diagnosis. As one worker noted on an agony aunt forum in 2001:

They said that unless I come back to work quickly (my GP signed me off for another three weeks) my present post would have to be given to someone else, and I would have to take whatever post was left when I go back.…If I don't go back I know I'll end up with the grotty job no-one else wants when I eventualy [sic] do. If I do go back I don't know if I can cope.…Why can't people leave me

[79] Alison Clements, 'Get a grip on your stressed-out staff', *Human Resources*, April 2008, pp. 30–; Tara Craig, 'Firing off…hard-up employees', *Personnel Today*, 9 December 2008, p. 28; Lucy Chamberlain and Nina Lakhani, 'Stress in the workplace', *Independent on Sunday*, 16 May 2010, pp. 10–11.
[80] Regional medical director of Chevron Texaco quoted in 'Rise in stress boosts EAPS', *Employee Benefits*, June 2003, p. 7.
[81] Peter Rose, 'Halt these bogus damages claims, says the police peer', *Daily Mail*, 22 June 1998, p. 30; Derren Hayes, 'Signing off the sick note?', *Community Care*, 8 May 2008, pp. 32–3; 'Absence rate still rising', *Employee Benefits*, August 2004, p. 14; 'Finance directors do not trust GPs' sicknote system', *Personnel Today*, 20 January 2004, p. 3; Mark Conrad, 'GPs tend to believe sick note requests', *Public Finance*, 15–21 July 2005, p. 15; 'GPs under fire for being no help', *Personnel Today*, 20 November 2007, p. 4.
[82] Sally Gainsbury, 'CBI joins in the criticism of GP opening hours', *Public Finance*, 21–7 September 2007, p. 11.
[83] Judith Hogarth, 'Pay less for stress', *Works Management*, 55 no. 8 (2002): p. 15.
[84] Clare Allan, 'It's my life', *Guardian*, 9 April 2008, p. 6.
[85] Sara Williams 'Gender change calls for caution', *GP*, 14 September 2007, p. 46; Irene Krechowiecka, 'Will previous health problems harm my chance of this job?', *Guardian*, 5 August 2006, p. 2; Judith Watson, 'Time off for fertility treatment', *Personnel Today*, 13 June 2006, p. 18; Amelia Hill, 'GPs rapped over eating disorders', *Observer*, 6 February 2005, p. 14.

alone? They knew [my husband], yet they understand so little about how it feels, and what they've done to me.[86]

Employers associated these diagnoses as 'problems' with equalities legislation under UK and European law, complaining of 'trading on eggshells' and how 'sacking slackers can be hard work'.[87] One expert advised having clear stress guidelines so that 'employees with *tactical* stress will have to move at your pace instead of being untouchable'.[88] The sick note did not help matters. Perhaps if a medical statement could provide more information, it would allow employers to help their employees back to work more safely and protect 'genuine' cases.

CBI criticisms of GPs were unwelcome, but doctors were equally unimpressed with their role. GPs did not want to be the police force for employers and DWP; they did not want to be in potential conflict with patients, who could leave for other doctors or, in some cases, become violent if denied a sick note; and they were especially critical at the workload demands of writing private notes for employers who refused to accept that self-certification had become standard for the first week of sickness.[89] They were also aware that sick notes were too crude, demanding certainty that was not always possible. One GP wrote to *The Times* about writing a statement recommending a worker could return to light duties who was then dismissed for not being fit enough to climb ladders.[90] Job Centres routinely asked for more definitive recommendations when presented with conditional notes.[91] Another doctor used the example of a wife who was in no emotional state to work because her husband had been diagnosed with terminal cancer. How could a sick note—which would need to maintain the confidentiality of the husband—express the genuine incapacity of the wife without opening her up to 'back to work interviews' or other forms of intervention from the employer for which she was not ready?[92] Even if they could provide certainty, there was simply not enough time (in aggregate or with each individual patient) to truly assess degrees of incapacity. The British Medical Association (BMA) asserted that

---

[86] Member of DearDenise Message Board, posted on 6 June 2001, accessed 3 December 2018, archived 15 July 2001, http://web.archive.org/web/20010715061955/http://www.linksolutions.co.uk:80/ubb/Forum2/HTML/000129-3.html.

[87] Laurie Mandy, 'ECJ ruling is bad for employers', *Personnel Today*, 22 September 2009, p. 4; 'Age laws threatening UK group life market', *Financial Adviser*, 1 May 2008; Ross Bentley, 'Treading on eggshells', *Personnel Today*, 25 September 2007, pp. 29–30; John O'Donnell, 'Sacking slackers can be hard work', *Sunday Times*, 29 July 2001, p. 60.

[88] Emphasis mine. Julie Quinn, 'Stress management – why bother?', *Personnel Today*, 11 March 2008, p. 11.

[89] See: 'GP has endured a decade of abuse and intimidation', *Pulse*, 20 March 1999, p. 12; Dr David Church letter to *Pulse*, 20 August 2005, p. 22; 'Return of the dreaded sicknote', *Pulse*, 3 April 1999, p. 57; Amelia Gentleman, 'BMA tells firms to cut demand for sick notes', *Guardian*, 23 November 1998, p. 7.

[90] Dr Neville Conway letter to *The Times*, 25 February 2008, p. 18.

[91] Anonymous letter to *Pulse*, 7 December 2006, p. 22; Dr David Church letter to *Pulse*, 20 August 2005, p. 22.

[92] Stuart Wavell, 'Liar, liar, you should be fired', *Sunday Times*, 2 May 2004, p. 9.

blaming GPs was a 'cop out' for the poor practices and low morale in British business, the real driver of absenteeism.[93] One surgery had even taken to providing template sick notes at reception for patients to fill in themselves and deliver to the employer, including the admonishment:

> We consider that any pressure by employers to coerce general practitioners into involvement in the policing of sick leave is an abuse of the National Health Service. Under no circumstances will we co-operate with any such system. Employers may, with the written consent of the patient, request a private medical report from this surgery.[94]

The presentation of sick notes in the media and the policing systems businesses employed had caused problems for doctors. However, not all coping strategies were targeted at those with power. It had become a trope that doctors all had weird and wonderful sick note stories. A column called 'Last Word' in the medical magazine *Pulse* had standard questions for doctors who had some connection to recent events, one of which was about the best excuse they had received for why their patient wanted a sick note. Examples included a criminal who did not want his work colleagues to see his ankle tag, and another who claimed he was dead.[95] *GP* magazine had its own feature, 'Plain tales from the surgery' ('£25 for each Plain Tale published') in which amusing stories would often feature a sick note of some kind: such as a shopping centre Father Christmas who claimed he only worked one day a year; and a sober man pretending to be an alcoholic so that he did not have to register for work at the local Job Centre.[96] These examples were relatively benign, as were those in the column by Catherine Laraman in *Pulse* in 2000. After expressing frustration at one patient, she explained 'Perhaps I wouldn't feel so irritated if I knew that those who were truly deserving were getting what they needed. Last week I spoke on the phone with a profoundly depressed lady who told me she had been refused [Disability Living Allowance] because she "could walk more than 100 yards and didn't need help with dressing".'[97] Nevertheless, some were simply nasty. Tony Copperfield wrote for *Doctor* and, later, *The Times* about his 'Neanderthal' patients who 'need a kick up the arse' rather than a sick note.[98] Phil Peverely expressed surprise at 'one of my call centre-employed patients who has an unusual – that is to say, a measurable – amount of

[93] Georgina Fuller, 'Doctors slam employers "cop out" over sicknotes', *Personnel Today*, 20 June 2006, p. 1; Deborah Orr, 'Our obsession with economic growth is producing dissatisfaction and unhappiness', *Independent*, 5 July 2006, p. 29.

[94] Dr Henry Tegner letter to *Pulse*, 7 March 1998, p. 45.

[95] 'Last Word', *Pulse*, 24 October 2007, p. 68 and 18 October 2007, p. 60.

[96] 'Plain tales from the surgery', *GP*, 27 April 2007, p. 68 and 20 April 2007, p. 88.

[97] Catherine Laraman, 'Life as a new principal', *Pulse*, 3 June 2000, p. 90.

[98] Tony Copperfield, 'The sick-note season opens', *The Times*, 29 December 2007, p. 4.

work ethic'.[99] Mary Selby scoffed at 'Mr Tired' who 'sees being bipolar as something rather fashionably artistic, like being a poet or a fan of Accrington Stanley';[100] and 'Mr Lazy' who 'would be devastated to the point of catatonia to realize that, in fact, he is a malingering freeloader'.[101]

While it is clear that these accounts were caricatures (perhaps even *Little Britain* style grotesques), with both the behaviour of the patient and the anger of the GP exaggerated for comedic effect, they were more than just the gallows humour of a profession letting off steam in the safe space of the trade magazine. Prejudices about patients had real-world medical and social effects.[102] A study in 2006 showed that decision making around sick notes for patients expressing the same symptoms was affected by the gender of the GP and the patient.[103] Such attitudes would disproportionately affect older women in part-time work, still the most likely demographic to need time off because of additional caring responsibilities and other factors that have been covered throughout this volume.[104] In part, this discrepancy in treatment was because of how people talked about sickness and the stresses in their lives. To demonstrate this point, a GP in Northern Ireland asked 'a gaggle of fourth year [medical] students' which patient they would most likely give a sick note to, 'the woman who needs a break from a job driving her insane or the man with a "bad back" during the World Cup?' The students chose the man. '"Why? I asked. "Because he gave a medical reason."'[105]

These representations of sick notes in the popular media and trade journals informed policy discussions and the way that medical certification was understood. One group remains largely absent from these accounts, however: the claimants themselves. If employers were demanding medical certificates from their workers, how did employees respond? Increased access to the World Wide Web from the late 1990s has left a trace of these responses in internet archives. Here we see resistance to surveillance and policing around absenteeism, but also how the sick note had become a ubiquitous part of illness in Britain by the new millennium.[106]

[99] Phil Peverely, 'Bacon vacations are a swine', *Pulse*, 4 November 2009, p. 44.

[100] Mary Selby, 'Not a lot of people have one of those', *GP*, 20 March 2009, p. 25.

[101] Mary Selby, 'It's time to drop the haloes', *GP*, 12 July 2004, p. 64.

[102] Carl Mclean, Catherine Campbell, and Flora Cornish, 'African-Caribbean interactions with mental health services in the UK: Experiences and expectations of exclusion as (re)productive of health inequalities', *Social Science & Medicine* 56, no. 3 (2003): pp. 657–69; Leigh Price, 'Wellbeing research and policy in the U.K.: Questionable science likely to entrench inequality', *Journal of Critical Realism* 16, no. 5 (2017): pp. 451–67; Kate Young, Jane Fisher, and Maggie Kirkman, '"Do mad people get endo or does endo make you mad?": Clinicians' discursive constructions of medicine and women with endometriosis', *Feminism & Psychology* (2018).

[103] 'Gender has impact on GP sicknote decision', *Pulse*, 16 February 2006, p. 16.

[104] Rhymer Rigby, 'Sick notes', *Human Resources*, January 2006, pp. 48–51.

[105] Ian Banks, *Chemist & Druggist*, 27 August 2005, p. 13.

[106] The following sources were found largely through the UK Web Archive's prototype web archive search engine *SHINE*. This allows users to perform rudimentary text and facet searches of data from the.uk domain from 1996 to April 2013. 'SHINE', UK Web Archive, accessed 22 February 2021, https://www.webarchive.org.uk/shine. Although this does not return a representative sample of all British web users, it does provide a series of illustrate examples that can be cross-referenced with other

Message boards and blogs gave new spaces for people to interact and share information in online communities that provided support and advice.[107] At a base level, it was a forum to vent frustration. One person complained about a GP who would not write sick notes for less than a week, which meant that 'thanks to the current fascist governmental absence policies, when I go back I'm going to have to go through an interview with my boss to find out why I'm sick so much (probably the amount of events I go to), and actually risk losing my job.'[108] However, stories on message boards for a range of medical conditions show it was more than a place to rant. Sick notes served a narrative purpose, representing the moment the storyteller understood that something might be wrong, explaining the diagnostic process, unveiling the instant at which illness was validated, or simply appearing as a trivial and necessary part of negotiating the bureaucracy of employment and benefits. Examples include experiences as diverse as chicken pox,[109] fertility treatment,[110] anorexia and self-harm,[111] post-natal depression,[112] elective gastric band surgery,[113] myalgic encephalomyelitis,[114] social anxiety,[115]

primary sources. For more on writing contemporary history using these archives, see: Gareth Millward, 'A history with web archives, not a history of web archives: A history of the British measles-mumps-rubella vaccine crisis, 1998–2004', in *SAGE Handbook of Web History*, edited by Niels Brügger and Ian Milligan (Thousand Oaks: SAGE, 2018), pp. 464–78; Niels Brügger, *The Archived Web: Doing History in the Digital Age* (Cambridge: MIT Press, 2018).

[107] Ian Milligan, 'Mining the "internet graveyard": Rethinking the historians' toolkit', *Journal of the Canadian Historical Association/Revue de La SociétéHistorique Du Canada* 23, no. 2 (2012): pp. 21–64; Josh Cowls, 'Cultures of the UK web', in *The Web as History: Using Web Archives to Understand the Past and the Present*, edited by Niels Brügger and Ralph Schroeder (London: UCL Press, 2017), pp. 220–37.

[108] Message on COWSARSE, 3 December 2002, accessed 31 August 2020, archived 4 January 2003, http://web.archive.org/web/20030104121038/http://www.cs.aston.ac.uk:80/~dorandw/phpboards/boards/ooc/board.php.

[109] Gareth Ashley, 'Adult chicken pox diary', 1998, accessed 9 November 2020, archived 7 December 1998, http://web.archive.org/web/19981207014243/http:/www.helpdesk.demon.co.uk:80/pox.htm.

[110] Multiple authorship, 'I've returned, but only just', discussion thread on ivf-infertility.co.uk, first post 20 November 2002, accessed 9 November 2020, archived 10 January 2003, http://web.archive.org/web/20030110234830/http://www.ivf-infertility.co.uk:80/cgi-bin/teemz/teemz.cgi?board=_master&action=opentopic&topic=424&forum=General_Forum.

[111] Jax, 'Diary - 2002', Silent Words, 2002, accessed 9 November 2020, archived 2 September 2004, http://web.archive.org/web/20040902080024/http:/www.silentwords.co.uk:80/2002.htm.

[112] Anon, 'Getting through post natal depression', Families Online, n.d., accessed 9 November 2020, archived 8 April 2005, http://web.archive.org/web/20050408201723/http://familiesonline.co.uk:80/index.php/article/static/419/.

[113] Multiple authorship, 'Life is great!', discussion thread on Weight Loss Surgery Information & Support, 25 December 2003, accessed 9 November 2020, archived 29 March 2005, http://web.archive.org/web/20050329034000/http://www.wlsinfo.org.uk:80/newweb2/forum/post.asp?method=ReplyQuote&REPLY_ID=29539&TOPIC_ID=3117&FORUM_ID=88.

[114] abeator81, 'Getting stuff done', Amy Loves Peccarys, 29 November 2004, accessed 9 November 2020, archived 22 March 2005, http://web.archive.org/web/20050322172433/http://journals.aol.co.uk:80/abeator81/AmyLovesPeccarys/entries/423.

[115] Multiple authorship, 'Member profiles', Social Anxiety UK, n.d., accessed 9 November 2020, archived 10 December 2004, http://web.archive.org/web/20041210162553/http:/www.social-anxiety.org.uk:80/members/browse.htm?page=1.

heart transplants,[116] and breast cancer.[117] Blogs also allowed people to show the importance of sick notes to personal identity, exemplified through 1990s and 2000s correspondents reflecting on prior decades. For one man remembering his early work life, his first sick note for getting flakes of steel in his eye during a summer job was transformative. He 'was now a mill hand. Branded by real steel. No longer some poncey student' in the eyes of his co-workers. The injury was the rite of passage but the 'sick note'—and his 'eye patch'—were integral to his war story.[118] Another man narrated his father's experience of cancer, demonstrating the agony he must have been in by referencing his willingness to work through pain in his younger years. He had lost an arm in a motorcycle accident and was once accidentally hit on his remaining hand by the son with a sledgehammer—'a lesser man would have cried and been off to the doctors for a sick note!'[119]

But if it was, at one time, 'the done thing' to battle through minor pain and injury, this could also engender feelings of guilt in those who could not. A woman signed off work to care for her child told work that she 'felt as though I was taking the piss a bit';[120] while another, later diagnosed with encephalitis, expressed feeling 'a bit guilty about having another two weeks off work' having just come back from holiday.[121] Others felt guilty because their inability to work exacerbated structural problems for their co-workers. For example, a student working in a shoe shop told the *Daily Mail*'s *Femail* message board that she '[felt] really bad…because one of the girls is leaving meaning only myself and the manager are left'. Her condition meant she could pull together the strength to deliver her sick note in person, which she acknowledged could reflect poorly upon her. But her condition was invisible and severe: 'constant abdominal pain and irregular bowel movements' meant she could not work. She was 'frustrated' that she was 'being made to feel guilty'.[122]

[116] Multiple authorship, 'Personal accounts', To Transplant and Beyond, n.d., 9 November 2020, archived 4 January 2003, http://web.archive.org/web/20030104072839/http://www.heart-transplant. co.uk:80/personal_accounts.htm.

[117] Monica, 'Monica's Diary, Part Two', Breast Cancer Care, 1997, accessed 9 November 2020, archived 6 January 2003, http://web.archive.org/web/20030106012844/http://www.breastcancercare. org.uk:80/Breastcancer/Practicalsupport/Monicasdiary/Parttwo?portal_skin=access.

[118] A reference to Scunthorpe United manager Ron Ashman suggests these events came from the late 1960s to early 1970s. Eric Jarvis, 'Cobble or Quits', www.ericjarvis.co.uk, 19 November 1999, accessed 31 August 2020, archived 15 February 2003, http://web.archive.org/web/20030215075418/ http://www.ericjarvis.co.uk:80/stories/cobble.html.

[119] Regan, 'This is my story', a1-health.co.uk, n.d., accessed 31 August 2020, archived 29 April 2005, http://web.archive.org/web/20050429182028/http://www.a1-health.co.uk:80/Myper cent20sto-ryFrame1Source1.htm.

[120] sarahc, 'Mummy's place to chat', post in discussion thread on Fertility Friends, 7 August 2004, accessed 9 November 2020, archived 4 October 2005, http://web.archive.org/web/20051004052852/ http://www.fertilityfriends.co.uk:80/forum/index.php/topic,11042.msg164286.html.

[121] Multiple authorship, 'Your stories', Encephalitis Information Resource, n.d., accessed 9 November 2020, archived 17 April 2003, http://web.archive.org/web/20030417090336/http://esg.org. uk:80/ESG/Support/recovery/YS.htm.

[122] vicky_just_vicky, 'SICK PAY problems', discussion thread on Femail, 19 March 2003, accessed 9 November 2020, archived 4 April 2003, http://web.archive.org/web/20030404005555/http://chat. femail.co.uk:80/femail/threadnonInd.jsp?forum=52&thread=9567387&message=9836865.

These narratives and on-line fora also offered opportunities for individual and collective resistance. Increased 'flexibility' in the labour market had influenced and been exacerbated by New Labour policy on employment and disability, as already discussed. But while irregular hours, short-term employment, out-sourcing, and the decline of traditional industries had weakened the ability of trades unions to recruit and organize, a different form of everyday resistance can be seen through the news stories and message boards. In part, this was aided by the equalities legislation that had left employers 'treading on eggshells'. People with experience and expertise could offer advice and link to organizations offering legal support. One claimant was able to gather information about his hip condition to help his claim to disability benefits from around the country; while many others chose to share their stories of poor behaviour from bosses on *i-resign.co.uk*.[123] High profile cases such as the victory for a Kwiksave employee who was sacked for not returning after her maternity leave, despite a sick note showing that complications had left her still unable to work, also showed that there was legal recourse against unreasonable bosses—if one could access it.[124] And yet, while it was easier for groups like Citizens Advice Bureaux in Scotland to publicize cases of poor practice,[125] it was also clear that people could express resistance against their co-workers' behaviour. Even if staff cutbacks had made it more difficult to get work done, people who were perceived to be absent without good cause needed to prove themselves. A middle manager told *Femail*:

> There is this guy in my work place who is just taking liberties. Already he has taken 21.5 days off this annual leave out of 25 and he still wants to go to Jamaica....The guy is now off work due to illness...wait for it...you'll like this...for a boil on his bum!...Thanks for the moan! I shall have to put up and shut up.[126]

That the manager had access to such detailed statistics says something about administrative practices in itself, but this attitude was not unique. Tesco introduced a new absence policy in which sick pay would not be paid for the first two days of illness unless it ran into a third day or was accompanied by an

[123] Sid, 'Working while on IB', discussion thread on Benefits Now, 20 August 2001, accessed 9 November 2020, archived 7 September 2003, http://web.archive.org/web/20030907082241/http://www.benefitsnowshop.co.uk/forum/display_message.asp?mid=1567; Jean, 'Need some advice', discussion thread on I Resign, 30 January 2003, accessed 9 November 2020, archived 20 March 2003, http://web.archive.org/web/20030320135044/http://www.i-resign.co.uk:80/uk/discussion/new_topic.asp?t=647.

[124] Amelia Gentleman, 'Ill mothers were sacked illegally', *Guardian*, 28 February 1998, p. 8; Peter Foster and Agnes Bell, 'Mothers wrongly sacked for being ill', *The Times*, 28 February 1998, p. 10; 'Victory for mothers', *Daily Mail*, 28 February 1998, p. 27.

[125] Una Bartley, 'Labour Pains – employment issues for pregnant women', Citizens Advice Scotland, June 2000, accessed 9 November 2020, archived 12 January 2003, http://web.archive.org/web/20030112230232/http://www.cas.org.uk:80/Change/Reports/LabPains/labpains.html.

[126] eragan, 'I'm so angry about one person....', discussion thread on Femail, 25 March 2003, accessed 9 November 2020, archived 4 April 2003, http://web.archive.org/web/20030404005231/http://chat.femail.co.uk:80/femail/threadnonInd.jsp?forum=52&thread=9568485&message=9846089.

acceptable sick note. The system appeared popular among larger retail businesses and was taken up Asda, Sainsbury's, Debenhams, and Next.[127] HR firm Ceridian produced a survey in 2006 suggesting two-thirds of workers 'strongly disapproved or felt it was unfair when a colleague had the audacity to invent an illness to enjoy life on the outside'.[128] No wonder some felt guilty about taking time off, even if they were legally and medically entitled to.

The 'Fit Note'

With these problems in the sick note system, the New Labour government and industry searched for ways to reduce absenteeism. The answer was to come in the form of the 'fit note' in 2010, though it was not the first option to be tried. On the government's part, similar political concerns to those in the 1950s reared their heads. New Labour had consciously sought to expand expenditure on the welfare state, albeit at a much slower pace than in 1945.[129] The associated growth in employment in the public sector (Figure 7.2) meant it could come under attack from the right if such spending could be painted as wasteful.[130]

Absenteeism, as we saw in Chapter 3, was something Labour had to be mindful of. Regular reports of higher levels of sick leave in the public sector than in private businesses continued to grace the press, particularly the *Daily Mail* and *The Times*.[131] Government departments invested in new absentee monitoring and rehabilitation systems, producing better metrics for public consumption as well as attempting to improve efficiency. The Royal Mail, just as in the 1950s, was particularly interested, garnering attention for its focus on occupational health provision for its workers.[132] While this might be seen as a return in some ways to its own medical service that had been established in the 1850s, some innovations were new—such as entering workers with exemplary attendance records into a lottery to win a car.[133] The Driver and Vehicle Licensing Authority and East Sussex County Council also brought in occupational health professionals, making

[127] Darren Behar and Liz Hull, 'More bosses get tough with staff over the growing sickies epidemic', *Daily Mail*, 20 May 2004, p. 10.
[128] Matt Keating, 'Can your boss dock your pay?', *Guardian*, 20 May 2006, p. 2.
[129] O'Hara and Parr, 'Conclusions'.   [130] 'The "sickie" habit', *Daily Mail*, 5 July 2004, p. 10.
[131] Paul Eastham and Gaby Hinsliff, 'Purge on the Civil Service sickness cheats', *Daily Mail*, 10 November 1998, p. 1; David Hughes, 'Blunkett's war on police who take 1.5m days off sick', *Daily Mail*, 3 December 2001, p. 2; Revecca Paveley, 'Why Monday means sickie day for staff down at the JobCentre', *Daily Mail*, 20 February 2003, p. 23; 'An ill wind keeps Civil service top of sick list', *The Times*, 9 December 2003, p. 3; Jim Sherman, 'No pay without a sick note for workers in public sector', *The Times*, 9 December 2004, p. 4; and passim.
[132] Louisa Peacock, 'Fist class delivery', *Personnel Today*, 17 June 2008, p. 6; John Carvel, 'Clinics at work cut sicknotes, says study', *Guardian*, 1 May 2008, p. 9. See also Chapter 3.
[133] Sam Greenhill, 'Come to work and you may win a car', *Daily Mail*, 6 August 2004, p. 17.

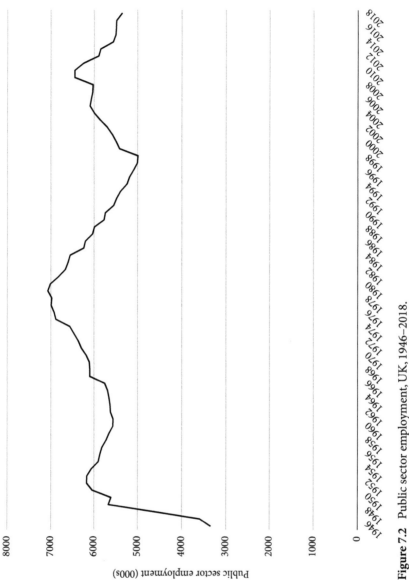

Figure 7.2 Public sector employment, UK, 1946–2018.

Source: Blessing Chiripanhura and Nikolas Wolf, 'Long-term trends in UK employment: 1861 to 2018', Office of National Statistics, 29 April 2019, accessed 24 November 2020, https://www.ons.gov.uk/economy/nationalaccounts/uksectoraccounts/compendium/economicreview/april2019/longtermtrendsinukemployment1861to2018.

changes to hours and workloads.[134] In doing so, these organizations followed a similar course to private companies. A growing service industry, occupational health consultancy offered the potential to tailor physiotherapy and psychological assessments of individual workers to the specific demands of their work. Both employers and GPs agreed that such professionals had more-relevant experience in making such judgments and would be more useful in determining 'real' levels of incapacity.[135] In negotiating concessions from both the worker and the employer, it was hoped that sick employees could return in a phased manner, reducing the amount of time taken off and the probability that the employee would have to resign on medical grounds. Direct contact would also, it was argued, make it easier to spot malingerers by reducing reliance upon the GP-written Med 3. But not everyone was convinced. Small businesses worried that they would not be able to afford such services in the way that larger organizations (public and private) could, echoing some of the collectivist arguments expressed around Statutory Sick Pay in the 1980s.[136] GPs also warned that the family doctor was an important port of call for workers to get trusted advice on conditions and psychological stresses that they might not feel comfortable sharing with a stranger—especially if they suspected the specialist's loyalties lay with the employer.[137]

For the government, these changes fit the logic around ESA and disability. By reducing the time spent off work and reducing the probability of early retirement or resignation on health grounds, economic inactivity, and the benefits bill could be cut. To begin with, several initiatives were tentatively launched to improve the existing system. Gordon Brown announced 'clamp downs' on civil servants' absenteeism in 1998 and 2004, with mixed success. Plans to remove self-certification, a key part of the Statutory Sick Pay reforms of the 1980s, were quickly shelved in part due to opposition from the BMA.[138] Attempts were made to reduce 'red tape' for GPs by encouraging nurses and accident and emergency doctors to write sick notes, saving a trip to the surgery; but the changes were poorly publicized and it had become so routine for workers to visit the GP for a sick note that they continued to do so anyway.[139] Proposals to use 'mystery shoppers' in surgeries to test whether GPs were too lax in their certification, creating

[134] Mat Snow, 'Absent without leave', *Guardian*, 8 March 2008, p. 1; Esther Cameron, 'Public eye: Sick of being stereotyped', *Guardian*, 19 March 2008, p. 10.
[135] A. Massey, *Sick-Note Britain: How Social Problems Became Medical Issues* (London: Hurst Publishers, 2019).
[136] 'Sick note changes cause industry alarm', *Hairdressers Journal International*, 19 December 2003, p. 9; Mark Vernon, 'A new chapter in outsourcing', *Financial Times*, 21 May 2003. See also Chapters 5 and 6.
[137] Mike Berry, 'Sicknote pilots fail as GPs bail out', *Personnel Today*, 21 November 2006, p. 11; Nic Patton, 'Sicknote alternatives fail to make an impact', *Personnel Today*, 14 November 2006, p. 3.
[138] 'Sick certificate scheme will add to GP workload', *Pulse*, 1 August 1998, p. 7.
[139] 'GPs scorn Government claims over red tape', *GP*, 28 January 2002, p. 12; Edward Davies, 'Sick note change hit by DoH delays', *GP*, 18 February 2005, p. 7; Cabinet Office, *Making a Difference: Reducing General Practitioner (GP) Paperwork* (London: Cabinet Office, 2001).

GP sick note 'league tables', or introducing performance-related pay for reducing the number of sick note written by a practice also went nowhere. Not only did GPs oppose the plans, but it was clear that sickness rates were so closely linked to the local economic climate that such weightings would be unfair and unworkable in disadvantaged areas.[140] Some success was found with pilots that placed occupational health experts in surgeries to give advice to patients. This reduced the number of sick notes written, saved time for GPs, and appeared to be appreciated by those patients surveyed.[141] Not all schemes were successful. Employers pulled out of a pilot that used nurses in call centres to discuss symptoms due to a lack of tangible results. In 2006 another collapsed after worker opposition, GP apathy and lack of buy in from employers.[142] The general principle, however, survived the setbacks and was central to the reforms proposed in 2008.

Carol Black's *Working for a Healthier Tomorrow* provided the catalyst for the end of the Med 3 and the creation of the 'fit note'.[143] Black argued for 'an expanded role for occupational health and its place within a broader collaborative and multidisciplinary service...available to all, whether they are entering work, seeking to stay in work, or trying to return to work without delay in the wake of illness or injury'.[144] Continuing with the biopsychosocial model approach that 'work is generally good for health and well-being',[145] Black proposed a framework that would reduce the amount of time workers spent sick and prevent long-term worklessness. Instead of focusing on a rigid delineation between 'capable' and 'incapable' as defined by a physical sick note, the Department of Health and DWP moved towards a new electronic system that encouraged patients and doctors to consider what the worker *could* do within the terms of employment. This addressed many of the concerns outlined earlier in the decade from employers about the lack of information on sick notes and the ease of which GPs handed them out. It provided a collectivized service through the NHS so that smaller businesses could continue to benefit from an occupational-health-style approach to assessing a worker, albeit still from the GP rather than a specialist.[146] The family doctor remained, reducing some cynicism from unions that the assessor would be

[140] '"Train GPs to refuse sicknotes" – Blunkett', *Pulse*, 13 August 2005, p. 3; 'GPs could be monitored and retrained on sick-note sign-offs', *Safety & Health Practitioner*, March 2005, p. 8; Abha Thakor, 'Ministers feud over GP sicknote plan', *Pulse*, 11 March 2000, p. 15; 'Why sicknote league tables of GPs won't work', *Pulse*, 11 March 2000, p. 29; 'GPs worry over sick note "spies" in the surgery', *Guardian*, 3 December 2004, p. 21.
[141] Gabby Hinsliff, 'GPs paid as job advisers', *Observer*, 22 January 2006, p. 4; Nerys Williams, 'Helping patients back to work', *GP*, 23 May 2008, p. 37.
[142] Mike Berry, 'Sicknote pilots fail as GPs bail out', *Personnel Today*, 21 November 2006, p. 11; Nic Patton, 'Sicknote alternatives fail to make an impact', *Personnel Today*, 14 November 2006, p. 3.
[143] Black, *Working for a Healthier Tomorrow*.
[144] Ibid., p. 4.
[145] Waddell and Burton, *Is Work Good for Your Health and Well-Being?*
[146] 'The fit note has landed', *Scottish Business Insider*, 21 April 2010, p. 108.

in the pay of the employer.[147] GPs would, it was argued, appreciate the opportunity to use their expertise to help the patient directly over the devalued and deskilled act of signing of a form that had been a bugbear since at least the 1910s.[148] And while there was scepticism that these changes would be anything more than cosmetic, there was also hope that reframing the nature of the interaction between a patient seeking a sick note and the GP would engender new attitudes to sick leave. Borrowing from behavioural psychology work around 'nudge theory', the idea was that workers would be placed in a position where they had to actively think about how much of their job they could do rather than focusing on the elements they could not.[149] 'The cynic in me thinks there'll be no change and I do suspect that initially many GPs will treat the fit note like the old sick note', wrote one occupational health doctor in 2010. 'But…in two to three years, this will start to change.'[150] Combined with the NHS's Improving Access to Psychological Therapies initiative, it was hoped that occupational and traditional health services would work with each other to reduce worklessness; although budgetary constraints in the wake of the 2007 financial crisis reduced the scope of the programme and, somewhat ironically, created higher rates of sickness and unemployment in the economic contraction that followed.[151]

While the new electronic fit note was welcomed both for its portability and finally doing away with the infamous 'doctors' handwriting', it had limitations.[152] This new system was only likely to make a difference with medium-to-long-term sickness. It could do nothing for the short bouts of viral infections, stomach bugs, or 'sickies' that continued to vex employers.[153] As had been the case throughout the postwar period, these were still the most prevalent forms of 'involuntary' absence, with most workers returning within a few weeks.[154] Industrial injuries might have reduced in relative importance, but workers were still essentially unpredictable, fallible cogs in the business machine. GPs were still not experts in occupational health, even if they could ask occupation-related questions. 'We need the CBI to stop moaning', declared the chair of the BMA's professional fees

[147] 'Flexible sick-leave policy is welcomed by industry', Motor Transport, 26 April 2010, p. 5.
[148] 'GPs welcome pilot to escape sick-note "rut"', Safety & Health Practitioner, July 2008, p. 7.
[149] Such approaches would become more common and overt in the following decade. For background, see: Cabinet Office and Institute for Government, MINDSPACE: Influencing Behaviour through Public Policy (London: Institute for Government, 2010); Simen Markussen, Knut Røed, and Ragnhild C. Schreiner, 'Can compulsory dialogues nudge sick-listed workers back to work?', Economic Journal 128, no. 610 (2018): pp. 1276–1303.
[150] Sam Barrett, 'Fitting the bill', Corporate Adviser, April 2010.
[151] Denis Campbell and Tracy McVeigh, 'Divorce counselling offered on NHS', Observer, 22 November 2009, p. 13; 'Sicknote? How about some CBT?', Pulse, 26 November 2005, p. 3; Jonathan Moules, 'Slowing economy blamed for increase in long-term sickness, says survey', Financial Times, 18 May 2009, p. 4.
[152] Virginia Matthews, 'Out of sight, out of mind', Personnel Today, 19 May 2009, pp. 16–18.
[153] Pat Hagan, 'A can-do culture', Commercial Motor 210, no. 5344 (2009): p. 24.
[154] Tracey Boles, 'Small firms count cost of sickness', Sunday Business, 11 August 2002, p. 1.

committee in 2008, 'and to encourage Government to invest in comprehensive occupational health services.'[155]

The fit note suited the New Labour market liberal approach to economic inactivity. Theoretically, it opened a hinterland between capacity and incapacity for sick and/or disabled employees. At the same time, it did little for short term sickness. It would not work without the active participation of GPs (to spend the time and energy to fully explore the fit note process), workers (to be willing to allow their bodies to be disciplined), and employers (to actively make changes to working conditions to adapt to the employee's needs). It also completely ignored the other side of the ledger. As the TUC argued in 2006, the idea of mass malingering was a 'myth'.[156] The Chartered Management Institute showed in 2008 that the average worker gave significantly more time to employers through unpaid overtime and working beyond their terms of employment than they 'took' though unscheduled absence.[157] Most importantly, these discussions often ignored the dangers of presenteeism—working through illness—which could lead to decreased productivity, burnout, exacerbated health conditions, and even infection of other workers.[158] Thus, with increasing hostility from employers, public and private, towards absentees, the fit note was like ESA. It created a system that *could* empower workers; but with the power imbalances between government, employer, and employee, this was by no means guaranteed.[159]

Conclusion

'Sick Note Britain' did not emerge in 1998 with *Daily Mail* headlines and a New Labour government. As this book demonstrates, many of the complaints bound up in 'Sick Note Britain', the 'sick note culture', and Britain's 'sick note capitals' existed throughout the postwar welfare state.[160] Britain was an uncompetitive

---

[155] 'GP "well-notes" to go ahead from next year', *Pulse*, 24 September 2008, p. 12.

[156] 'Malingering "myth" debunked by TUC report', *Safety & Health Practitioner*, February 2005, p. 7; TUC, 'Countering an urban legend: Sicknote Britain?', TUC, 7 January 2005, accessed 2 September 2020, archived 8 November 2005, http://web.archive.org/web/20051108200505/http://www.tuc.org.uk/welfare/tuc-9208-f0.cfm.

[157] Les Worrall, 'Absence of common sense blights "sickie" debate', *Personnel Today*, 20 May 2008, p. 18; Bruce Hayward, Barry Fong, and Alex Thornton, *The Third Work-Life Balance Employer Survey: Main Findings* (London: Department for Business, Enterprise and Regulatory Reform, 2007); Hülya Hooker et al., *The Third Work-Life Balance Employee Survey: Main Findings* (London: Department of Trade and Industry, 2007).

[158] Gary Johns, 'Presenteeism in the workplace: A review and research agenda', *Journal of Organizational Behavior* 31, no. 4 (2010): pp. 519–42; Hugh Wilson, 'Go with the flu – and stay away', *Guardian*, 22 November 2004, p. 5. See also Chapter 8.

[159] Taylor et al., 'Too scared to go sick'.

[160] Jones, 'Sign up here for Sick-note Britain'; Kamal Ahmed and Gaby Hinsliff, 'Blair launches attack on Britain's "sick note" culture', *Observer*, 9 June 2002, p. 4; 'Sick-note city', *The Times*, 6 February 2006, p. 4.

country, brought to its financial and moral knees by malingerers and work-shy scroungers who were, at best, misguided people who needed to be shown the salvation found in a good day's work, or, at worst, deliberately stealing a living from a state that had made it too easy to find excuses. The sick note itself was emblematic of those excuses. It was a failed device, one that workers were too eager to seek, employers too eager to lean on, GPs too eager to issue, and governments too eager to leave untouched. The whole welfare state was culpable. As one GP succinctly put it:

> We know it's a crock, they know it's a crock, whatever faceless individual receives the sick note knows it's a crock. We know they know and they know we know they know, but as long as it is not an overly outrageous and detectable fib, nobody will rock the boat.[161]

Shifts in attitudes from the New Labour government, employers, and the evolution of the global economy changed the way Britain talked about these issues. Now visible as 'Sick Note Britain', such problems could be discussed and policy responses could be formulated. This mobilized attacks on absenteeism while also providing ways that workers could respond within these same frameworks. Increased equalities protections infuriated employers, but could provide protection for those with the knowledge, finance, and other resources to press their rights. The internet and increased research into absenteeism increased the flow of information among employers and private companies offering ways to curb sickness while also giving a venue for workers to express their frustrations and provide support to each other. Still, ESA and the fit note provided the building blocks for the problems that workers and benefit claimants would experience in the 2010s and during the coronavirus pandemic—which will be disused in the following, final chapter.

* * *

Despite all the problems with the sick note—evident since at least the 1940s—it chugged on. The new testing regimes for disability benefits still contained the provision to sign individuals off work. There remained a 'common sense' level at which it was unreasonable for the government to expect a sick person to work, even if the measurement of that level was couched in 'objective' terms.[162] The 'fit note', despite its claims to focus on phased returns to work, could be, and often was, simply used as a way to sign people off work. It still used the relationship between the GP and the patient; it still came in the form of a certificate; and it was still tied into the gatekeeping procedures for sickness and disability benefits in the

---

[161] Liam Farrell, 'GPs, the gatekeepers of justice', *GP*, 31 May 2004, p. 17.
[162] Gulland, *Gender, Work and Social Control.*

public and private sectors. Employers, despite their complaints, continued to demand 'proof' that their workers were not stealing time and sick pay from them. Employees retained the need to protect themselves and give validation to their symptoms and provide access to sickness-related benefits. The government kept its role as a semi-independent referee of sickness through the provision of NHS doctors, as well as policing its own boundaries of who qualified for benefits. At any one time, each of these groups would experience the limitations of the sick note and complain vociferously. The revelation that sick notes did not work would be publicized, and there would be demands for something to be done. And then it would be forgotten, to be rediscovered by the next generation allowing the cycle to continue. In the end, the sick note was the tried and tested option, the least terrible solution that worked just well enough, enough of the time, for no one alternative to ever take hold. It could adapt to circumstances just well enough to remain relevant. That is, perhaps, the perfect metaphor for the welfare state itself.

8

Conclusion

This book has been about Britain's sickness system—the intersection of employment, social security and health policy designed to control sick pay and sick leave. That sick note came to represent how that system was policed. The previous chapters explored how both the note and the system evolved over the postwar period. Bringing these themes together, *Sick Note* ends by considering how these themes have endured through the COVID-19 crisis.

Chapter 2 showed how persistent the sick note has been. Medical certification in some form or another has existed since the early modern period.[1] The 1948 National Insurance 'Med 1' was a direct descendent of systems created for interwar National Health Insurance. Moreover, despite the many complaints from doctors about the workload certification created (and the compromising gatekeeping position it put them in with regard to their patients), the system survived the negotiations over the National Health Service Acts. Grievances did not disappear in the following decades, but, crucially, neither did the sick note. Even after the reforms outlined in Chapter 5, the creation of new tests of long-term incapacity in Chapter 6 and the introduction of the 'fit note' in Chapter 7, there remained a belief that it was possible to certify the border between sickness and health—at least for social security purposes. This has continued into the 2020s.

The need for such a border was not simply about state benefits. It was tied to the wider productionist goals of the postwar welfare state.[2] Chapter 3 introduced how the British sickness system has wrestled with concepts of absenteeism. Gatekeeping procedures needed to be robust enough to ensure workers did not take excessive leave, while also safeguarding their health by preventing overwork and 'presenteeism'. This was a constant tension in the welfare state, as seen in the concerns of business groups over self-certification in Chapter 5 and the increase in sickness policing in Chapter 7. Media coverage also suggested that scepticism about people in possession of a sick note was not a new phenomenon in the 1980; nor has it gone away.

---

[1] James C. Riley, 'Sickness in an early modern workplace', *Continuity and Change* 2, no. 3 (1987): pp. 363–85.

[2] John Pickstone, 'Production, community and consumption: The political economy of twentieth-century medicine', in *Medicine in the Twentieth Century*, edited by Roger Cooter and John Pickstone (Abingdon: Routledge, 2003), pp. 1–20.

Still, these gatekeeping procedures were designed to triage a particular type of claimant whose desert and qualification were otherwise not in doubt. As seen through the experiences of newly-arrived migrants and women in the sickness system, sick notes, and sickness status were not the overriding factor as to whether people economically affected by ill health would be able to gain access to support. Chapter 4 thus showed for whom the welfare state was designed by examining who was excluded. Not only did this indicate that there were demographics that had been shown little consideration when the Poor Laws were replaced; it demonstrated that Britain continued to change over the postwar period. Its welfare systems did not always keep pace with those economic, political, and cultural shifts. It was this change over time that produced the need for and allowed the reforms to short- and long-term sickness benefit from the 1980s as explored in Chapters 5 and 6. But it also re-emphasised the assumptions made about nuclear households and male, British-born 'breadwinners' that had been central to the postwar reconstruction projects described in Chapter 3.[3] Britain continued to evolve over the twentieth century; and as this chapter will go on to show, the sickness system had to adapt quickly to a major shock in March 2020.

Chapter 5 showed that reforms to sick notes did not remove the gatekeeping principles that underlay them. Employers and government departments still needed to police the boundary of sickness, meaning workers and benefit claimants still needed to prove their medical status. In turn, doctors would remain key experts, even if their legal obligations were reduced for very short-term illness. The same principles outlined in Chapter 2 endured. Even as new tests were introduced for chronic sickness and disability in Chapter 6 and the fit note in Chapter 7, the system could not escape its need for gatekeeping. Reformed or not, the basic tenets of the sick note continued.

Because of that continuity, 'sick note' had become a shorthand for the gatekeeping system by the 1980s. Jokes and media coverage reflected cynicism about the effectiveness of those systems. Chapter 6 showed how the sick note could be a technically-correct-but-morally-dubious excuse to evade obligation, a sense that gatekeeping did not adequately weed out the deserving from the undeserving. At the same time, official scepticism about long-term claimants allowed the Conservative government to introduce new 'objective' testing regimes to determine 'incapacity'.[4] Productionist concerns, as expressed in Chapters 2 and 3, were reformulated around newer ideas about disability, rehabilitation, and the right (as well as the obligation) to work in a deindustrialized society. It also stressed that chronic and acute sickness had always presented different challenges

---

[3] Jane Lewis, 'Gender and the development of welfare regimes', *Journal of European Social Policy* 2, no. 2 (1992): pp. 159–73.

[4] Jackie Gulland, *Gender, Work and Social Control: A Century of Disability Benefits* (London: Palgrave Macmillan, 2019).

to the welfare state—even if the state continued to believe it was possible to certificate the boundary between capacity and incapacity.

Finally, Chapter 7 demonstrated that New Labour's 'third way' conception of work and its 'active labour market policy' contributed to the increased policing of absenteeism and sickness into the twenty-first century.[5] The jokes from previous decades remained, as did the gatekeeping procedures. But the economic shifts of the late-twentieth century had created a workforce that was much more diverse and precariously employed than that of the 1960s and 1970s. Just as had been shown in Chapter 4, the sickness system was not designed to deal with 'flexible' employment practices and active labour policies built around contradictory features. Low pay and short-term contracts clashed with policies that forced people with health conditions and caring responsibilities into full-time unsuitable work under threat of sanctions. The 'fit note' was designed to tailor work more appropriately, working with occupational health services to reduce absenteeism, lower the workload on GPs, increase the employability of marginalized groups and rebuild faith in the gatekeeping procedure. But while the fit note and new Work Capability Assessment introduced more 'grey areas' in the margins between capacity and incapacity, sick-note thinking remained. There still was a boundary. It still needed to be policed. People still referred to 'the sick note'. 'Sick Note Britain' was here to stay.

The Afterlife of the Sick Note

Sick-note thinking lived on in the 2010s. Sarah Dorrington's research has shown how many doctors and patients have continued to use the fit note in much the same way as it Med 3 predecessor. The ritual of getting evidence from the doctor remains the same, and the lack of time or faith that adjustments will be made means that, in effect, it remains primarily a document designed to give access to sick leave and sick pay.[6] Besides, headlines and book titles using the term 'sick note Britain' have continued long after the Black Report.[7] More pertinently, the

---

[5] Peter Hill, 'Working hard or hardly working? Evaluating New Labour's active labour market policy' (PhD thesis, University of Warwick, 2016).

[6] I am grateful to Sarah Dorrington for advanced copies of her PhD research. For published work, see: Sarah Dorrington et al., 'Multimorbidity and fit note receipt in working-age adults with long-term health conditions', *Psychological Medicine* (2020); Sarah Dorrington et al., 'Demographic variation in fit note receipt and long-term conditions in South London', *Occupational and Environmental Medicine* 77, no. 6 (2020): pp. 418–26. See also: Carol Coole et al., *Getting the Best from the Fit Note: Investigating the Use of the Statement of Fitness for Work* (Leicester: IOSH, 2015).

[7] For examples, spread across the 2000s and 2010s, see: TUC, 'Countering an urban legend: Sicknote Britain?', TUC, 7 January 2005, accessed 2 September 2020, archived 8 November 2005, http://web. archive.org/web/20051108200505/ http://www.tuc.org.uk/welfare/tuc-9208-f0.cfm; WalesOnline. '"Rip up sick-note Britain"', *Wales Online*, 13 November 2007, accessed 23 November 2020, https://www. walesonline.co.uk/news/wales-news/rip-up-sick-note-britain-2217280; Laura Donnell, 'The "terrible

sickness benefit system persists. Short-term sickness still relies upon a formal employer–employee relationship and stable work. Long-term sickness has moved away from the sick note itself (especially after the Conservative–Liberal Democrat coalition government's attempts to restrict access to benefit) but continues to draw arbitrary lines for the border between capacity and incapacity.[8] Ultimately, the perceived need for medical gatekeeping remains. Whether enacted through self-certification, sick visiting, doctors' signatures, or occupational health examinations, sick-note thinking will continue.

When the funding application was submitted in 2016 for the research that eventually became this book, I had therefore expected to end by discussing the structural changes in the British economy and welfare state that had undermined and would continue to erode the sickness system. Governments could continue to tinker with the sick note itself, but the core problems were in the wider welfare state. The phrase 'Sick-note Britain' obscured these structural issues by focusing on the representative slip of paper rather than the underlying economic and bureaucratic edifice.

More people had become reliant on what had become known as the 'gig economy'—performing individual tasks solicited via online platforms—with little job security and no access to Statutory Sick Pay (SSP).[9] 'Automation', reflected in the increased visibility of self-service checkouts, online banking, and other 'artificial intelligence' solutions in service industries, risked making employment ever more precarious and low paid, particularly for women, part-time workers, and those without recognized experience or qualifications.[10] Zero-hours contracts added to these problems by taking away the concept of a regular wage, making SSP unworkable even for those not reliant upon gig economy work.[11] Freelancing

legacy" of sick-note Britain', *Daily Telegraph*, 9 March 2008; Maria Tadeo, 'Sick note Britain: Employees face four week health check under new scheme', *Independent*, 13 February 2014, accessed 23 November 2020, https://www.independent.co.uk/news/business/news/sick-note-britain-employees-face-four-week-health-check-under-new-scheme-9126201.html; Sophie Borland, 'Sicknote Britain: One in four visits to a GP is avoidable because they are taken up with form-filling or minor ailments', *Mail Online*, 29 June 2017, accessed 23 November 2020, https://www.dailymail.co.uk/health/article-4648904/Sicknote-Britain-One-four-visits-GP-avoidable.html; Adrian Massey, *Sick-Note Britain: How Social Problems Became Medical Issues* (London: Hurst Publishers, 2019).

[8] Gareth Millward and Peter Border, *Assessing Capacity for Work (PN 413)* (London: Parliamentary Office of Science and Technology, 2012); Chris Grover, 'The end of an era? The resignation of Iain Duncan Smith, Conservatism and social security benefits for disabled people', *Disability & Society* 31, no. 8 (2016): pp. 1127–31; Gulland, *Gender, Work and Social Control*.

[9] Geraint Johnes, 'The gig economy in the UK: A regional perspective', *Journal of Global Responsibility* 10, no. 3 (2019): pp. 197–210.

[10] Mark Skilton and Felix Hovsepian, *The 4th Industrial Revolution: Responding to the Impact of Artificial Intelligence on Business* (Cham: Springer, 2017); Trades Union Congress, *How Industrial Change Can Be Managed to Deliver Better Jobs* (London: Trades Union Congress, 2019); Office for National Statistics, 'Which occupations are at the highest risk of being automated?', Office for National Statistics, 25 March 2019, accessed 17 November 2020, https://www.ons.gov.uk/employmentandlabourmarket/peopleinwork/employmentandemployeetypes/articles/whichoccupationsareathighestriskofbeingautomated/2019-03-25.

[11] Doug Pyper and Daniel Harari, *Zero-Hours Contracts (SN/BT/6553)* (London: House of Commons Library, July 2013).

became ever more common, not necessarily by choice but because of the way companies turned to piece work rather than paying regular salaries and benefits to full employees.[12] Technically employed (or self-employed), people on such contracts could not claim Job Seeker's Allowance or Universal Credit if work dried up for sickness or other reasons. All this combined to put pressure on workers to labour even when ill, whether because they feared losing their jobs or because they did not have access to any other funds. Even businesses recognized the problem, with reports on 'presenteeism'—the opposite of 'absenteeism'— beginning to proliferate.[13] The 'flexible' employment practices described in Chapters 6 and 7 had exacerbated problems that had been known for decades.[14] If people were less willing or able to take time off work, did the data coming from the Labour Force Survey (see Figure 1.2) suggest that there was a cultural *deflation* of morbidity, at least for short-term sickness for employed people?[15]

The history of sick notes and sick pay has a lot to contribute to this discussion.[16] It shows those underlying economic, political, cultural, and bureaucratic processes that created and maintained a system that has, in the popular imagination, been reduced to simply 'the sick note'. History demonstrates how the current system was built on the assumption of full employment—not just *a lack of unemployment*, but a formal, stable relationship between an employer and an employee. Self-employed workers had therefore always posed difficulties, but the belief in the 1940s was that such individuals would be a minority, mostly business owners (see Figure 8.1). Sick notes and eligibility for benefit were difficult to define because 'the man who glories in being his own master has such freedom over his own time and the way he works (or directs other people to work) that it is hard to say whether on a particular day he is in fact working or not'.[17] In such a world, the distinction between 'voluntary' and 'involuntary' absenteeism was

[12] Amy Genders, *An Invisible Army: The Role of Freelance Labour in Bristol's Film and Television Industries* (Bristol: University of the West of England Bristol, 2019); Will Sutherland et al., 'Work precarity and gig literacies in online freelancing', *Work, Employment and Society* 34, no. 3 (2020): pp. 457–75.

[13] Gary Johns, 'Presenteeism in the workplace: A review and research agenda', *Journal of Organizational Behavior* 31, no. 4 (2010): pp. 519–42, Gail Kinman, 'Sickness presenteeism at work: Prevalence, costs and management', *British Medical Bulletin* 129, no. 1 (2019): pp. 69–78.

[14] Il-Ho Kim et al., 'Welfare states, Flexible employment, and health: A critical review', *Health Policy* 104, no. 2 (2012): pp. 99–127; Jill Rubery, Arjan Keizer, and Damian Grimshaw, 'Flexibility bites back: The multiple and hidden costs of flexible employment policies', *Human Resource Management Journal* 26, no. 3 (2016): pp. 235–51; Hill, 'Working hard or hardly working?'

[15] Office for National Statistics, 'Sickness absence in the UK labour market', *gov.uk*, 3 March 2021, accessed 13 July 2021, https://www.ons.gov.uk/employmentandlabourmarket/peopleinwork/ employmentandemployeetypes/datasets/sicknessabsenceinthelabourmarket; Martin Gorsky et al., 'The "cultural inflation of morbidity" during the English mortality decline: A new look', *Social Science & Medicine* 73 (2011): pp. 1775–83.

[16] In this vein, historians' responses to *History & Policy* have been valuable resources in understanding the link between historical research and modern-day policy concerns. *History & Policy*, accessed 23 November 2020, http://www.historyandpolicy.org/.

[17] 'Towards Social Security', *The Lancet* 247, no. 6392 (1946): pp. 320–1.

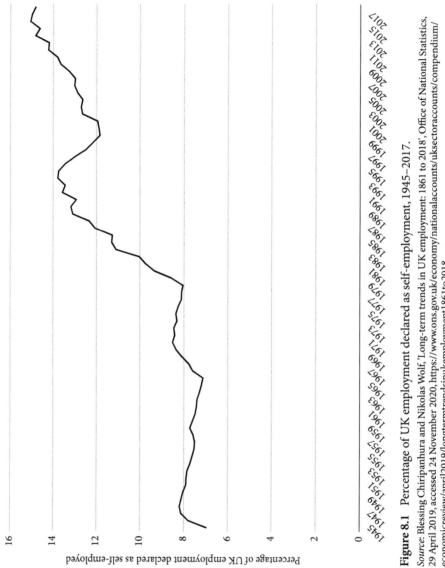

Figure 8.1 Percentage of UK employment declared as self-employment, 1945–2017.

Source: Blessing Chiripanhura and Nikolas Wolf, 'Long-term trends in UK employment: 1861 to 2018', Office of National Statistics, 29 April 2019, accessed 24 November 2020, https://www.ons.gov.uk/economy/nationalaccounts/uksectoraccounts/compendium/economicreview/april2019/longtermtrendsinukemployment1861to2018.

difficult to draw.[18] As self-employment became more common, especially among those with either low incomes or inconsistent work, it became more clear that 'the discussion of the "sick note culture" forgets those who work when they are ill because their income is stopped if they don't'.[19]

It seemed these questions would remain in the news throughout the research project. In July 2017, the government published the Taylor review entitled *Good Work* to address concerns about the quality of employment and long-term prospects in the globalized, twenty-first century, post-Fordist economy.[20] Meanwhile, workers for gig economy platforms such as Uber and Deliveroo continued to demand better pay and conditions—including the right to sick pay.[21] Sick notes, if they ever did fully work, did so for those regularly-employed male breadwinners with short-term conditions, as discussed in Chapter 4. These changes neatly demonstrated the point as precarity intensified.

*   *   *

Then came COVID-19. The effects of the virus on employment, the health system, and social security were impossible to ignore. I was fortunate. The archival research for this project was completed before 'lockdown' went into effect. The Wellcome Trust extended my funding (and therefore my employment) by nine months. And while there were no guarantees that new paid work would be available at the end of my contract given the massive disruption to teaching and research at universities across the globe, I did at least have a steady income, a reliable internet connection, a spare bedroom, a partner whose job had also survived, no caring responsibilities, and helpful colleagues on the other end of a video conference call. This was not the case for all, and the fragility of Britain's sickness system became immediately apparent when the usual structures for handling illness were disrupted for the middle classes as well as the precariat.[22] This was exacer-

[18] See Chapter 3.
[19] Rev Paul Nicolson, letter to *The Times*, 4 February 2005, p. 18. See also Fay Weldon, 'The rise of the egonarchy', *New Statesman*, 17 April 2000, pp. 25–7.
[20] Matthew Taylor et al., *Good Work: The Taylor Review of Modern Working Practices* (London: Department for Business, Energy and Industrial Strategy, July 2017).
[21] Arianna Tassinari and Vincenzo Maccarrone, 'Riders on the storm: Workplace solidarity among gig economy couriers in Italy and the UK', *Work, Employment and Society* 34, no. 1 (2020): pp. 35–54; Sky News, 'Uber loses Supreme Court battle on drivers' rights in gig economy test', 19 February 2021, accessed 22 February 2021, https://news.sky.com/story/uber-loses-supreme-court-battle-on-drivers-rights-in-gig-economy-test-12222531. For local examples, see: Tristan Cork, 'Deliveroo riders announce all-out strike in Bristol', *BristolLive*, 14 January 2019, accessed 17 November 2020, https://www.bristol-post.co.uk/whats-on/food-drink/deliveroo-riders-announce-out-strike-2428691; Julia Kollewe, 'Uber drivers strike over pay and conditions', *Guardian*, 8 May 2019, accessed 17 November 2020, https://www.theguardian.com/technology/2019/may/08/uber-drivers-strike-over-pay-and-conditions; Robert Cumber, 'Deliveroo couriers stage strike in Sheffield', *The Star*, 3 September 2019, accessed 17 November 2020, https://www.thestar.co.uk/business/deliveroo-couriers-stage-strike-sheffield-busiest-day-493657; Sonia Sharma, 'This is why Deliveroo drivers went on strike in Newcastle', *Chronicle Live*, 20 September 2020, accessed 17 November 2020, https://www.chroniclelive.co.uk/news/north-east-news/deliveroo-drivers-went-strike-newcastle-16946640.
[22] Ruth Patrick, 'Covid has exposed the decade-long lie that benefits are a lifestyle choice', *Guardian*, 3 November 2020, accessed 20 November 2020, https://www.theguardian.com/society/2020/nov/03/

bated by decades of reduced eligibility for state benefits and the system's reliance upon solvent employers, regular salaries, education as a provider of school-age childcare, and/or plentiful supplies of 'gig economy' work.[23]

More importantly than this, however, was the realization that Britain's sickness system was not just a safety net, or, as the Disablement Income Group described disability benefits in the 1960s, 'the ambulance waiting at the bottom of the cliff' to prevent destitution.[24] Nor was it simply a Beveridgean, productionist, collectivized attempt to ensure worker fitness and economic output, as discussed in Chapter 2. It was a vital public health tool. The discourse around *Good Work* had focused on the individual risks of poverty, underemployment, and unemployment.[25] Now people wondered what would happen if infectious people were forced to go to the workplace. Making it affordable to stay at home was going to be critical to staying alert, controlling the virus, and saving lives. If the system could not do this, could Britain cope?

COVID-19 was not the first epidemic or pandemic to put strain on Britain's sickness systems. An influenza epidemic at the turn of the 1970s had forced the Department of Health and Social Security to allow claimants to self-certificate to reduce the demand on GPs' time and discourage individuals from making unnecessary trips to doctors' surgeries.[26] In the late 2000s, H1N1 influenza (commonly known as 'swine flu') caused similar anxieties. Self-certification was now the norm for short bouts of illness, but people with symptoms were encouraged to avoid work and keep the spread of the disease under control. The Department of Health suggested that self-certification for up to a fortnight for those with influenza symptoms would free up doctor's surgeries and slow infection rates, a proposal that was defeated when employers protested that absenteeism would accelerate and devastate the economy.[27] The use of telediagnosis on NHS telephone lines and websites seemed to be an acceptable compromise, although this also came with economic consequences. A snide column from a GP talked about workers faking a 'bacon vacation' or 'hog holiday' to take additional leave, albeit with the risk that an actual bout of swine flu would

covid-decade-long-lie-benefits-lifestyle-choice-george-osborne-free-school-meals. On the precariat and other class groupings in twenty-first-century Britain, see: Michael Savage, *Social Class in the 21st Century* (London: Pelican, 2015).

[23] Unemployment remained historically low in Britain after the 2008 financial crash, although underemployment was a major economic and social problem across the 2010s. See: David N. F. Bell and David G. Blanchflower, 'Underemployment in the UK Revisited', *National Institute Economic Review* 224, no. 1 (May 2013): pp. F8–F22; Victoria Mousteri, Michael Daly, and Liam Delaney, 'Underemployment and psychological distress: Propensity score and fixed effects estimates from two large UK samples', *Social Science & Medicine* 244 (2020).

[24] Pat Healy, 'Disabled to press for early allowance', *The Times*, 1 February 1969, p. 2.

[25] Taylor et al., *Good Work*.

[26] See Chapter 5 and TNA: PIN 35/116, K. J. Wright to N. W. Cossins, 10 February 1970.

[27] 'Don't waste the calm before the second swine flu wave', *Pulse*, 5 August 2009, p. 16.

expose the lie.[28] Whether real or an exaggerated vignette on surgery life,[29] finding the true spread of the disease was difficult, since telediagnosis did not produce reliable verification of the virus.[30] It seemed logical that increased access to sick leave would result in higher absenteeism—though as discussed in Chapter 3, it was impossible to assess how much of that was 'legitimate'.

In the end, neither of these influenza crises forced the devolved British public health authorities to declare 'lockdown'. They did, however, show that in emergencies the need for medical proof—the sick note—could be superseded by bureaucratic and public health concerns. That is to say, short-term economic contraction was less important than affordable restricted movement. COVID-19 presented the same conundrum but with much higher stakes. The United States had already found with swine flu that its lack of sick leave protection had contributed to the spread of the H1N1 virus.[31] With the UK in March 2020, similar questions were raised.[32] SSP paid £95.85 per week, but only to those whose regular incomes were above £120 per week.[33] The Trades Union Congress (TUC) estimated a living wage to be around £320 per week.[34] But, as the OECD declared in July 2020:

> paid sick leave can only effectively help to contain the spread of the virus, absorb the economic shock and facilitate an orderly de-confinement if it is widely available to large parts of the labour force.…The cost to society of providing paid sick leave to these workers…is small in comparison to the cost of them not isolating and spreading the virus further.…Paid sick leave continues to function as a protective device to workers and societies at-large.[35]

[28] Phil Peverley, 'Bacon vacations are a swine', *Pulse*, 4 November 2009, p. 44.

[29] See GPs insulting remarks in columns about patients in Chapter 7.

[30] Sarah Standing, 'The swine flu panic will turn us into a national sickie', *Spectator*, 25 July 2009, accessed 16 November 2020, https://www.spectator.co.uk/article/the-swine-flu-panic-will-turn-into-a-national-sickie. Of course, an in-person visit would not necessarily produce scientific results either, though it would give an opportunity for a test to be administered. This was a problem with sick notes seen in Chapters 2 and 5. See: TNA: PIN 35/435/1, Cutting from *General Practitioner*, 5 July 1974; R. S. Brock, 'Disqualification under the Bill', *British Medical Journal* 1, no. 4449 (1946): p. 585.

[31] Robert Drago and Kevin Miller, 'Sick at work: Infected employees in the workplace during the H1N1 pandemic' (Washington, D.C.: Institute for Women's Policy Research, January 2011).

[32] Natasha Koshnitsky and Eleanor Lynch, 'COVID-19 puts the spotlight on the UK's Statutory Sick Pay', Kingsley Napley, 6 November 2020, accessed 19 November 2020, https://www.kingsleynapley.co.uk/insights/blogs/employment-law-blog/covid-19-puts-the-spotlight-on-the-uks-statutory-sick-pay.

[33] The average post-tax household income in 2019/20 was around £592 per week. See: Office for National Statistics, 'Average household income, UK: financial year ending 2020 (provisional)', Office for National Statistics, 22 July 2020, accessed 19 November 2020, https://www.ons.gov.uk/peoplepopulationandcommunity/personalandhouseholdfinances/incomeandwealth/bulletins/householddisposableincomeandinequality/financialyearending2020provisional.

[34] TUC, 'TUC calls on government to tackle coronavirus with immediate #SickPayForAll', TUC, 3 March 2020, accessed 19 November 2020, https://www.tuc.org.uk/news/tuc-calls-government-tackle-coronavirus-immediate-sickpayforall.

[35] OECD, 'Paid sick leave to protect income, health and jobs through the COVID-19 crisis', OECD, 2 July 2020, accessed 19 November 2020, https://www.oecd.org/coronavirus/policy-responses/paid-sick-leave-to-protect-income-health-and-jobs-through-the-covid-19-crisis-a9e1a154/.

In September, the British government did increase access to funds, providing £500 to those asked to isolate (though this was difficult to access).[36] The waiting period for SSP had also been dropped in March in an attempt to get payments to workers quicker.[37] Beyond this, there was the wider Coronavirus Job Retention Scheme—commonly known as 'furlough'—which was agreed in April and designed to avoid mass unemployment during the partial economic lockdown invoked to control the spread of the virus.[38] Formal employment, even if financed by the state, was considered the quickest and most efficient use of existing bureaucratic structures to ensure support got to as many people as possible. These changes were at the heart of health, social security, and employment policy. But unlike traditional sickness in normal times, it was assumed to affect everyone. There was no need for a sick note here.

Despite the words of warning from the OECD and the desire of public health officials to control the 'R' number, there were still voices among business leaders and the government urging for a loosening of economic restrictions. For some, their attitudes proved a public relations disaster. Boohoo lost £1 billion from its stock value after a Leicester clothes factory it used was found to have breached a series of labour laws and became an epicentre for the virus.[39] For others, 'presenteeism' had become a literal problem: the idea that workers must 'present' themselves, in person, to perform their work. A culture had developed among management where working and being present through sickness had become a badge of honour and supposed 'leading by example' to subordinates—much like how Tony Blair's recovery from heart surgery was used in Chapter 7.[40] While in a number of occupations there was a material need to be present, many in office-based work found that jobs could performed remotely. This did not help the bottom line of office landlords and takeaway coffee chains; but it did allow sections of the economy to continue to function.[41] This posed significant problems

[36] Prime Minister's Office, 'New package to support and enforce self-isolation', gov.uk, 20 September 2020, accessed 19 November 2020, https://www.gov.uk/government/news/new-package-to-support-and-enforce-self-isolation; Rob Merrick, 'Only a few hundred people told to self-isolate receive £500 help pledged by Boris Johnson in most cities', Independent, 6 December 2020, accessed 22 February 2021, https://www.independent.co.uk/news/uk/politics/self-isolate-payment-discretionary-fund-boris-johnson-b1766402.html.
[37] For reasons discussed in Chapters 3 and 5, the normal waiting period was three days. This was eliminated entirely. Department for Work and Pensions and Boris Johnson, 'Sick pay from day one for those affected by coronavirus', gov.uk, 4 March 2020, accessed 19 November 2020, https://www.gov.uk/government/news/sick-pay-from-day-one-for-those-affected-by-coronavirus.
[38] Treasury, 'Coronavirus Job Retention Scheme up and running', gov.uk, 20 April 2020, accessed 19 November 2020, https://www.gov.uk/government/news/coronavirus-job-retention-scheme-up-and-running.
[39] Rob Davies and Annie Kelly, 'More than £1 billion wiped off Boohoo value as it investigates Leicester factory', Guardian, 6 July 2020, accessed 19 November 2020, https://www.theguardian.com/business/2020/jul/06/boohoo-leicester-factory-conditions-covid-19.
[40] Monojit Chatterji and Colin J. Tilley, 'Sickness, absenteeism, presenteeism, and sick pay', Oxford Economic Papers 54, no. 4 (2002): pp. 669–87.
[41] Jim Pickard, 'Business calls for clarity on where people should work', FT.com, 28 August 2020, accessed 20 November 2020, https://www.ft.com/content/ac66a7ba-ba32-411f-a7fb-3ee0dde0d1c2.

for management that had become used to surveillance and policing of absenteeism. On the one hand, how could workers be monitored to ensure they were being productive during their contracted hours? On the other, if 'working from home' had replaced the need for commuting or the risk of infection, there was a risk of employees continuing to labour while sick; a sort of remote presenteeism.[42] In some ways, the 'fit note' logic of reasonable adjustments could allow partial working at home.[43] But when working from home was less of a 'choice' than a public health mandate, generating new guidelines and codes of conduct became tricky.[44] The perceived need for gatekeeping sick leave and benefits remained, but the traditional tools—direct supervision and the doctor's note—were beyond reach in a public health emergency.

Not everyone had the option of working at home. Some were furloughed. Some did not have access to the necessary technological equipment. Still others were in occupations that required a physical presence. The concept of 'key workers' became a way of emphasizing the importance of jobs that were vital to the running of public and private services such as food supply chains, manufacturing, healthcare, refuse collection, education, and so on. As Kevin Siena shows using evidence from early modern Europe, such jobs have historically been reserved for the poor. Risky jobs did not pay well, and yet they were supposedly vital to maintaining the social and economic order. People took them because there was not much other choice.[45] Now, this narrative was skewed somewhat by the presence of middle- and working-class labourers in amongst the precariat: nurses, doctors, police officers, university lecturers, and teachers. For a little while, the nation showed its appreciation by going onto the streets to 'Clap for Carers.'[46] Still, the idea of a shared or collectivized risk of sickness was warped. In some ways, what was left of the sickness system would provide some pay for these workers who were (for the most part) fully employed. Yet the rhetoric of

[42] Alison Collins, 'Why you should call in sick more often than you think – even if working from home', *Management Today*, 29 September 2020, accessed 20 November 2020, https://www.management-today.co.uk/why-call-sick-often-think-per centE2per cent80 per cent93-even-working-home/food-for-thought/article/1695823.

[43] See, for example, this blog post written before 2020 focusing on employees who might take advantage of 'working from home' to avoid eating into sick pay entitlements and remain on full pay. Nicola Goodridge, 'Employees too sick to come to the office yet well enough to work from home..... sound familiar?!', Good HR, 1 October 2020, accessed 20 November 2020, http://www.goodhr.co.uk/employees-too-sick-to-come-to-the-office-yet-well-enough-to-work-from-home-sound-familiar/.

[44] CBI, 'Factsheet: supporting employees to work from home', CBI, 5 May 2020, accessed 20 November 2020, https://www.cbi.org.uk/articles/factsheet-supporting-employees-to-work-from-home-1/; TUC, 'TUC advice for people working at home during the coronavirus outbreak', TUC, 18 March 2020, accessed 20 November 2020, https://www.tuc.org.uk/news/tuc-advice-people-working-home-during-coronavirus-outbreak.

[45] Kevin Siena, 'Epidemics and "essential work" in early modern Europe', *History & Policy*, 25 March 2020, accessed 17 November 2020, http://www.historyandpolicy.org/opinion-articles/articles/epidemics-and-essential-work-in-early-modern-europe.

[46] BBC News, 'Clap for Carers: UK applauds NHS staff and key workers', *BBC News*, 2 April 2020, accessed 20 November 2020, https://www.bbc.co.uk/news/av/uk-52143223.

'heroes' was seen by some to reflect the nation's cynical view that the risks taken by such workers were simply 'what they signed up for'.[47] Even if the financial risks of sickness had been somewhat collectivized, some individuals—who were also disproportionately economically marginalized in other ways—were taking on much greater health risks without necessarily the material support to do so safely. But perhaps, as we saw in Chapter 4, the sickness system was never designed to overcome those obstacles.

While some focused on public health, for others the principle of retaining freedom of movement and keeping businesses open took precedence. Iain Duncan Smith accused the government of '"giving in" to scientific advisers and "marching" England back into lockdown' when a second set of economic restrictions were imposed in November.[48] There were protests throughout the year.[49] Opinion polling suggested Duncan Smith and the protestors were in the minority.[50] Regardless, the sick note and sick leave were not a viable solution. The strength of the gatekeeping was moot for those who did not believe a gate should exist in the first place. Regardless of pros or antis, the crisis exposed deeper failings in the welfare state. In a parallel with the 1940s, lower paid workers who relied most upon state benefit were most at risk. Only 26 per cent of UK employees relied upon SSP when sick because, in a trend that had been noted in the 1980s, most employers provided their own schemes that were far more generous.[51] The issues with self-employment and the gig economy that had reared their head with swine flu and in the intervening decade became more acute. Neither the state nor individuals had reserves to fall back on. Food bank use had increased markedly before COVID-19 and would accelerate still further in the economic contraction that followed.[52] Homelessness had increased, a problem solved in the short-term

---

[47] Olivia Peter, 'Coronavirus: Don't call NHS workers "heroes", says new mental health guide', *Independent*, 30 April 2020, accessed 20 November 2020, https://www.independent.co.uk/life-style/coronavirus-nhs-mental-health-workers-heroes-a9492341.html.

[48] Alan McGuinness, 'Coronavirus: Boris Johnson accused by ex-Tory leader of "giving in" to scientific advisers and "marching" England back into lockdown', *Sky News*, 1 November 2020, accessed 19 November 2020, https://news.sky.com/story/coronavirus-boris-johnson-accused-by-ex-tory-leader-of-giving-in-to-scientific-advisers-and-marching-england-back-into-lockdown-12120759.

[49] For a curated list, see: Multiple authorship, 'COVID-19 anti-lockdown protests in the United Kingdom', Wikipedia, accessed 19 November 2020, https://en.wikipedia.org/wiki/COVID-19_anti-lockdown_protests_in_the_United_Kingdom.

[50] Connor Ibbetson, 'Brits support new lockdown rules, but many think they don't go far enough', YouGov, 23 September 2020, accessed 19 November 2020, https://yougov.co.uk/topics/politics/articles-reports/2020/09/23/brits-support-new-lockdown-rules-many-think-they-d.

[51] Koshnitsky and Lynch, 'COVID-19'. Using data from Department for Work and Pensions and Department of Health and Social Care, 'Health in the workplace – patterns of sickness, absence, employer support and employment retention', 15 July 2019, accessed 19 November 2020, https://assets.publishing.service.gov.uk/government/uploads/system/uploads/attachment_data/file/817124/health-in-the-workplace-statistics.pdf. See also Chapter 5 and Department of Health and Social Security, *Income during Initial Sickness: A New Strategy (Cmnd 7864)* (London: HMSO, 1980).

[52] Rachel Loopstra and Doireann Lalor, *Financial Insecurity, Food Insecurity, and Disability: The Profile of People Receiving Emergency Food Assistance from The Trussell Trust Foodbank Network in Britain* (Trussell Trust: Salisbury, 2017); Patrick Butler, 'Growing numbers of "newly hungry" forced to

on public health grounds but there seemed little appetite to continue to provide accommodation once coronavirus had subsided.[53] Debt was a growing problem, accrued through legitimate means, 'pay day lenders' who charged large amounts of interest, and the black market.[54]

As lockdown eased, it was clear that many of the cultural responses to sick notes would also remain. Fay Weldon opined at the turn of the millennium that sick notes were part of the 'ergonarchy'—the rule of work—so insidious in society that one of the first things taught to school children is that they can only avoid work if they give a sick note to teacher.[55] Teenagers certainly understood how to undermine those who had authority over them. Using social media networks, they taught each other how to use lemon juice to produce false positives on COVID-19 tests, and therefore get out of class.[56] Meanwhile, the uneasy position of professional sport as simultaneously one of the few live entertainment outlets and a potential vector of disease gave professional contrarians opportunities to continue the sort of rhetoric all too familiar to people like Stephen Fry and Martine McCutcheon. When Simone Biles and Naomi Osaka both withdrew from major events citing mental health concerns, their reasoning was debated online, fuelled by pronouncements from public figures.[57]

*   *   *

It also became obvious that neither the inadequacies in the sickness system nor the effects of COVID-19 were going away any time soon. DWP had begun a consultation on the future of SSP before the pandemic. The Fabian Society and other think tanks used this as an opportunity to put forward proposals for significant reforms to sick pay, without which, they argued, productivity and public health would suffer.[58] In addition, growing recognition of 'long covid', the chronic post-

use UK food banks', *Guardian*, 1 November 2020, accessed 19 November 2020, https://www.theguard-ian.com/society/2020/nov/01/growing-numbers-newly-hungry-forced-use-uk-food-banks-covid.

[53] Francisco Garcia, 'Coronavirus nearly ended homelessness in the UK. Why can't we end it for good?', *Guardian*, 11 June 2020, accessed 19 November 2020, https://www.theguardian.com/commentisfree/2020/jun/11/coronavirus-homelessness-uk-rough-sleepers-lockdown-tories; Brian Lund, *Housing Politics in the United Kingdom: Power, Planning and Protest* (Bristol: Policy Press, 2016), esp. pp. 272–4.

[54] Simon Szreter, 'Covid-19 is not a Black Swan: Predictable shocks need fully-funded, resilient public services', *History & Policy*, 1 May 2020, accessed 17 November 2020, http://www.historyandpolicy.org/opinion-articles/articles/covid-19-is-not-a-black-swan-predictable-shocks-need-fully-funded-resilient-public-services.

[55] Fay Weldon, 'The rise of the egonarchy', *New Statesman*, 17 April 2000, pp. 25–7.

[56] John Dunne, 'TikTok crackdown on teens sharing tips on faking Covid-19 tests', *Evening Standard*, 1 July 2021, accessed 2 September 2021, https://www.standard.co.uk/news/uk/teenagers-fake-covid-tests-tiktok-b943711.html.

[57] Mel Evans, 'Piers Morgan sparks outrage as he dubs Simone Biles' withdrawal from Olympics final a 'joke' over mental health issues', *Metro*, 27 July 2021, accessed 2 September 2021, https://metro.co.uk/2021/07/27/tokyo-olympics-piers-morgan-dubs-simone-biles-withdrawal-a-joke-14997440/.

[58] Kevin Rawlinson, 'Lack of sick pay for all threatens Covid plan, UK thinktank warns', *Guardian*, 8 July 2021, accessed 2 September 2021, https://www.theguardian.com/world/2021/jul/08/lack-of-sick-pay-for-all-threatens-covid-plan-uk-thinktank-warns; Andrew Harrop, 'Statutory Sick Pay: Options

viral effects of the disease among a significant minority of infected people, made it obvious that claim to sickness and disability related benefits would come as a direct result of the pandemic. The nature of the diagnosis-based, sick-note inspired industrial injuries system meant that the TUC felt the need to campaign for the condition to be recognised officially as an occupational disease.[59] Would such reforms be enough, or would more radical changes to work, social security, and employment be required. Was Britain ready, as Mike Savage argued, for a 'new Beveridge Report'?[60]

* * *

Sick Note has traced the evolution of Britain's sickness system and the sick note. But while it is clear that the changes made over the past fifty years or so have undermined the welfare state's ability to respond to the acute challenges posed by COVID-19, this book is not about 'decline'.[61] Nor is it about a need to 'return' to a 'golden age'. The 1940s system was designed to cope with people in unsecure employment by providing sick pay through state National Insurance, so perhaps it does offer answers to present-day precarious employment. The principle of collectivized risk it represented spread the costs of ill health among workers and employers, giving protection to 'key workers' and those most at risk of economic shocks. Yet even in the 'classic welfare state' the sickness system failed many people. Chapter 4 especially showed just how *National* Insurance built for 'breadwinners' in nuclear family households excluded those who did not fit the interwar, liberal, Beveridgean template. Guy Standing's work on the precariat shows that there is little desire among young left-wing radicals to return to the secure employment model of the 1970s which tied people to industries and modes of thinking that have been superseded by a globalized, service-based economy.[62]

Indeed, COVID-19 appears to offer exactly the sort of crisis that gives an opportunity to build new anti-discrimination responses to our shared risks.[63] The sense, at least until the illusion was shattered by Dominic Cummings'

for reform', *Fabian Society*, June 2021, accessed 2 September 2021, https://www.tuc.org.uk/sites/default/files/SSPreport.pdf.

[59] TUC, 'TUC calls for long Covid to be urgently recognised as a disability to prevent "massive" discrimination', 20 June 2021, accessed 2 September 2021, https://www.tuc.org.uk/news/tuc-calls-long-covid-be-urgently-recognised-disability-prevent-massive-discrimination.

[60] Mike Savage, 'Call for new Beveridge report as number of destitute UK households doubles during Covid', *Guardian*, 20 February 2021, accessed 2 September 2021, https://amp.theguardian.com/society/2021/feb/20/call-for-new-beveridge-report-as-number-of-destitute-uk-households-doubles-during-covid.

[61] See Chapter 1 and Jim Tomlinson, 'De-industrialization not decline: A new meta-narrative for post-war British history', *Twentieth Century British History* 27, no. 1 (2016): pp. 76–99.

[62] Guy Standing, *The Precariat: The New Dangerous Class* (London: Bloomsbury, 2014).

[63] Lucy Delap, D.-M. Withers, and Margaretta Jolly, 'Not business as usual: A feminist map for the post-Covid future', *History & Policy*, 15 June 2020, accessed 17 November 2020, http://www.history-andpolicy.org/opinion-articles/articles/not-business-as-usual-a-feminist-map-for-the-post-covid-future; Savage, 'Call for new Beveridge report'.

eyesight-testing drive to Barnard Castle,[64] was that Britons were 'all in this together'.[65] Perhaps there is room for new (or *renewed*) understandings of our shared vulnerabilities to economic shocks and the need to provide both safety nets and prophylactics against ill health and poverty.[66] Regardless, the basic tenets of sick-note thinking will remain. While resources are finite, employers and social security authorities will continue to gatekeep the boundaries of sickness. And gatekeepers need something to perform the job of validating sickness. Proponents of a Universal Basic Income might argue that the provision of a statutory minimum, regardless of employment status, will allow states to be less worried about whether an individual is 'really' sick and give less incentive to 'force' people back to work in unsuitable jobs. It would also re-collectivize some of those risks of sickness that disproportionately hit certain industrial sectors and geographic regions.[67] Yet it is difficult to imagine, having seen their behaviour over the course of this volume, that employers are going to abandon disciplinary procedures designed to ensure predictable attendance, even if they are no longer directly responsible for sick pay. More pertinently, many supporters of UBI's supposed 'universalism' still propose *selective* extra-costs and loss-of-earnings benefits for disabled people. These must inevitably contain medical rules for who does and does not qualify.[68] Despite many constituencies' best efforts, the least objectionable and most widely understood tool that can help in these matters is still the humble sick note. However, just like it has for over a century, it will have to adapt to new forms of employment, health systems, and social security. So too will Britain and its welfare state.

---

[64] Chris Curtis, 'How Dominic Cummings' lockdown travels changed public opinion', YouGov, 29 May 2020, accessed 20 November 2020, https://yougov.co.uk/topics/politics/articles-reports/2020/05/29/how-dominic-cummings-lockdown-travels-changed-publ.

[65] Patrick, 'Covid has exposed the decade-long lie that benefits are a lifestyle choice'.

[66] For this, see the ahistorical invocation of 'Blitz spirit' and critique from historians. Henry Irving and Marc Wiggam, 'Loosening lockdown: Lesson from the blackout', *History & Policy*, 15 May 2020, accessed 17 November 2020, http://www.historyandpolicy.org/opinion-articles/articles/loosening-lockdown-lessons-from-the-blackout; Henry Irving, Rosemary Cresswell, Barry Doyle, Shane Ewen, Mark Roodhouse, Charlotte Thomas, and Marc Wiggam, 'The real lessons of the Blitz for Covid-19', *History & Policy*, 3 April 2020, accessed 20 November 2020, http://www.historyandpolicy.org/policy-papers/papers/the-real-lessons-of-the-blitz-for-covid-19.

[67] See: Peter Sloman, Daniel Zamora Vargas, and Pedro Ramos Pinto, 'Introduction'. In *Universal Basic Income in Historical Perspective*, edited by Peter Sloman, Daniel Zamora Vargas, and Pedro Ramos Pinto (London: Palgrave Macmillan, forthcoming 2021). I am grateful to Peter Sloman for an advanced copy of this chapter.

[68] Guy Standing, *Basic Income as Common Dividends: Piloting a Transformative Policy* (London: Progressive Economy Forum, 2019); Green Party, 'Basic income: A detailed proposal', Green Party, April 2015, accessed 20 November 2020, https://policy.greenparty.org.uk/assets/files/Policyper cent20files/Basicper cent20Incomeper cent20Consultationper cent20Paper.pdf.

Bibliography

It is the nature of contemporary history that the lines between 'primary' and 'secondary' sources are blurred. A sociological journal article from 1987, for example, might provide secondary interpretation of research data; at the same time, it is primary evidence of how knowledge circulated in 1980s Britain. For simplicity, this bibliography categorizes official publications, newspapers, and archival holdings (manuscript and digital) as 'primary sources'—and any monographs, articles published in peer-reviewed journals, and edited book chapters are classed as 'secondary sources'. This includes editorial and research articles published in contemporary medical and professional journals such as *The Lancet* and *British Medical Journal*.

Primary Sources

Archives

The Modern Records Centre, University of Warwick, Coventry
The National Archives, London
The Peter Townsend Collection, Albert Sloman Library, University of Essex, Colchester
British Library Oral History Collection, London

Newspapers/Periodicals

British Medical Journal.
Chemist & Druggist.
Commercial Motor.
Corporate Adviser.
Daily Express.
Daily Mail.
Daily Telegraph.
Employee Benefits.
Financial Times.
Guardian.
GP.
Hairdressers Journal International.
Human Resources.
Independent.
Independent on Sunday.
New Statesman.
Manchester Guardian.
Motor Transport.
Observer.
Personnel Today.
Police Review.
Public Finance.

Pulse.
Safety & Health Practitioner.
Scottish Business Insider.
Sunday Business.
Sunday Times.
The Economist.
The Lancet.
The Times.
Works Management.

Legislation and Legal Decisions

Disabled Persons (Employment) Act 1944.
European Council, Council Directive 79/7/EEC, 19 December 1978.
European Council, Council Directive 92/85/EEC, 19 October 1992.
Social Security Pensions Act 1975.

Government and Parliamentary Publications

Beveridge, William H. *Social Insurance and Allied Services (Cmd. 6404)* (London: HMSO, 1942).
Black, Carol. *Working for a Healthier Tomorrow* (London: TSO, 2008).
Black, Carol Mary, and David Frost. *Health at Work: An Independent Review of Sickness Absence* (London: TSO, 2011).
Buzzard, R. B., and F. D. K. Liddell. *Coalminers' Attendance at Work* (London: National Coal Board, 1963).
Cabinet Office. *Making a Difference: Reducing General Practitioner (GP) Paperwork* (London: Cabinet Office, 2001).
Cabinet Office and Institute for Government. *MINDSPACE: Influencing Behaviour through Public Policy* (London: Institute for Government, 2010).
Central Statistical Office. *Annual Abstract of Statistics, No. 92* (London: HMSO, 1955).
Central Statistical Office. *Annual Abstract of Statistics, No. 102* (London: HMSO, 1965).
Central Statistical Office. *Annual Abstract of Statistics, No. 105* (London: HMSO, 1968).
Central Statistical Office. *Annual Abstract of Statistics 1971, No. 108* (London: HMSO, 1971).
Central Statistical Office. *Annual Abstract of Statistics 1974* (London: HMSO, 1974).
Central Statistical Office. *Annual Abstract of Statistics 1977* (London: HMSO, 1977).
Chiripanhura, Blessing, and Nikolas Wolf. 'Long-term trends in UK employment: 1861 to 2018', Office of National Statistics, 29 April 2019, accessed 24 November 2020, https://www.ons.gov.uk/economy/nationalaccounts/uksectoraccounts/compendium/economicreview/april2019/longtermtrendsinukemployment1861to2018.
Committee of Public Accounts. *First, Third and Fourth Reports from the Committee of Public Accounts Together with the Proceedings of the Committee, Minutes of Evidence, Appendices and Index (HC 71-I, 78-I, 138-I (1950))* (London: HMSO, 1950).
Committee on Restrictions Against Disabled People. *Report by the Committee on Restrictions Against Disabled People* (London: HMSO, 1982).
Department of Health. *A Report of the CFS/ME Working Group: Report to the Chief Medical Officer of an Independent Working Group* (London: Department of Health, January 2002).
Department of Health and Social Security. *Income during Initial Sickness: A New Strategy (Cmnd 7864)* (London: HMSO, 1980).
Department of Health and Social Security. *Review of the Household Duties Test* (London: HMSO, 1983).

Department of Social Security. *A New Contract for Welfare (Cm 3805)* (London: TSO, 1998).

Department of Health and Social Security. *Disability Benefits: The Delivery of Disability Living Allowance and Disability Working Allowance Reply by the Government to the Third Report from the Social Security Committee (Cm 2282)* (London: HMSO, 1993).

Department for Work and Pensions. *A New Deal for Welfare: Empowering People to Work (Cm 6730)* (London: TSO, 2006).

Department for Work and Pensions. *A New Deal for Welfare: Empowering People to Work. Consultation Report (Cm 6859)* (London: TSO, 2006).

Department for Work and Pensions. 'Benefit expenditure tables', March 2013, accessed 17 July 2020, http://statistics.dwp.gov.uk/asd/asd4/expenditure_tables_Budget_2013.xls.

Department for Work and Pensions. *Five Year Strategy: Opportunity and Security Throughout Life (Cm 6447)* (London: TSO, 2005).

Department for Work and Pensions. 'Spring budget 2020: Expenditure and caseload forecasts', *gov.uk*, 20 March 2020, accessed 13 July 2021, https://www.gov.uk/government/publications/benefit-expenditure-and-caseload-tables-2020.

Department for Work and Pensions and Boris Johnson. 'Sick pay from day one for those affected by coronavirus', gov.uk, 4 March 2020, accessed 19 November 2020, https://www.gov.uk/government/news/sick-pay-from-day-one-for-those-affected-by-coronavirus.

Department for Work and Pensions and Department of Health and Social Care. 'Health in the workplace – patterns of sickness, absence, employer support and employment retention', 15 July 2019, accessed 19 November 2020, https://assets.publishing.service.gov.uk/government/uploads/system/uploads/attachment_data/file/817124/health-in-the-workplace-statistics.pdf.

Disability Rights Commission. *Annual Report and Accounts April to September 2007 (HC 753 (2008-09))*' (London: TSO, 2009).

Ethel, Lawrence (ed.). *Annual Abstract of Statistics 1980* (London: HMSO, 1980).

Ethel, Lawrence (ed.). *Annual Abstract of Statistics 1983* (London: HMSO, 1983).

Fisher, Henry. *Report of the Committee on Abuse of Social Security Benefits (Cmnd 5228)* (London: HMSO, 1972).

Harrington, Malcolm. *An Independent Review of the Work Capability Assessment* (London: TSO, 2010).

Hayward, Bruce, Barry Fong, and Alex Thornton. *The Third Work-Life Balance Employer Survey: Main Findings* (London: Department for Business, Enterprise and Regulatory Reform, 2007).

Hooker, Hülya, Fiona Neathy, Jo Casebourne, and Miranda Munro. *The Third Work-Life Balance Employee Survey: Main Findings* (London: Department of Trade and Industry, 2007).

House of Commons Official Report (Hansard).

House of Lords Official Report (Hansard).

Kennedy, Stephen, and Wendy Wilson. *The Welfare Reform Bill (RP 06/39)* (London: House of Commons Library, 2006).

Litchfield, Paul. *An Independent Review of the Work Capability Assessment – Year Five* (London: TSO, 2014).

Millward, Gareth, and Peter Border. *Assessing Capacity for Work (PN 413)* (London: Parliamentary Office of Science and Technology, 2012).

Ministry of National Insurance. *National Insurance (Medical Certification) Regulations, 1948 (HC 149 (1947–48))* (London: HMSO, 1948).

Ministry of Reconstruction. *Social Insurance Part II: Workmen's Compensation. Proposals for an Industrial Injury Insurance Scheme (Cmd. 6551)* (London: HMSO, 1944).

Ministry of Social Security. *Report of the Ministry of Social Security for the Year 1966 (Cmnd 3338)* (London: HMSO, 1967).

Morton, Fergus. *Royal Commission on Marriage and Divorce (Cmd. 9678)* (London: HMSO, 1956).

National Assistance Board. *Report of the National Assistance Board for the Year Ended 31st December 1948 (Cmd. 7767)* (London: HMSO, 1949).

National Audit Office. *Invalidity Benefit: Report by the Comptroller and Auditor General (HC 91 (1989–90))* (London: HMSO, 1989).

National Insurance Advisory Committee. *National Insurance (Maternity Benefit) Regulations 1948: Report (HC 147 (1947–48))* (London: HMSO, 1948).

National Insurance Advisory Committee. *Maternity Benefits (Cmd. 8446)* (London: HMSO, 1952).

National Insurance Advisory Committee. *Report of the National Insurance Advisory Committee on the Question of Contribution Conditions and Credit Provisions (Cmd. 9854)* (London: HMSO, 1956).

National Insurance Advisory Committee. *Report of the National Insurance Advisory Committee on the Question of Doctors' and Midwives' Certificates for National Insurance Purposes (Cmnd 1021)* (London: HMSO, 1960).

National Insurance Advisory Committee. *National Insurance (Medical Certification) Amendment Regulations 1966. Report of the National Insurance Advisory Committee (Cmnd 2875)* (London: HMSO, 1966).

NHS Digital. 'Health survey for England – Health social care and lifestyles', *NHS Digital*, 2 March 2021, accessed 17 August 2021, https://digital.nhs.uk/data-and-information/areas-of-interest/public-health/health-survey-for-england-health-social-care-and-lifestyles.

Office for National Statistics. 'UK Population Estimates 1851 to 2014', 6 July 2015, accessed 2 August 2021, https://www.ons.gov.uk/peoplepopulationandcommunity/populationandmigration/populationestimates/adhocs/004356ukpopulationestimates1851to2014.

Office for National Statistics. 'Which occupations are at the highest risk of being automated?', Office for National Statistics, 25 March 2019, accessed 17 November 2020, https://www.ons.gov.uk/employmentandlabourmarket/peopleinwork/employmentandemployeetypes/articles/whichoccupationsareathighestriskofbeingautomated/2019-03-25.

Office for National Statistics. 'Average household income, UK: financial year ending 2020 (provisional)', Office for National Statistics, 22 July 2020, accessed 19 November 2020, https://www.ons.gov.uk/peoplepopulationandcommunity/personalandhouseholdfinances/incomeandwealth/bulletins/householddisposableincomeandinequality/financialyearending2020provisional.

Office for National Statistics. 'Sickness absence in the UK labour market', *gov.uk*, 3 March 2021, accessed 13 July 2021, https://www.ons.gov.uk/employmentandlabourmarket/peoplein-work/employmentandemployeetypes/datasets/sicknessabsenceinthelabourmarket.

Poor Law Commissioners. *Report from His Majesty's Commissioners for Inquiring into the Administration and Practical Operation of the Poor Laws* (London: B. Fellowes, 1834).

Priestley, Raymond E. *Royal Commission on the Civil Service 1953–55. Report (Cmd. 9613)* (London: HMSO, 1955).

Prime Minister's Office, 'New package to support and enforce self-isolation', gov.uk, 20 September 2020, accessed 19 November 2020, https://www.gov.uk/government/news/new-package-to-support-and-enforce-self-isolation.

Prime Minister's Strategy Unit. *Improving the Life Chances of Disabled People* (London: Prime Minister's Strategy Unit, 2005).

Pyper, Doug, and Daniel Harari. *Zero-Hours Contracts (SN/BT/6553)* (London: House of Commons Library, July 2013).

Ross, William David. *Royal Commission on the Press 1947–1949. Report (Cmd. 7700)* (London: HMSO, 1949).

Schuster, Claud. *Report of the Departmental Committee on Sickness Benefit Claims Under the National Insurance Act (Cd. 7687)* (London: HMSO, 1914).

Select Committee on Estimates. *Seventh Report from the Select Committee on Estimates (HC 200 (1947–48))* (London: HMSO, 1948).

Select Committee on Estimates. *Fifth Report from the Select Committee on Estimates (HC 141 (1948–49))* (London: HMSO, 1949).

Taylor, Matthew, Greg Marsh, Diane Nicol, and Paul Broadbent. *Good Work: The Taylor Review of Modern Working Practices* (London: Department for Business, Energy and Industrial Strategy, 2017).

Treasury. 'Coronavirus Job Retention Scheme up and running', gov.uk, 20 April 2020, accessed 19 November 2020, https://www.gov.uk/government/news/coronavirus-job-retention-scheme-up-and-running.

Waddell, Gordon, and Mansel Aylward. *The Scientific and Conceptual Basis of Incapacity Benefits* (London: TSO, 2005).

Waddell, Gordon, and A. Kim Burton. *Is Work Good for Your Health and Well-Being?* (London: TSO, 2006).

Williams, Wendy. *Windrush Lessons Learned Review HC 93 (2019–20)* (London: TSO, March 2020).

Wyatt, S., R. Marriott, and D. E. R. Hughes. *A Study of Absenteeism among Women* (London: HMSO, 1943).

Film, television, and audio

BBC. *A Life on Screen – Stephen Fry*, broadcast BBC Four, 14 July 2018.

BBC. *Little Britain – Bath of Beans*, broadcast BBC Three, 16 September 2003.

Boyce, Max. '9-3', *Live at Treorchy* (EMI, 1974).

Gillespie, Craig (dir.). *I, Tonya* (Neon, 2017).

Loach, Ken (dir.). *I, Daniel Blake* (BFI, 2016).

Ministry of National Insurance, 'Industrial Accidents – Trailer', British Pathé, 1948, accessed 20 February 2021, https://www.britishpathe.com/video/industrial-accidents-trailer.

Archived Websites

abeator81. 'Getting stuff done', Amy Loves Peccarys, 29 November 2004, accessed 9 November 2020, archived 22 March 2005, http://web.archive.org/web/20050322172433/http:/journals.aol.co.uk:80/abeator81/AmyLovesPeccarys/entries/423.

Anon. 'Getting through post natal depression', Families Online, n.d., accessed 9 November 2020, archived 8 April 2005, http://web.archive.org/web/20050408201723/http:/familiesonline.co.uk:80/index.php/article/static/419/.

Anon. Message on COWSARSE, 3 December 2002, accessed 31 August 2020, archived 4 January 2003, http://web.archive.org/web/20030104121038/http://www.cs.aston.ac.uk:80/~dorandw/phpboards/boards/ooc/board.php.

Ashley, Gareth. 'Adult chicken pox diary', 1998, accessed 9 November 2020, archived 7 December 1998, http://web.archive.org/web/19981207014243/http:/www.helpdesk.demon.co.uk:80/pox.htm.

Bartley, Una. 'Labour Pains – employment issues for pregnant women', Citizens Advice Scotland, June 2000, accessed 9 November 2020, archived 12 January 2003, http://web. archive.org/web/20030112230232/http://www.cas.org.uk:80/Change/Reports/ LabPains/labpains.html.

eragan. 'I'm so angry about one person...', discussion thread on Femail, 25 March 2003, accessed 9 November 2020, archived 4 April 2003, http://web.archive.org/web/ 20030404005231/http://chat.femail.co.uk:80/femail/threadnonInd.jsp?forum=52&threa d=9568485&message=9846089.

Jarvis, Eric. 'Cobble or Quits', www.ericjarvis.co.uk, 19 November 1999, accessed 31 August 2020, archived 15 February 2003, http://web.archive.org/web/20030215075418/ http://www.ericjarvis.co.uk:80/stories/cobble.html.

Jax. 'Diary - 2002', Silent Words, 2002, accessed 9 November 2020, archived 2 September 2004, http://web.archive.org/web/20040902080024/http:/www.silentwords.co.uk:80/2002.htm.

Jean. 'Need some advice', discussion thread on I Resign, 30 January 2003, accessed 9 November 2020, archived 20 March 2003, http://web.archive.org/web/20030320135044/ http://www.i-resign.co.uk:80/uk/discussion/new_topic.asp?t=647.

Member of DearDenise Message Board, posted on 6 June 2001, accessed 3 December 2018, archived 15 July 2001, http://web.archive.org/web/20010715061955/http://www. linksolutions.co.uk:80/ubb/Forum2/HTML/000129-3.html.

Monica. 'Monica's Diary, Part Two', Breast Cancer Care, 1997, accessed 9 November 2020, archived 6 January 2003, http://web.archive.org/web/20030106012844/http:/www. breastcancercare.org.uk:80/Breastcancer/Practicalsupport/Monicasdiary/Parttwo? portal_skin=access.

Multiple authorship. 'I've returned, but only just', discussion thread on ivf-infertility.co.uk, first post 20 November 2002, accessed 9 November 2020, archived 10 January 2003, http:// web.archive.org/web/20030110234830/http:/www.ivf-infertility.co.uk:80/cgi-bin/teemz/ teemz.cgi?board=_master&action=opentopic&topic=424&forum=General_Forum.

Multiple authorship. 'Life is great!', discussion thread on Weight Loss Surgery Information & Support, 25 December 2003, accessed 9 November 2020, archived 29 March 2005, http:// web.archive.org/web/20050329034000/http:/www.wlsinfo.org.uk:80/newweb2/forum/ post.asp?method=ReplyQuote&REPLY_ID=29539&TOPIC_ID=3117&FORUM_ID=88.

Multiple authorship. 'Member profiles', Social Anxiety UK, n.d., accessed 9 November 2020, archived 10 December 2004, http://web.archive.org/web/20041210162553/http:/www. social-anxiety.org.uk:80/members/browse.htm?page=1.

Multiple authorship. 'Personal accounts', To Transplant and Beyond, n.d., 9 November 2020, archived 4 January 2003, http://web.archive.org/web/20030104072839/http:/www. heart-transplant.co.uk:80/personal_accounts.htm.

Multiple authorship. 'Your stories', Encephalitis Information Resource, n.d., accessed 9 November 2020, archived 17 April 2003, http://web.archive.org/web/20030417090336/ http://esg.org.uk:80/ESG/Support/recovery/YS.htm.

Regan. 'This is my story', a1-health.co.uk, n.d., accessed 31 August 2020, archived 29 April 2005, http://web.archive.org/web/20050429182028/http://www.a1-health.co.uk:80/My%20 storyFrame1Source1.htm.

sarahc. 'Mummy's place to chat', post in discussion thread on Fertility Friends, 7 August 2004, accessed 9 November 2020, archived 4 October 2005, http://web.archive.org/web/ 20051004052852/http://www.fertilityfriends.co.uk:80/forum/index.php/topic,11042. msg164286.html.

Sargent, Louise. 'A short history of myalgic encephalomyelitis', M.E. Support, accessed 16 July 2020, archived 17 March 2016, https://web.archive.org/web/20160317130141/ http://mesupport.co.uk/index.php?page=a-short-history-of-m-e.

Shenton, Mark. 'Interview with Rik Mayall', Theatre.com, 11 January 2007, accessed 24 November 2020, archived 24 November 2020, https://web.archive.org/web/20070513082433/http://www.theatre.com/story/id/3005429/.

Sid. 'Working while on IB', discussion thread on Benefits Now, 20 August 2001, accessed 9 November 2020, archived 7 September 2003, http://web.archive.org/web/20030907082241/http://www.benefitsnowshop.co.uk/forum/display_message.asp?mid=1567.

TUC. 'Countering an urban legend: Sicknote Britain?', TUC, 7 January 2005, accessed 2 September 2020, archived 8 November 2005, http://web.archive.org/web/20051108200505/http://www.tuc.org.uk/welfare/tuc-9208-f0.cfm.

vicky_just_vicky. 'SICK PAY problems', discussion thread on Femail, 19 March 2003, accessed 9 November 2020, archived 4 April 2003, http://web.archive.org/web/20030404005555/http://chat.femail.co.uk:80/femail/threadnonInd.jsp?forum=52&thread=9567387&message=9836865.

Contemporary Websites

BBC News. 'Clap for Carers: UK applauds NHS staff and key workers', BBC News, 2 April 2020, accessed 20 November 2020, https://www.bbc.co.uk/news/av/uk-52143223.

Borland, Sophie. 'Sicknote Britain: One in four visits to a GP is avoidable because they are taken up with form-filling or minor ailments', Mail Online, 29 June 2017, accessed 23 November 2020, https://www.dailymail.co.uk/health/article-4648904/Sicknote-Britain-One-four-visits-GP-avoidable.html.

British Postal Museum and Archive Blog. '#MuseumCats Day: "Industrial chaos in the Post Office cat world"', The British Postal Museum and Archive Blog, 30 July 2014, accessed 16 July 2019, https://postalheritage.wordpress.com/2014/07/30/museumcats-day-industrial-chaos-in-the-post-office-cat-world.

Butler, Patrick. 'Growing numbers of "newly hungry" forced to use UK food banks', Guardian, 1 November 2020, accessed 19 November 2020, https://www.theguardian.com/society/2020/nov/01/growing-numbers-newly-hungry-forced-use-uk-food-banks-covid.

CBI. 'Factsheet: supporting employees to work from home', CBI, 5 May2020, accessed 20 November2020, https://www.cbi.org.uk/articles/factsheet-supporting-employees-to-work-from-home-1/.

Collins, Alison. 'Why you should call in sick more often than you think – even if working from home', Management Today, 29 September 2020, accessed 20 November 2020, https://www.managementtoday.co.uk/why-call-sick-often-think-%E2%80%93-even-working-home/food-for-thought/article/1695823.

Cork, Tristan. 'Deliveroo riders announce all-out strike in Bristol', BristolLive, 14 January 2019, accessed 17 November 2020, https://www.bristolpost.co.uk/whats-on/food-drink/deliveroo-riders-announce-out-strike-2428691.

Cumber, Robert. 'Deliveroo couriers stage strike in Sheffield', The Star, 3 September 2019, accessed 17 November 2020, https://www.thestar.co.uk/business/deliveroo-couriers-stage-strike-sheffield-busiest-day-493657.

Curtis, Chris. 'How Dominic Cummings' lockdown travels changed public opinion', YouGov, 29 May 2020, accessed 20 November 2020, https://yougov.co.uk/topics/politics/articles-reports/2020/05/29/how-dominic-cummings-lockdown-travels-changed-publ.

Davies, Rob, and Annie Kelly. 'More than £1 billion wiped off Boohoo value as it investigates Leicester factory', Guardian, 6 July 2020, accessed 19 November 2020, https://www.theguardian.com/business/2020/jul/06/boohoo-leicester-factory-conditions-covid-19.

Delap, Lucy, D.-M. Withers and Margaretta Jolly. 'Not business as usual: A feminist map for the post-Covid future', *History & Policy*, 15 June 2020, accessed 17 November 2020, http://www.historyandpolicy.org/opinion-articles/articles/not-business-as-usual-a-feminist-map-for-the-post-covid-future.

Dunne, John. 'TikTok crackdown on teens sharing tips on faking Covid-19 tests', *Evening Standard*, 1 July 2021, accessed 2 September 2021, https://www.standard.co.uk/news/uk/teenagers-fake-covid-tests-tiktok-b943711.html.

Evans, Mel. 'Piers Morgan sparks outrage as he dubs Simone Biles' withdrawal from Olympics final a "joke" over mental health issues', *Metro*, 27 July 2021, accessed 2 September 2021, https://metro.co.uk/2021/07/27/tokyo-olympics-piers-morgan-dubs-simone-biles-withdrawal-a-joke-14997440/.

Fox, Nikki. 'The Disability Discrimination Act: 20 years on', *BBC News*, 6 November 2015, accessed 24 November 2020, https://www.bbc.co.uk/news/av/health-34743197.

Garcia, Francisco. 'Coronavirus nearly ended homelessness in the UK. Why can't we end it for good?', *Guardian*, 11 June 2020, accessed 19 November 2020, https://www.theguardian.com/commentisfree/2020/jun/11/coronavirus-homelessness-uk-rough-sleepers-lockdown-tories.

Goodridge, Nicola. 'Employees too sick to come to the office yet well enough to work from home.....sound familiar?!', Good HR, 1 October 2020, accessed 20 November 2020, http://www.goodhr.co.uk/employees-too-sick-to-come-to-the-office-yet-well-enough-to-work-from-home-sound-familiar/.

Green Party. 'Basic income: A detailed proposal', Green Party, April 2015, accessed 20 November 2020, https://policy.greenparty.org.uk/assets/files/Policy%20files/Basic%20Income%20Consultation%20Paper.pdf.

Harrop, Andrew. 'Statutory Sick Pay: Options for reform', *Fabian Society*, June 2021, accessed 2 September 2021, https://www.tuc.org.uk/sites/default/files/SSPreport.pdf.

History & Policy. 'History & Policy', accessed 23 November 2020, http://www.historyandpolicy.org/.

Ibbetson, Connor. 'Brits support new lockdown rules, but many think they don't go far enough', YouGov, 23 September 2020, accessed 19 November 2020, https://yougov.co.uk/topics/politics/articles-reports/2020/09/23/brits-support-new-lockdown-rules-many-think-they-d.

Irving, Henry, and Marc Wiggam. 'Loosening lockdown: Lesson from the blackout', *History & Policy*, 15 May 2020, accessed 17 November 2020, http://www.historyandpolicy.org/opinion-articles/articles/loosening-lockdown-lessons-from-the-blackout.

Irving, Henry, Rosemary Cresswell, Barry Doyle, Shane Ewen, Mark Roodhouse, Charlotte Thomas, and Marc Wiggam. 'The real lessons of the Blitz for Covid-19', *History & Policy*, 3 April 2020, accessed 20 November 2020, http://www.historyandpolicy.org/policy-papers/papers/the-real-lessons-of-the-blitz-for-covid-19.

Jolly, Debbie. 'A tale of two models: Disabled people vs Unum, Atos, government and disability charities', Disabled People Against Cuts, 8 April 2012, accessed 24 November 2020, http://dpac.uk.net/2012/04/a-tale-of-two-models-disabled-people-vs-unum-atos-government-and-disability-charities-debbie-jolly/.

Kollewe, Julia. 'Uber drivers strike over pay and conditions', *Guardian*, 8 May 2019, accessed 17 November 2020, https://www.theguardian.com/technology/2019/may/08/uber-drivers-strike-over-pay-and-conditions.

Koshnitsky, Natasha, and Eleanor Lynch. 'COVID-19 puts the spotlight on the UK's Statutory Sick Pay', Kingsley Napley, 6 November 2020, accessed 19 November 2020, https://www.kingsleynapley.co.uk/insights/blogs/employment-law-blog/covid-19-puts-the-spotlight-on-the-uks-statutory-sick-pay.

McGuinness, Alan. 'Coronavirus: Boris Johnson accused by ex-Tory leader of "giving in" to scientific advisers and "marching" England back into lockdown', *Sky News*, 1 November 2020, accessed 19 November 2020, https://news.sky.com/story/coronavirus-boris-johnson-accused-by-ex-tory-leader-of-giving-in-to-scientific-advisers-and-marching-england-back-into-lockdown-12120759.

Merrick, Rob. 'Only a few hundred people told to self-isolate receive £500 help pledged by Boris Johnson in most cities', *Independent*, 6 December 2020, accessed 22 February 2021, https://www.independent.co.uk/news/uk/politics/self-isolate-payment-discretionary-fund-boris-johnson-b1766402.html.

Multiple authorship. 'Bert "Sicknote" Quigley', Fandom – London's Burning Wiki, accessed 31 January 2019, https://londons-burning.fandom.com/wiki/Bert_%27Sicknote%27_Quigley.

Multiple authorship. 'COVID-19 anti-lockdown protests in the United Kingdom', Wikipedia, accessed 19 November 2020, https://en.wikipedia.org/wiki/COVID-19_anti-lockdown_protests_in_the_United_Kingdom.

Murray, Andrew. 'A warning for Mourinho? Anderton bemoans having to pay through injury', *FourFourTwo*, 9 November 2016, accessed 31 January 2019, www.fourfourtwo.com/features/be-careful-forcing-players-play-through-injury-mou-darren-anderton-told-us.

NHS at 70. 'NHS at 70', accessed 17 September 2020, www.nhs70.org.uk.

OECD. 'Paid sick leave to protect income, health and jobs through the COVID-19 crisis', OECD, 2 July 2020, accessed 19 November 2020, https://www.oecd.org/coronavirus/policy-responses/paid-sick-leave-to-protect-income-health-and-jobs-through-the-covid-19-crisis-a9e1a154/.

Patrick, Ruth. 'Covid has exposed the decade-long lie that benefits are a lifestyle choice', *Guardian*, 3 November 2020, accessed 20 November 2020, https://www.theguardian.com/society/2020/nov/03/covid-decade-long-lie-benefits-lifestyle-choice-george-osborne-free-school-meals.

Peter, Olivia. 'Coronavirus: Don't call NHS workers "heroes", says new mental health guide', *Independent*, 30 April 2020, accessed 20 November 2020, https://www.independent.co.uk/life-style/coronavirus-nhs-mental-health-workers-heroes-a9492341.html.

Pickard, Jim. 'Business calls for clarity on where people should work', FT.com, 28 August 2020, accessed 20 November 2020, https://www.ft.com/content/ac66a7ba-ba32-411f-a7fb-3ee0dde0d1c2.

PwC. 'Rising sick bill is costing UK business £29bn a year – PwC research', PwC, 15 July 2013, accessed 19 July 2019, https://pwc.blogs.com/press_room/2013/07/rising-sick-bill-is-costing-uk-business-29bn-a-year-pwc-research.html.

Rawlinson, Kevin. 'Lack of sick pay for all threatens Covid plan, UK thinktank warns', *Guardian*, 8 July2021, accessed 2 September 2021, https://www.theguardian.com/world/2021/jul/08/lack-of-sick-pay-for-all-threatens-covid-plan-uk-thinktank-warns.

Savage, Michael. 'Call for new Beveridge report as number of destitute UK households doubles during Covid', *Guardian*, 20 February 2021, accessed 2 September 2021, https://amp.theguardian.com/society/2021/feb/20/call-for-new-beveridge-report-as-number-of-destitute-uk-households-doubles-during-covid.

Sharma, Sonia. 'This is why Deliveroo drivers went on strike in Newcastle', *Chronicle Live*, 20 September 2020, accessed 17 November 2020, https://www.chroniclelive.co.uk/news/north-east-news/deliveroo-drivers-went-strike-newcastle-16946640.

Siena, Kevin. 'Epidemics and "essential work" in early modern Europe', *History & Policy*, 25 March 2020, accessed 17 November 2020, http://www.historyandpolicy.org/opinion-articles/articles/epidemics-and-essential-work-in-early-modern-europe.

Sky News. 'Uber loses Supreme Court battle on drivers' rights in gig economy test', 19 February 2021, accessed 22 February 2021, https://news.sky.com/story/uber-loses-supreme-court-battle-on-drivers-rights-in-gig-economy-test-12222531.

Smith, Mikey. 'Alan Johnson reveals he was very nearly Secretary of State for PENIS', *Mirror*, 11 September 2016, accessed 17 August 2020, https://www.mirror.co.uk/news/uk-news/alan-johnson-reveals-very-nearly-8812242.

Snow, Stephanie, and Angela Whitecross. 'Connecting voices in a time of crisis: NHS at 70 and Covid-19', *Oral History Review*, 5 May 2020, accessed 17 September 2020, http://oralhistoryreview.org/current-events/nhs-70-covid-19/.

Szreter, Simon. 'Covid-19 is not a Black Swan: Predictable shocks need fully-funded, resilient public services', *History & Policy*, 1 May 2020, accessed 17 November 2020, http://www.historyandpolicy.org/opinion-articles/articles/covid-19-is-not-a-black-swan-predictable-shocks-need-fully-funded-resilient-public-services.

Tadeo, Maria. 'Sick note Britain: Employees face four week health check under new scheme', *Independent*, 13 February 2014, accessed 23 November 2020, https://www.independent.co.uk/news/business/news/sick-note-britain-employees-face-four-week-health-check-under-new-scheme-9126201.html.

TUC. 'TUC advice for people working at home during the coronavirus outbreak', TUC, 18 March 2020, accessed 20 November 2020, https://www.tuc.org.uk/news/tuc-advice-people-working-home-during-coronavirus-outbreak.

TUC. 'TUC calls for long Covid to be urgently recognised as a disability to prevent "massive" discrimination', 20 June 2021, accessed 2 September 2021, https://www.tuc.org.uk/news/tuc-calls-long-covid-be-urgently-recognised-disability-prevent-massive-discrimination.

TUC. 'TUC calls on government to tackle coronavirus with immediate #SickPayForAll', TUC, 3 March 2020, accessed 19 November 2020, https://www.tuc.org.uk/news/tuc-calls-government-tackle-coronavirus-immediate-sickpayforall.

UK Web Archive. 'SHINE', UK Web Archive, accessed 22 February 2021, https://www.webarchive.org.uk/shine.

WalesOnline. '"Rip up sick-note Britain"', Wales Online, 13 November 2007, accessed 23 November 2020, https://www.walesonline.co.uk/news/wales-news/rip-up-sick-note-britain-2217280.

Secondary Sources

Articles and chapters

Andersen, Jørgen Goul, and Tor Bjørklund. 'Structural change and new cleavages: The progress parties in Denmark and Norway'. *Acta Sociologica* 33, no. 3 (1990): pp. 195–217.

Anon. 'British Medical Association Annual Representative Meeting', *The Lancet* 246 no. 6362 (1945): pp. 148–50.

Anon. 'Industrial medicine: A report by the Social and Preventive Medicine Committee of the Royal College of Physicians of London'. *British Journal of Industrial Medicine* 2, no. 1 (1945): pp. 51–5.

Anon. 'Medicine and the law'. *The Lancet* 245, no. 6343 (1945): pp. 381–2.

Anon. 'The panel conference'. *The Lancet* 246, no. 6378 (1945): pp. 684–6.

Anon. 'In England now'. *The Lancet* 248, no. 6428 (1946): pp. 691–2.

Anon. 'Industrial medical services'. *The Lancet* 248, no. 6418 (1946): pp. 321–2.

Anon. 'Proceedings of the Association of Industrial Medical Officers'. *British Journal of Industrial Medicine* 3, no. 1 (1946): pp. 48–54.

Anon. 'Towards Social Security'. *The Lancet* 247, no. 6392 (1946): 320–1.

Anon. 'Towards Social Security'. *The Lancet* 247, no. 6393 (1946): 356.

Anon. 'The act in action'. *The Lancet* 252, no. 6534 (1948): pp. 823–5.

Anon. 'Annual Conference of Representatives of Local Medical Committees'. *British Medical Journal* 2, no. 5660 (1969): pp. 155–65.

Anon. 'Annual Representative Meeting, Aberdeen, 1969'. *British Medical Journal* 3, no. 5662 (1969): pp. 9–67.

Anon. 'A.R.M. round up'. *British Medical Journal* 3, no. 5770 (1971): pp. 319–20.

Anon. 'Conference of Representatives of L.M.C.s'. *British Medical Journal* 3, no, 5922 (1974): pp. 57–63.

Aronsson, Gunnar, Klas Gustafsson, and Margareta Dallner. 'Sick but yet at work. An empirical study of sickness presenteeism'. *Journal of Epidemiology & Community Health* 54, no. 7 (2000): pp. 502–9.

Asher, Robert. 'Experience counts: British workers, accident prevention and compensation, and the origins of the welfare state'. *Journal of Policy History* 15 (2003): 359–88.

Beecham, Linda. 'Gordon Macpherson: Editor who bridged the gap between the BMJ and the BMA'. *British Medical Journal* 366 (2019).

Bell, David N. F., and David G. Blanchflower. 'Underemployment in the UK revisited'. *National Institute Economic Review* 224, no. 1 (2013): pp. F8–22.

Berridge, Virginia. 'Jerry Morris'. *International Journal of Epidemiology* 30, no. 5 (2001): pp. 1141–5.

Betz, Hans-Georg. 'Facets of nativism: A heuristic exploration'. *Patterns of Prejudice* 53, no. 2 (2019): pp. 111–35.

Billings, Mark, and John Wilson. '"Breaking New Ground": The National Enterprise Board, Ferranti, and Britain's prehistory of privatization'. *Enterprise & Society* 20, no. 4 (2019): pp. 907–38.

Bransby, E. R. 'Comparison of the rates of sick absence of Metropolitan policemen before and after the war'. *Monthly Bulletin of the Ministry of Health and the Public Laboratory Service* 8 (1949): pp. 31–6.

Bransby, E. R., and D. Thomson. 'Sick absence in the Metropolitan Police, especially that due to respiratory infections'. *Monthly Bulletin of the Ministry of Health and the Public Laboratory Service* 12 (1953): pp. 32–42.

British Medical Association. 'A charter for the family doctor service'. *British Medical Journal* 1, no. 5436 (1965): pp. S89–91.

Brooke, Stephen. 'Gender and working class identity in Britain during the 1950s'. *Journal of Social History* 34, no. 4 (2001): pp. 773–95.

Brooke, Stephen. 'Space, emotions and the everyday: The affective ecology of 1980s London'. *Twentieth Century British History* 28, no. 1 (2017): pp. 110–42.

Buzzard, R. B. 'Attendance and absence in industry: The nature of the evidence'. *The British Journal of Sociology* 5, no. 3 (1954): pp. 238–52.

Buzzard, R. B., and W. J. Shaw. 'An analysis of absence under a scheme of paid sick leave'. *British Journal of Industrial Medicine* 9, no. 4 (1952): pp. 282–95.

Carne, Stuart. 'Sick absence certification. Analysis of one group practice in 1967'. *British Medical Journal* 1, no. 5637 (1969): pp. 147–9.

Carruthers, Susan L. '"Manning the Factories": Propaganda and policy on the employment of women, 1939–1947'. *History* 75, no. 244 (1990): pp. 232–56.

Chatterji, Monojit, and Colin J. Tilley. 'Sickness, absenteeism, presenteeism, and sick pay'. *Oxford Economic Papers* 54, no. 4 (2002): pp. 669–87.

Clarke, John. 'Going public: The act of complaining'. In *Complaints, Controversies and Grievances in Medicine: Historical and Social Science Perspectives*, edited by Jonathan Reinartz and Rebecca Wynter (London: Routledge, 2014), pp. 259–69.

Claussen, Bjørgulf. 'Physicians as gatekeepers: Will they contribute to restrict disability benefits?' *Scandinavian Journal of Primary Health Care* 16, no. 4 (1999): pp. 199–203.

Cohen, Nissim. 'How culture affects street-level bureaucrats' bending the rules in the context of informal payments for health care: The Israeli case'. *The American Review of Public Administration* 48, no. 2 (2018): pp. 175–87.

Cowls, Josh. 'Cultures of the UK Web'. In *The Web as History: Using Web Archives to Understand the Past and the Present*, edited by Niels Brügger and Ralph Schroeder (London: UCL Press, 2017), pp. 220–37.

Devane, Ed. 'Pilgrim's progress: The landscape of the NHS hospital, 1945–70'. *Twentieth Century British History* 32, no. 4 (2021): 534–52.

Digby, Anne, and Nick Bosanquet. 'Doctors and patients in an era of National Health Insurance and private practice, 1913–1938'. *Economic History Review* 41, no. 1 (1988): pp. 74–94.

Dorrington, Sarah, Ewan Carr, Sharon A. M. Stevelink, Alex Dregan, Charlotte Woodhead, Jayati Das-Munshi, Mark Ashworth, et al. 'Multimorbidity and fit note receipt in working-age adults with long-term health conditions'. *Psychological Medicine* (2020).

Dorrington, Sarah, Ewan Carr, Sharon A. M. Stevelink, Alexandru Dregan, David Whitney, Stevo Durbaba, Mark Ashworth, et al. 'Demographic variation in fit note receipt and long-term conditions in south London'. *Occupational and Environmental Medicine* 77, no. 6 (2020): pp. 418–26.

Drake, Robert F. 'Charities, authority and disabled people: A qualitative study'. *Disability & Society* 11 (1996): pp. 5–23.

Edgerton, David. 'C. P. Snow as anti-historian of British science: Revisiting the technocratic moment, 1959–1964'. *History of Science* 43, no. 2 (2005): pp. 187–208.

Elizabeth, Hannah J. 'Love carefully and without "over-bearing fears": The persuasive power of authenticity in late 1980s British AIDS education material for adolescents'. *Social History of Medicine* 34, no. 4 (2020): pp. 1317–42.

Elizabeth, Hannah J., Gareth Millward, and Alex Mold. '"Injections-While-You-Dance": Press advertisements and poster promotion of the polio vaccine to British publics, 1956–1962'. *Cultural and Social History* 16, no. 3 (2019): pp. 315–36.

Feldman, David. 'Migrants, immigrants and welfare from the Old Poor Law to the welfare state'. *Transactions of the Royal Historical Society*, 13 (2003): pp. 79–104.

Fielding, Steven. 'What did "the people" want?: The meaning of the 1945 General Election'. *The Historical Journal* 35, no. 3 (1992): pp. 623–39.

Finkelstein, Vic. 'Phase 2: Discovering the person in "disability" and "rehabilitation"'. *Magic Carpet*, 27 (1975): pp. 31–8.

Finlayson, Geoffrey. 'A moving frontier: Voluntarism and the state in British social welfare 1911–1949'. *Twentieth Century British History* 1, no. 2 (1990): pp. 183–206.

Foote, Stephanie. 'Making sport of Tonya: Class performance and social punishment'. *Journal of Sport and Social Issues* 27, no. 1 (2003): pp. 3–17.

Gale, Arthur H. '"I stuffed their mouths with gold"'. *Missouri Medicine* 114, no. 1 (2017): pp. 13–15.

Giles, Audrey C. 'Railway accidents and nineteenth-century legislation: "Misconduct, want of caution or causes beyond their control?"' *Labour History Review* 76, no. 2 (2011): pp. 121–42.

Gillam, Stephen. 'The Family Doctor Charter: 50 years on'. *British Journal of General Practice* 67, no. 658 (2017): pp. 227–8.

Gleeson, B. J. 'Disability studies: A historical materialist view'. *Disability & Society* 12 (2010): pp. 179–202.

Goerke, Laszlo. 'Sick pay reforms and health status in a unionised labour market'. *Scottish Journal of Political Economy* 64, no. 2 (2017): pp. 115–42.

Gorsky, M. 'The growth and distribution of English friendly societies in the early nineteenth century'. *Economic History Review* 51 (1998): pp. 489–511.

Gorsky, Martin, Aravinda Guntupalli, Bernard Harris, and Andrew Hinde. 'The "cultural inflation of morbidity" during the English mortality decline: A new look'. *Social Science & Medicine* 73, no. 12 (2011): pp. 1775–83.

Grdešić, Marko. 'Neoliberalism and welfare chauvinism in Germany: An examination of survey evidence'. *German Politics & Society* 37, no. 2 (2019): pp. 1–22.

Grover, C., and L. Piggott. 'Disabled people, the reserve army of labour and welfare reform'. *Disability & Society* 20 (2005): pp. 705–17.

Grover, C., and L. Piggott. 'Social security, employment and incapacity benefit: Critical reflections on A New Deal for Welfare'. *Disability & Society* 22 (2007): pp. 733–46.

Grover, Chris. 'The end of an era? The resignation of Iain Duncan Smith, conservatism and social security benefits for disabled people'. *Disability & Society* 31, no. 8 (2016): pp. 1127–31.

Gulland, Jackie. 'Extraordinary housework: Women and claims for sickness benefit in the early twentieth century'. *Women's History Magazine* 71 (2013): pp. 23–30.

Gulland, Jackie. 'Conditionality in social security: Lessons from the Household Duties Test'. *Journal of Social Security Law* 26, no. 2 (2019): pp. 62–78.

Hall, Alice, and Hannah Tweed. 'Curating care: Creativity, women's work, and the Carers UK archive'. *Journal of Contemporary Archive Studies* 6 (2019).

Hall, Stuart. 'The great moving right show'. In *The Politics of Thatcherism*, edited by Stuart Hall and Martin Jacques (London: Lawrence & Wishart, 1983), pp. 19–39.

Handy, L. J. 'Absenteeism and attendance in the British coal-mining industry: An examination of post-war trends'. *British Journal of Industrial Relations* 6, no. 1 (1968): pp. 27–50.

Hanley, James G. 'The public's reaction to public health: Petitions submitted to Parliament, 1847–1848'. *Social History of Medicine* 15, no. 3 (2002): pp. 393–411.

Harris, Bernard, Martin Gorsky, Aravinda Meera Guntupalli, and Andrew Hinde. 'Long-term changes in sickness and health: further evidence from the Hampshire Friendly Society'. *The Economic History Review* 65, no. 2 (2012): pp. 719–45.

Haug, Marie R. 'The deprofessionalization of everyone?' *Sociological Focus* 8, no. 3 (1975): pp. 197–213.

Hay, Colin. 'Chronicles of a death foretold: The Winter of Discontent and construction of crisis of British Keynesianism'. *Parliamentary Affairs* 63 (2010): pp. 446–70.

Hay, Colin. 'Whatever happened to Thatcherism?' *Political Studies Review* 5, no. 2 (2007): pp. 183–201.

Hayes, Nick. 'Did we really want a National Health Service? Hospitals, patients and public opinions before 1948'. *The English Historical Review* 127, no. 526 (2012): pp. 625–61.

Heller, Michael. 'The National Insurance Acts 1911–1947, the Approved Societies and the Prudential Assurance Company'. *Twentieth Century British History* 19, no. 1 (2008): pp. 1–28.

Henrekson, Magnus, and Mats Persson. 'The effects on sick leave of changes in the sickness insurance system'. *Journal of Labor Economics* 22, no. 1 (2004): 87–113.

Hewitt, Martin. 'New Labour and social security'. In *New Labour, New Welfare State? The 'Third Way' in British Social Policy*, edited by Martin A. Powell (Bristol: Policy Press, 1999), pp. 149–70.

Hicks, Marie. 'Hacking the cis-tem: Transgender citizens and the early digital state'. *IEEE Annals of the History of Computing* 4, no. 1 (2019): pp. 20–33.

Hilton, Matthew, Chris Moores, and Florence Sutcliffe-Braithwaite. 'New Times revisited: Britain in the 1980s'. *Contemporary British History* 31, no. 2 (2017): pp. 145–65.

Holmes, G. P., J. E. Kaplan, N. M. Gantz, A. L. Komaroff, L. B. Schonberger, S. E. Straus, J. F. Jones, R. E. Dubois, C. Cunningham-Rundles, and S. Pahwa. 'Chronic fatigue syndrome: A working case definition'. *Annals of Internal Medicine* 108, no. 3 (1988): pp. 387–9.

Holroyde, Andy. 'Sheltered employment and mental health in Britain: Remploy c. 1945–1981'. In *Healthy Minds in the Twentieth Century: In and Beyond the Asylum*, edited by Steven J. Taylor and Alice Brumby (Cham: Springer International Publishing, 2020), pp. 113–35.

Horrell, Sara. 'The household and the labour market'. In *Work and Pay in 20th Century Britain*, edited by Nicholas Crafts, Ian Gazeley, and Andrew Newell (Oxford: Oxford University Press, 2007), pp. 117–41.

Hughes, J. P. W. 'Sickness absence recording in industry'. *British Journal of Industrial Medicine* 9, no. 4 (1952): pp. 264–74.

Insurance Committee Secretary, An. 'The white paper reviewed'. *The Lancet* 243, no. 6289 (1944): p. 350.

Jackson, Ben. 'Free markets and feminism: The neo-liberal defence of the male breadwinner model in Britain, c. 1980–1997'. *Women's History Review* 28, no. 2 (2019): pp. 297–316.

Johnes, Geraint. 'The gig economy in the UK: A regional perspective'. *Journal of Global Responsibility* 10, no. 3 (2019): pp. 197–210.

Johns, Gary. 'Presenteeism in the workplace: A review and research agenda'. *Journal of Organizational Behavior* 31, no. 4 (2010): pp. 519–42.

Johnston, Ronnie, and Arthur McIvor. 'Marginalising the body at work? Employers' occupational health strategies and occupational medicine in Scotland c. 1930–1974'. *Social History of Medicine* 21, no. 1 (2008): pp. 127–44.

Kane-Galbraith, Adrian. 'Male breadwinners of "doubtful sex": Trans men and the welfare state, 1945–1969'. In *Twentieth Century British Masculinities* (Manchester: Manchester University Press (under review)).

Kelly, Marisa. 'Theories of justice and street-level discretion'. *Journal of Public Administration Research and Theory* 4, no. 2 (1994): pp. 119–40.

Kim, Il-Ho, Carles Muntaner, Faraz Vahid Shahidi, Alejandra Vives, Christophe Vanroelen, and Joan Benach. 'Welfare states, flexible employment, and health: A critical review'. *Health Policy* 104, no. 2 (2012): pp. 99–127.

Kimber, Nick. 'Race and equality'. In *Unequal Britain: Equalities in Britain since 1945*, edited by Pat Thane (Oxford: Oxford University Press, 2010), pp. 29–51.

King, Laura. 'How men valued women's work: Labour in and outside the home in post-war Britain'. *Contemporary European History* 28, no. 4 (2019): pp. 454–68.

Kinman, Gail. 'Sickness presenteeism at work: Prevalence, costs and management'. *British Medical Bulletin* 129, no. 1 (2019): pp. 69–78.

Klein, R. 'The state and the profession: The politics of the double bed.' *British Medical Journal* 301, no. 6754 (1990): pp. 700–2.

Langhamer, Claire. 'Feelings, women and work in the long 1950s'. *Women's History Review* 26, no. 1 (2017): pp. 77–92.

Langhamer, Claire. '"Who the hell are ordinary people?" Ordinariness as a category of historical analysis'. *Transactions of the Royal Historical Society* 28 (2018): pp. 175–95.

Lawrence, Jon. 'Class, "affluence" and the study of everyday life in Britain, c. 1930–64'. *Cultural and Social History* 10, no. 2 (2013): pp. 273–99.

Leeworthy, Daryl. 'A diversion from the new leisure: Greyhound racing, working-class culture, and the politics of unemployment in inter-war South Wales'. *Sport in History* 32, no. 1 (2012): pp. 53–73.

Lewis, Jane. 'Gender and the development of welfare regimes'. *Journal of European Social Policy* 2, no. 2 (1992): pp. 159–73.

Lewis, Jane. 'The medical profession and the state: GPs and the GP contract in the 1960s and the 1990s'. *Social Policy & Administration* 32, no. 2 (1998): pp. 132–50.

Liddell, F. D. K. 'Attendance in the coal-mining industry'. *The British Journal of Sociology* 5, no. 1 (1954): pp. 78–86.

Liebowitz, S. J., and Stephen E. Margolis. 'The fable of the keys'. *The Journal of Law & Economics* 33, no. 1 (1990): pp. 1–25.

Long, Vicky, and Victoria Brown. 'Conceptualizing work-related mental distress in the British coalfields (c. 1900–1950)'. *Palgrave Communications* 4, no. 1 (2018): pp. 1–10.

Lowe, Rodney. 'The rediscovery of poverty and the creation of the Child Poverty Action Group'. *Contemporary Record* 9 (1995): pp. 602–11.

Machin, Stephen. 'Union decline in Britain'. *British Journal of Industrial Relations* 38, no. 4 (2000): pp. 631–45.

Markussen, Simen, Knut Røed, and Ragnhild C. Schreiner. 'Can compulsory dialogues nudge sick-listed workers back to work?' *Economic Journal* 128, no. 610 (2018): pp. 1276–1303.

McCarthy, Helen. 'Social science and married women's employment in post-war Britain'. *Past & Present* 233, no. 1 (2016): pp. 269–305.

McCarthy, Helen. 'Women, marriage and paid work in post-war Britain'. *Women's History Review* 26, no. 1 (2017): pp. 46–61.

McIvor, Arthur. 'Body talk: Oral history methodology in the study of occupational health and disability in twentieth century British coalmining'. In *Santé et Travail à la Mine: XIXe–XXIe Siècle*, edited by J Rainhorn, translated by Arthur McIvor (Rennes: Presses Universitaires du Septentrion, 2014), pp. 238–61.

Mclean, Carl, Catherine Campbell, and Flora Cornish. 'African-Caribbean interactions with mental health services in the UK: Experiences and expectations of exclusion as (re) productive of health inequalities'. *Social Science & Medicine* 56, no. 3 (2003): pp. 657–69.

Meiklejohn, A. 'Doctor and workman'. *British Journal of Industrial Medicine* 7, no. 3 (1950): pp. 105–16.

Milligan, Ian. 'Mining the "internet graveyard": Rethinking the historians' toolkit'. *Journal of the Canadian Historical Association / Revue de La Société Historique Du Canada* 23, no. 2 (2012): pp. 21–64.

Millward, Gareth. 'A history with web archives, not a history of web archives: A history of the British measles-mumps-rubella vaccine crisis, 1998–2004'. In *SAGE Handbook of Web History*, edited by Niels Brügger and Ian Milligan (Thousand Oaks: SAGE, 2018), pp. 464–78.

Millward, Gareth. '"A matter of commonsense": The Coventry poliomyelitis epidemic 1957 and the British public'. *Contemporary British History* 31, no. 3 (2017): 384–406.

Millward, Gareth. 'Social security policy and the early disability movement – Expertise, disability and the government, 1965–1977'. *Twentieth Century British History* 26, no. 2 (2015): pp. 274–97.

Montgomerie, Margaret Anne. 'Visibility, empathy and derision: Popular television representations of disability'. *Alter* 4, no. 2 (April 2010): 94–102.

Morrice, Andrew. '"Strong combination": The Edwardian BMA and contract practice'. In *Financing Medicine: The British Experience since 1750*, edited by Martin Gorsky and Sally Sheard (London: Routledge, 2006), pp. 165–81.

Mousteri, Victoria, Michael Daly, and Liam Delaney. 'Underemployment and psychological distress: Propensity score and fixed effects estimates from two large UK samples'. *Social Science & Medicine* 244 (2020).

Nevers, Jeppe, and Thomas Paster. 'Business and the Nordic welfare states, 1890–1970'. *Scandinavian Journal of History* 44, no. 5 (2019): pp. 535–51.

Noordegraaf, Mirko. 'From "pure" to "hybrid" professionalism: Present-day professionalism in ambiguous public domains'. *Administration & Society* 39, no. 6 (2007): pp. 761–85.

Nullmeier, Frank, and Franz-Xaver Kaufmann. 'Post-war welfare state development'. In *The Oxford Handbook of the Welfare State*, edited by Francis G. Castles, Stephan Leibfried, Jane Lewis, Herbert Obinger, and Christopher Pierson (Oxford: Oxford University Press, 2010), pp. 81–102.

Offer, Avner. 'The market turn: From social democracy to market liberalism'. *Economic History Review* 70, no. 4 (2017): pp. 1051–71.

O'Hara, Glen, and Helen Parr. 'Conclusions: Harold Wilson's 1964–70 governments and the heritage of "New" Labour'. *Contemporary British History* 20 (2006): pp. 477–89.

Oliver, Mike. 'The disability movement is a New Social Movement!' *Community Development Journal* 32 (1997): pp. 244–51.

Paterson, Laura. '"I didn't feel like my own person": Paid work in women's narratives of self and working motherhood, 1950–1980'. *Contemporary British History* 33, no. 3 (2019): pp. 405–26.

Payling, Daisy. '"The people who write to us are the people who don't like us:" Public responses to the Government Social Survey's Survey of Sickness, 1943–1952'. *Journal of British Studies* 59, no. 2 (2020): pp. 315–42.

Payne, Reginald T. 'The National Health Service Act'. *British Medical Journal* 1, no. 4489 (1947): pp. 102–6.

Pemberton, Hugh. 'WASPI's is (mostly) a campaign for inequality'. *The Political Quarterly* 88, no. 3 (2017): pp. 510–16.

Pickstone, John. 'Production, community and consumption: The political economy of twentieth-century medicine'. In *Medicine in the Twentieth Century*, edited by Roger Cooter and John Pickstone (Abingdon: Routledge, 2003), pp. 1–20.

Pierson, Paul. 'Increasing returns, path dependence, and the study of politics'. *The American Political Science Review* 94 (2000): pp. 251–67.

Powell, Martin A. 'Introduction'. In *New Labour, New Welfare State? The 'Third Way' in British Social Policy*, edited by Martin A. Powell (Bristol: Policy Press, 1999), pp. 1–28.

Practitioner. 'The doctor's wife'. *The Lancet* 251, no. 6508 (1948): pp. 811–12.

Price, Leigh. 'Wellbeing research and policy in the U.K.: Questionable science likely to entrench inequality'. *Journal of Critical Realism* 16, no. 5 (2017): pp. 451–67.

Reed, R. R., and D. Evans. 'The deprofessionalization of medicine. Causes, effects, and responses'. *Journal of the American Medical Association* 258, no. 22 (1987): pp. 3279–82.

Riley, James C. 'Ill health during the English mortality decline: The friendly societies' experience'. *Bulletin of the History of Medicine* 61, no. 4 (1987): pp. 563–88.

Riley, James C. 'Sickness in an early modern workplace'. *Continuity and Change* 2, no. 3 (1987): pp. 363–85.

Roberts, Cecil. 'Post Office medical services and morbidity statistics'. *Monthly Bulletin of the Ministry of Health and the Public Laboratory Service* 7 (1948): pp. 184–201.

Rubery, Jill, Arjan Keizer, and Damian Grimshaw. 'Flexibility bites back: The multiple and hidden costs of flexible employment policies'. *Human Resource Management Journal* 26, no. 3 (2016): pp. 235–51.

Ryan Johansson, S. 'The health transition: the cultural inflation of morbidity during the decline of mortality'. *Health Transition Review* 1, no. 1 (1991): pp. 39–68.

Safford, Archibald. 'The creation of case law under the National Insurance and National Insurance (Industrial Injuries) Acts'. *Modern Law Review* 17, no. 3 (1954): pp. 197–210.

Saunders, Robert. '"Crisis? What crisis?" Thatcherism and the seventies'. In *Making Thatcher's Britain*, edited by Ben Jackson and Robert Saunders (Cambridge: Cambridge University Press, 2012), pp. 25–42.

Saurel-Cubizolles, M.-J., P. Romito, and J. Garcia. 'Description of maternity rights for working women in France, Italy and in the United Kingdom'. *European Journal of Public Health* 3, no. 1 (1993): pp. 48–53.

Savage, Mike. 'Working-class identities in the 1960s: Revisiting the affluent worker study'. *Sociology*, no. 5 (2005): pp. 929–46.

Seaton, Andrew. 'Against the "sacred cow": NHS opposition and the Fellowship for Freedom in Medicine, 1948–72'. *Twentieth Century British History* 26, no. 3 (2015): pp. 424–49.

Shakespeare, Tom, Nicholas Watson, and Ola Abu Alghaib. 'Blaming the victim, all over again: Waddell and Aylward's biopsychosocial (BPS) model of disability'. *Critical Social Policy* 37, no. 1 (2017): pp. 22–41.

Sher, George. 'Health care and the "deserving poor"'. *The Hastings Center Report* 13 (1983): pp. 9–12.

Sirrs, Christopher. 'Accidents and apathy: The construction of the "Robens Philosophy" of occupational safety and health regulation in Britain, 1961–1974'. *Social History of Medicine* 29, no. 1 (2016): pp. 66–88.

Sloman, Peter. 'Redistribution in an age of neoliberalism: Market economics, "poverty knowledge", and the growth of working-age benefits in Britain, c. 1979–2010'. *Political Studies* 67, no. 3 (2019): pp. 732–51.

Sloman, Peter, Daniel Zamora Vargas, and Pedro Ramos Pinto, 'Introduction' in *Universal Basic Income in Historical Perspective*, edited by Peter Sloman, Daniel Zamora Vargas, and Pedro Ramos Pinto (London: Palgrave Macmillan, forthcoming).

Smith, Lewis Charles. 'Marketing modernity: Business and family in British Rail's "Age of the Train" campaign, 1979–84'. *The Journal of Transport History* 40, no. 3 (2019): pp. 363–94.

Stone, Deborah A. 'Physicians as gatekeepers'. *Public Policy* 27 (1979): pp. 227–54.

Sutherland, Will, Mohammad Hossein Jarrahi, Michael Dunn, and Sarah Beth Nelson. 'Work precarity and gig literacies in online freelancing'. *Work, Employment and Society* 34, no. 3 (2020): pp. 457–75.

Tassinari, Arianna, and Vincenzo Maccarrone. 'Riders on the storm: Workplace solidarity among gig economy couriers in Italy and the UK'. *Work, Employment and Society* 34, no. 1 (2020): pp. 35–54.

Taylor, P. J. 'Individual variations in sickness absence'. *British Journal of Industrial Medicine* 24, no. 3 (1967): pp. 169–77.

Taylor, P. J. 'Self-certification for brief spells of sickness absence'. *British Medical Journal* 1, no. 5637 (1969): pp. 144–7.

Taylor, Phil, Ian Cunningham, Kirsty Newsome, and Dora Scholarios. '"Too scared to go sick" – Reformulating the research agenda on sickness absence'. *Industrial Relations Journal* 41, no. 4 (2010): pp. 270–88.

Taylor, Stephen. 'The Survey of Sickness, 1943–52: Was our survey really necessary?'. *The Lancet* 271, no. 7019 (1958): pp. 521–3.

Thane, P. M. 'The debate on the declining birth-rate in Britain: The "menace" of an ageing population, 1920s–1950s'. *Continuity & Change* 5, no. 2 (1990): pp. 238–305.

Thane, Pat. 'Family life and "normality" in postwar British culture'. In *Life after Death: Approaches to a Cultural and Social History of Europe During the 1940s and 1950s*, edited by Richard Bessel and Dirk Schumann (Cambridge: Cambridge University Press, 2003), pp. 193–210.

Thane, Pat. 'Voluntary action in Britain since Beveridge'. In *Beveridge and Voluntary Action in Britain and the Wider British World*, edited by Melanie Oppenheimer and Nicholas Deakin (Manchester: Manchester University Press, 2011), pp. 121–34.

Tomlinson, Jim. 'De-industrialization not decline: A new meta-narrative for post-war British history'. *Twentieth Century British History* 27, no. 1 (2016): pp. 76–99.

Tomlinson, Jim. 'De-industrialization: Strengths and weaknesses as a key concept for understanding post-war British history'. *Urban History* 47, no. 2 (2020): pp. 199–219.

Tomlinson, Jim, Jim Phillips, and Valerie Wright. 'De-industrialization: A case study of Dundee, 1951–2001, and its broad implications'. *Business History* 64, no. 1 (2019): pp. 28–54.

Vernon, James. 'Heathrow and the making of neoliberal Britain'. *Past & Present* 252, no. 1 (2021): pp. 213–37.

Viet-Wilson, John. 'The National Assistance Board and the "rediscovery" of poverty'. In *Welfare Policy in Britain: The Road from 1945*, edited by Helen Fawcett and Rodney Lowe (Basingstoke: Macmillan, 1999), pp. 116–57.

Waal, Jeroen Van Der, Willem De Koster, and Wim Van Oorschot. 'Three worlds of welfare chauvinism? How welfare regimes affect support for distributing welfare to immigrants in Europe'. *Journal of Comparative Policy Analysis: Research and Practice* 15, no. 2 (2013): pp. 164–81.

Ward, Jacob. 'Computer models and Thatcherist futures: From monopolies to markets in British Telecommunications'. *Technology & Culture* 61, no. 3 (2020): pp. 843–70.

Ward, Jacob. 'Financing the information age: London TeleCity, the legacy of IT-82, and the selling of British Telecom'. *Twentieth Century British History* 30, no. 3 (2019): pp. 424–46.

Warren, Jon, Kayleigh Garthwaite, and Clare Bambra. 'After Atos Healthcare: Is the Employment and Support Allowance fit for purpose and does the Work Capability Assessment have a future?' *Disability & Society* 29, no. 8 (2014): pp. 1319–23.

Watermeyer, B. 'Claiming loss in disability'. *Disability & Society* 24 (2009): pp. 91–102.

Webster, Charles. 'Doctors, public service and profit: General practitioners and the National Health Service'. *Transactions of the Royal Historical Society* 40 (1990): pp. 197–216.

Weston, Janet. 'Managing mental incapacity in the 20th century: A history of the Court of Protection of England & Wales'. *International Journal of Law and Psychiatry* 68 (2020).

Whiteside, Noel. 'L'assurance sociale en Grande Bretagne: La genèse de l'état providence'. In *Les assurances sociales en Europe*, translated by Noel Whiteside (Rennes: Presses Universitaires de Rennes, 2009), pp. 127–58.

Williams, Simon J. 'Parsons revisited: From the sick role to…?' *Health* 9, no. 2 (2005): pp. 123–44.

Williamson, Clifford. '"To remove the stigma of the Poor Law": The "comprehensive" ideal and patient access to the municipal hospital service in the city of Glasgow, 1918–1939'. *History* 99, no. 334 (2014): pp. 73–99.

Wilson, Dolly Smith. 'A new look at the affluent worker: The good working mother in post-war Britain'. *Twentieth Century British History* 17, no. 2 (2006): pp. 206–29.

Young, Kate, Jane Fisher, and Maggie Kirkman. '"Do mad people get endo or does endo make you mad?": Clinicians' discursive constructions of medicine and women with endometriosis'. *Feminism & Psychology* 29, no. 3 (2018): pp. 337–56.

Books and PhD Theses

Abel-Smith, Brian, and Peter Townsend. *The Poor and the Poorest: A New Analysis of the Ministry of Labour's Family Expenditure Surveys of 1953–54 and 1960* (London: Bell, 1965).

Anderson, Julie. *War, Disability and Rehabilitation in Britain: 'Soul of a Nation'* (Manchester: Manchester University Press, 2011).

Armstrong, David. *Political Anatomy of the Body: Medical Knowledge in Britain in the Twentieth Century* (Cambridge: Cambridge University Press, 1983).

Arnoldi, Jakob. *Risk: An Introduction* (Cambridge: Polity, 2009).

Baggini, Julian. *Complaint: From Minor Moans to Principled Protests* (London: Profile, 2010).

Bailkin, Jordanna. *The Afterlife of Empire* (Berkeley: University of California Press, 2012).

Baldwin, Peter. *The Politics of Social Solidarity: Class Bases of the European Welfare State 1875–1975* (Cambridge: Cambridge University Press, 1990).

Beatty, Christina, Stephen Fothergill, Tony Gore, and Anne Green. *Hidden Unemployment in the East Midlands* (Sheffield: Centre for Regional Economic and Social Research, Sheffield Hallam University, 2002).

Beck, Ulrich. *World at Risk* (Cambridge: Polity, 2009).

Berkovitch, Israel. *Coal on the Switchback: The Coal Industry since Nationalisation* (London: Routledge, 2017).

Berridge, Virginia. *Marketing Health* (Oxford: Oxford University Press, 2007).

Berthoud, Richard. *Invalidity Benefit: Where Will the Savings Come From?* (London: Policy Studies Institute, 1993).

Berthoud, Richard. *Trends in the Employment of Disabled People in Britain* (Colchester: Institute for Social & Economic Research, 2011).

Bevan, S., and S. Hayday. *Costing Sickness Absence in the UK* (Brighton: Institute for Employment Studies, 2001).

Beveridge, William H. *Voluntary Action: A Report on Methods of Social Advance* (London: George Allen & Unwin, 1948).

Bivins, Roberta E. *Contagious Communities: Medicine, Migration, and the NHS in Post-War Britain* (Oxford: Oxford University Press, 2015).

Blair, Tony. *Tony Blair: A Journey* (London: Stanley Paul, 2010).

Bohata, Kirsti, Alexandra Jones, Mike Mantin, and Steven Thompson. *Disability in Industrial Britain* (Manchester: Manchester University Press, 2020).

Bolderson, Helen. *Social Security, Disability and Rehabilitation* (London: Jessica Kingsley, 1991).

Brazier, Alex. *A Double Deficiency? A Report on the Social Security Act 1986 and People with Acquired Immune Deficiency Syndrome (AIDS), AIDS Related Complex (ARC) and HIV Infection* (London: Terrence Higgins Trust, 1989).

Brügger, Niels. *The Archived Web: Doing History in the Digital Age* (Cambridge, Massachusetts: MIT Press, 2018).

Burney, Ian A. *Bodies of Evidence: Medicine and the Politics of the English Inquest, 1830-1826* (Baltimore: Johns Hopkins University Press, 1999).

Burton, Michael. *The Politics of Public Sector Reform: From Thatcher to the Coalition* (Basingstoke: Palgrave Macmillan, 2013).

Campbell, Jane, and Michael Oliver. *Disability Politics: Understanding Our Past, Changing Our Future* (London: Routledge, 1996).

CBI. *On the Path to Recovery: Absence and Workplace Health Survey 2010* (London: CBI, 2010).

Centre for Economics and Business Research. *The Benefits of Early Intervention and Rehabilitation* (London: Centre for Economics and Business Research, 2015).

Chartered Institute of Personnel Development. *Health and Well-Being at Work* (London: Chartered Institute of Personnel Development, 2019).

Collins, Tony. *Sport in Capitalist Society: A Short History* (New York: Routledge, 2013).

Confederation of British Industry. *Absence from Work: A Survey of Non-Attendance and Sickness Absence* (London: Confederation of British Industry, 1987).

Conservative Party. *1979 Conservative Party General Election Manifesto* (London: Conservative Party, 1979).

Conservative Party, *A Better Tomorrow* (London: Conservative Party, 1970).

Coole, Carol, Avril Drummond, Paul Watson, Fiona Nouri, and Iskra Potgieter. *Getting the Best from the Fit Note: Investigating the Use of the Statement of Fitness for Work* (Leicester: IOSH, 2015).

Corker, Mairian, and Tom Shakespeare. *Disability/Postmodernity: Embodying Disability Theory* (London: Continuum, 2002).

Crane, Jennifer. *Child Protection in England, 1960–2000: Expertise, Experience, and Emotion* (London: Palgrave Macmillan, 2018).

Cronin, A. J. *The Citadel* (Basingstoke: Bello, 2013).

Daunton, Martin J. *Royal Mail: The Post Office since 1840* (London: Athlone Press, 1985).

Digby, Anne. *British Welfare Policy: Workhouse to Workfare* (London: Faber, 1989).

Donnison, David Vernon. *The Politics of Poverty* (Oxford: Robertson, 1982).

Douglas, Mary, and Aaron Wildavsky. *Risk and Culture* (Berkeley: University of California Press, 1983).

Drago, Robert, and Kevin Miller. *Sick at Work: Infected Employees in the Workplace During the H1N1 Pandemic* (Washington: Institute for Women's Policy Research, 2011).

Drakeford, Mark, and Ian Butler. *Scandal, Social Policy and Social Welfare*. 2nd ed. (Bristol: Policy Press, 2006).

Duncan, Alan, Iain Duncan-Smith, Bernard Jenkin, Barry Legg, and John Whittingdale. *Who Benefits? A Plan for Social Security: Reinventing Welfare* (London: No Turning Back Group, 1993).

Edgerton, David. *The Rise and Fall of the British Nation: A Twentieth-Century History* (London: Allen Lane, 2018).

Esping-Andersen, Gøsta. *The Three Worlds of Welfare Capitalism* (Cambridge: Polity, 1990).

Floud, Roderick, Kenneth W. Wachter, and Annabel Gregory. *Height, Health, and History: Nutritional Status in the United Kingdom, 1750–1980* (Cambridge: University Press, 1990).

Foucault, Michel. *Discipline and Punish: The Birth of the Prison* (New York: Pantheon Books, 1977).

Foucault, Michel. *The Birth of the Clinic: An Archaeology of Medical Perception* (London: Tavistock, 1973).

Foxhall, Katherine. *Migraine: A History* (Baltimore: Johns Hopkins University Press, 2019).

Fraser, Derek. *The Evolution of the British Welfare State – A History of Social Policy since the Industrial Revolution*. 4th ed. (Basingstoke: Palgrave Macmillan, 2009).

Freidson, Eliot. *Professionalism: The Third Logic* (Cambridge: Polity, 2001).

Genders, Amy. *An Invisible Army: The Role of Freelance Labour in Bristol's Film and Television Industries* (Bristol: University of the West of England Bristol, 2019).

Giddens, Anthony. *Beyond Left and Right: The Future of Radical Politics* (Cambridge: Polity Press, 1994).

Gordon, Richard. *Doctor at Large* (London: Michael Joseph, 1955).

Gough, Ian. *The Political Economy of the Welfare State* (London: Macmillan, 1979).

Gray, Helen, Richard Dorsett, and Getinet Haile. *The Impact of Pathways to Work* (Leeds: Corporate Document Services, 2007).

Gulland, Jackie. *Gender, Work and Social Control: A Century of Disability Benefits* (London: Palgrave Macmillan, 2019).

Hadjipateras, Angela, and Marilyn Howard. *Worried Sick: Reactions to the Government's Plans for Invalidity Benefit* (London: Disability Benefits Consortium, 1993).

Hampton, Jameel. *Disability and the Welfare State in Britain: Changes in Perception and Policy 1948–1979* (Bristol: Policy Press, 2016).

Hardwick, Charles. *The History, Present Position, and Social Importance of Friendly Societies* (London: Routledge, Warne and Routledge, 1859).

Harris, Bernard. *The Origins of the British Welfare State: Society, State and Social Welfare in England and Wales, 1800–1945* (Basingstoke: Palgrave Macmillan, 2004).

Hill, Peter. 'Working Hard or Hardly Working? Evaluating New Labour's Active Labour Market Policy' (PhD thesis, University of Warwick, 2016).

Hilton, Matthew, Nick Crowson, Jean-François Mouhot, and James McKay. *A Historical Guide to NGOs in Britain: Charities, Civil Society and the Voluntary Sector since 1945* (Basingstoke: Palgrave Macmillan, 2012).

Holroyde, Andrew. 'Sheltered Employment and Disability in the Classic Welfare State: Remploy c. 1944–1979' (PhD thesis, University of Huddersfield, 2019).

Honigsbaum, Frank. *The Division in British Medicine: A History of the Separation of General Practice from Hospital Care 1911–1968* (London: Kogan Page, 1979).

Hsu, Madeline Yuan-yin. *The Good Immigrants: How the Yellow Peril Became the Model Minority* (Princeton: Princeton University Press, 2017).

Industrial Society, The. *Studies of Absence Rates and Control Policies* (London: The Industrial Society, 1987).

Jackson, Mark, ed. *Stress in Post-War Britain, 1945-85* (Abingdon: Routledge, 2013).

Kersbergen, Kees van, and Barbara Vis. *Comparative Welfare State Politics: Development, Opportunities, and Reform* (Cambridge: Cambridge University Press, 2014).

Kingdon, John W., and James A. Thurber. *Agendas, Alternatives, and Public Policies* (Boston: Longman, 2011).

Kirby, Jill. *Feeling the Strain: A Cultural History of Stress in Twentieth-Century Britain* (Manchester: Manchester University Press, 2019).

Klein, Rudolf. *The New Politics of the NHS*. 7th edn (London: CRC Press, 2013).

Labour Party. *Towards Equality: Women and Social Security* (London: Labour Party, 1969).

Lawson, Nigel. *The View from No. 11: Memoirs of a Tory Radical* (London: Bantam, 1992).

Levitas, Ruth. *The Inclusive Society?* (London: Palgrave Macmillan UK, 2005).

Lipsky, Michael. *Street-Level Bureaucracy: Dilemmas of the Individual in Public Services* (New York: Russell Sage Foundation, 1980).

Long, Vicky. *The Rise and Fall of the Healthy Factory: The Politics of Industrial Health in Britain, 1914–60* (Basingstoke: Palgrave Macmillan, 2010).

Loopstra, Rachel and Doireann Lalor. *Financial Insecurity, Food Insecurity, and Disability: The Profile of People Receiving Emergency Food Assistance from The Trussell Trust Foodbank Network in Britain* (Trussell Trust: Salisbury, 2017).

Lowe, Rodney. *The Welfare State in Britain since 1945* (Basingstoke: Palgrave Macmillan, 2005).

Lund, Brian. *Housing Politics in the United Kingdom: Power, Planning and Protest* (Bristol: Policy Press, 2016).

Mandler, Peter. *The Crisis of the Meritocracy: Britain's Transition to Mass Education since the Second World War* (Oxford: Oxford University Press, 2020).

Marshall, T. H. *Citizenship and Social Class, and Other Essays* (Cambridge: Cambridge University Press, 1950).

Massey, Adrian. *Sick-Note Britain: How Social Problems Became Medical Issues* (London: Hurst Publishers, 2019).

McCarthy, Helen. *Double Lives: A History of Working Motherhood in Modern Britain* (London: Bloomsbury, 2020).

McKay, Stephen, and Karen Rowlingson. *Social Security in Britain* (Basingstoke: Macmillan, 1999).

Millward, Gareth. 'Invalid Definitions, Invalid Responses: Disability and the Welfare State, 1965–1995' (PhD thesis, London School of Hygiene and Tropical Medicine, 2014).

Millward, Gareth. *Vaccinating Britain: Mass Vaccination and the Public since the Second World War* (Manchester: Manchester University Press, 2019).

Mold, Alex. *Making the Patient-Consumer: Patient Organisations and Health Consumerism in Britain* (Manchester: Manchester University Press, 2015).

Mold, Alex, Peder Clark, Gareth Millward, and Daisy Payling. *Placing the Public in Public Health in Postwar Britain* (London: Palgrave Macmillan, 2019).

Moore, Martin D. *Managing Diabetes, Managing Medicine: Chronic Disease and Clinical Bureaucracy in Post-War Britain* (Manchester: Manchester University Press, 2019).

Newlands, Emma. *Civilians into Soldiers: War, the Body and British Army Recruits, 1939–45* (Manchester: Manchester University Press, 2014).

Newman, Janet, and John Clarke. *Publics, Politics and Power: Remaking the Public in Public Services* (London: Sage, 2009).

Office of Health Economics. *The Work of Primary Medical Care* (London: Office of Health Economics, 1974).

Office of Health Economics. *Work Lost through Sickness* (London: Office of Health Economics, 1965).

Oliver, Michael, and Colin Barnes. *The New Politics of Disablement* (Basingstoke: Palgrave Macmillan, 2012).

Ortolano, Guy. *Thatcher's Progress: From Social Democracy to Market Liberalism through an English New Town* (Cambridge: Cambridge University Press, 2019).

Parkhurst, Justin. *The Politics of Evidence: From Evidence-Based Policy to Good Governance of Evidence* Routledge Studies in Governance and Public Policy (Abingdon: Routledge, 2017).

Parsons, Talcott. *The Social System.* (Glencoe: Free Press, 1951).

Pierson, Paul. *Dismantling the Welfare State?: Reagan, Thatcher, and the Politics of Retrenchment* (Cambridge: Cambridge University Press, 1994).

Pikó, Lauren. *Milton Keynes in British Culture: Imagining England* (Abingdon: Routledge, 2019).

Porter, Dorothy. *Health Citizenship: Essays in Social Medicine and Biomedical Politics* (Berkeley: University of California Press, 2011).

Puar, Jasbir K. *The Right to Maim: Debility, Capacity, Disability* (Durham: Duke University Press, 2017).

Renwick, Chris. *Bread for All: The Origins of the Welfare State* (London: Penguin, 2018).

Riley, James C. *Sick, Not Dead: The Health of British Working Men During the Mortality Decline* (Baltimore: Johns Hopkins University Press, 1997).

Ritchie, Jane, Kit Ward, and Wendy Duldig. *A Qualitative Study of the Role of General Practitioners in the Award of Invalidity Benefit* (London: Social and Community Planning Research, 1993).

Rivett, Geoffrey. *From Cradle to Grave: Fifty Years of the NHS* (London: King's Fund, 1998).

Savage, Michael. *Identities and Social Change in Britain since 1940: The Politics of Method* (Oxford: Oxford University Press, 2010).

Savage, Michael. *Social Class in the 21ˢᵗ Century* (London: Pelican, 2015).

Shakespeare, Tom. *Disability Rights and Wrongs* (Abingdon: Routledge, 2006).

Sheard, Sally. *The Passionate Economist: How Brian-Abel Smith Shaped Global Health and Social Welfare* (Bristol: Policy Press, 2013).

Shukla, Nikesh, ed. *The Good Immigrant* (London: Unbound, 2016).

Simpson, Julian M. *Migrant Architects of the NHS: South Asian Doctors and the Reinvention of British General Practice (1940s–1980s)* (Manchester: Manchester University Press, 2018).

Skilton, Mark, and Felix Hovsepian. *The 4th Industrial Revolution: Responding to the Impact of Artificial Intelligence on Business* (Cham: Springer, 2017).

Standing, Guy. *The Precariat: The New Dangerous Class* (London: Bloomsbury Academic, 2014).

Standing, Guy. *Basic Income as Common Dividends: Piloting a Transformative Policy* (London: Progressive Economy Forum, 2019).

Stone, Deborah. *The Disabled State* (Philadelphia: Temple University Press, 1984).

Sutcliffe-Braithwaite, Florence. *Class, Politics, and the Decline of Deference in England, 1968–2000* (Oxford: Oxford University Press, 2018).

Thane, Pat, and Tanya Evans. *Sinners? Scroungers? Saints?: Unmarried Motherhood in Twentieth-Century England* (Oxford: Oxford University Press, 2012).

Timmins, Nicholas. *The Five Giants: A Biography of the Welfare State*. 2nd edn (London: Harper Collins, 2001).

Trades Union Congress. *How Industrial Change Can Be Managed to Deliver Better Jobs* (London: Trades Union Congress, 2019).

Treble, John, and Tim Barmby. *Worker Absenteeism and Sick Pay* (Cambridge: Cambridge University Press, 2011).

Virdee, Satnam. *Racism, Class and the Racialized Outsider* (Basingstoke: Palgrave Macmillan, 2014).

Walker, Carol. *Managing Poverty: The Limits of Social Assistance* (London: Routledge, 1993).

Walt, Gill. *Health Policy: An Introduction to Process and Power* (London: Zed Books, 1994).

Webster, Charles. *National Health Service: A Political History*. 2nd revised edn (Oxford: Oxford University Press, 2002).

Welshman, John. *Underclass: A History of the Excluded, 1880–2000* (London: Hambledon Continuum, 2007).

Westerbeek, Hans, and Aaron Smith. *Sport Business in the Global Marketplace* (London: Palgrave Macmillan, 2003).

Whiteley, Paul, and Steve Winyard. *Pressure for the Poor: The Poverty Lobby and Policy Making* (London: Methuen, 1987).

Index